The Atlas of
Ankle
Replacements

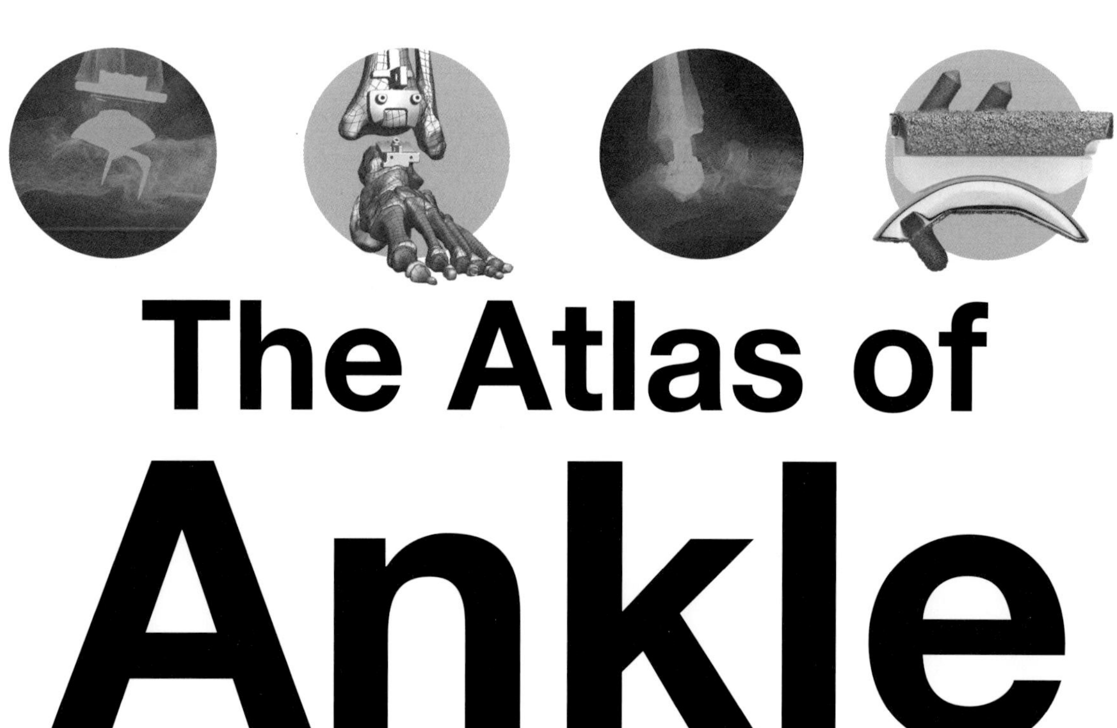

The Atlas of Ankle Replacements

Editors

Andrew J. Goldberg OBE

Director, London Ankle & Arthritis Centre, The Wellington Hospital, London, UK

Paul H. Cooke

Director of the Oxford Centre for Foot & Ankle Medicine, UK

World Scientific

NEW JERSEY · LONDON · SINGAPORE · BEIJING · SHANGHAI · HONG KONG · TAIPEI · CHENNAI · TOKYO

Published by

World Scientific Publishing Europe Ltd.

57 Shelton Street, Covent Garden, London WC2H 9HE

Head office: 5 Toh Tuck Link, Singapore 596224

USA office: 27 Warren Street, Suite 401-402, Hackensack, NJ 07601

Library of Congress Cataloging-in-Publication Data

Names: Goldberg, Andrew, editor. | Cooke, Paul (Orthopedic surgeon), editor.
Title: The atlas of ankle replacements / edited by: Andrew J. Goldberg OBE (The Wellington Hospital, London, UK)
    and Paul H. Cooke (The Oxford Centre for Foot & Ankle Medicine, UK).
Description: New Jersey : World Scientific, 2020. | Includes bibliographical references and index.
Identifiers: LCCN 2019003537 | ISBN 9781786346230 (hc : alk. paper) | ISBN 9781786349712 (pbk : alk. paper) |
    ISBN 9781786346247 (ebook) | ISBN 9781786346254 (ebook other)
Subjects: | MESH: Arthroplasty, Replacement, Ankle--methods | Atlas
Classification: LCC RD562 | NLM WE 17 | DDC 617.5/84059--dc23
LC record available at https://lccn.loc.gov/2019003537

British Library Cataloguing-in-Publication Data
A catalogue record for this book is available from the British Library.

For any available supplementary material, please visit
https://www.worldscientific.com/worldscibooks/10.1142/Q0186#t=suppl

Desk Editors: Anthony Alexander/Jennifer Brough/Shi Ying Koe

Typeset by Stallion Press
Email: enquiries@stallionpress.com

Printed in Singapore

FOREWORD

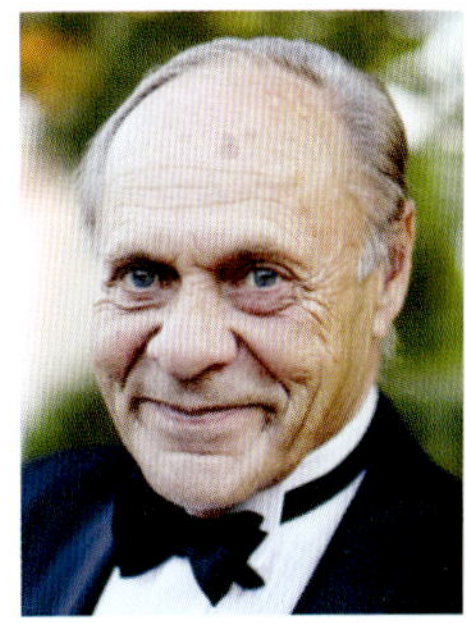

I started my work on ankle replacements in 1978, more than forty years ago, and since then I have seen numerous implants and theories come and go.

I am excited to write a foreword for *The Atlas of Ankle Replacements*, a resource written by many of the world's leading ankle arthritis experts across Europe, the US, and further afield. The senior editors are to be congratulated on pulling together this vast experience into a single resource.

This textbook is a culmination of years of trial and error, research, and collaboration in an important field where there is a proliferation of new implant designs on the market, each with limited published outcome data. Although I am proud to be the inventor of one of the oldest implants still on the market, and one with the highest level of supportive evidence, it is important in such a fast-growing market that we take a step back to evaluate the evidence critically and learn from history and from past mistakes.

There is clearly a renewed interest in ankle replacement and the role of the FDA and European regulators is becoming increasingly important as will be the introduction of unique implant identification numbers and collaborative joint registers.

There is a need for an authoritative, objective, and independent text, and I believe *The Atlas of Ankle Replacements* will become an essential reference source for foot and ankle surgeons as well as industry.

Hakon Kofoed

Consultant Foot and Ankle Orthopaedic Surgeon (Ret),
Kysthospitalet, Skodsborg, Denmark
Professor of Orthopaedics at University of Copenhagen, Denmark

PREFACE

The journey to create this Atlas began in 2007. It began from frustration of how difficult it was to find information on each of the implants on the market and a chance discussion between a fellow and his boss on how an Atlas of every implant on the market may be the missing link. The difficulty was that new implants seemed to be coming to the market with increasing frequency and it begged the question how we could find reliable information on every implant. We both relished the challenge and so hatched a plan to involve surgeons from all around the world, whose expertise and knowledge was unparalleled. The journey involved a travelling fellowship to visit every contributing author as well as finding World Scientific who are superb publishers and that kindly agreed to come with us on our journey. We never anticipated that the project would be delayed by numerous obstructions, from computer crashes to stock market crashes, and from personal illness and family events to global pandemics, but like all good journeys, despite delays we finally reached the end and we hope you enjoy the results.

ABOUT THE EDITORS

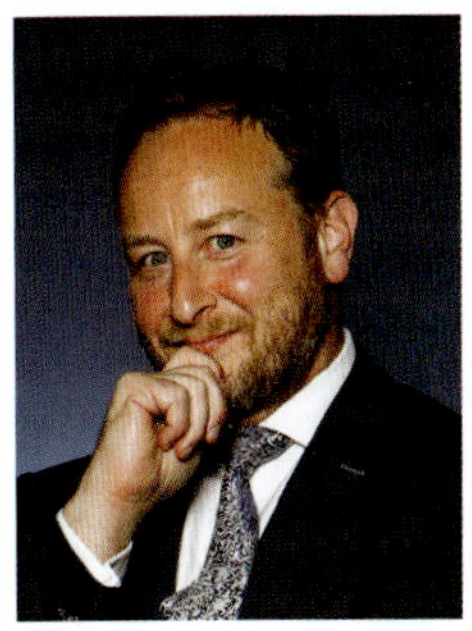

Andrew J. Goldberg OBE is a translational researcher, translating exciting ideas into medical practice and meaningful health outcomes. He graduated from St Mary's Hospital Medical School (Imperial College) in 1994 before completing his specialist training in trauma and orthopaedics in London, UK, with a specialist fellowship in complex foot and ankle disorders in Oxford, as well as overseas in centres of excellence across the USA and Europe.

He was awarded an MD from the University of London in 2006 in Stem Cells in Articular Cartilage Repair. In 2009, he was appointed as a Consultant Orthopaedic Surgeon in Northampton prior to moving to London in 2010 as a Clinical Senior Lecturer at UCL as well as an Honorary Consultant Orthopaedic Surgeon at the Royal National Orthopaedic Hospital NHS Trust in Stanmore, UK.

Andy helped raise more than £10m in research grants for health informatics, first-in-man studies into stem cell therapies (ASCAT), and NIHR HTA multicentre RCTs comparing ankle replacement against ankle fusion (TARVA); he also helped in examining and supervising PhD students. In 2011, he was awarded an OBE for services to medicine. In 2018 he moved into independent practice as a founding Director of the London Ankle & Arthritis Centre at the Wellington Hospital in London as well as a Visiting Professor in Orthopaedics at Imperial College London.

Andy has a major interest in innovation, having created the Medical Futures Innovation Awards which helped fund and recognise several hundred healthcare ideas. He sits on the outcomes committee for BOFAS, the National Joint Registry (NJR) Editorial and Medical Advisory Committees representing BOFAS, and the AOFAS editorial board for Foot and Ankle Orthopaedics (FAO).

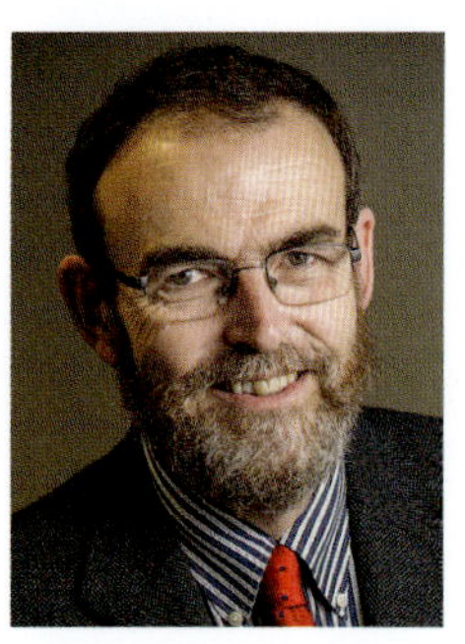

Paul H. Cooke worked as a consultant orthopaedic surgeon at the Nuffield Orthopaedic Centre in Oxford for 28 years. He founded the Foot and Ankle Unit and had a special interest in the surgical management of ankle deformity and arthritis. As well as describing new techniques (and developing implants for these) for open fusion, he pioneered arthroscopic ankle fusion. He was also one of the first surgeons in the UK to build up a practice in ankle replacement and was actively involved in the design of implants and instrumentation over many years. He led the first practical course in ankle replacement in the UK and continued to demonstrate and teach techniques throughout his career – including to many fellows. He encouraged the formation of the National Joint Register for ankles and the world's first randomised study comparing ankle fusion against ankle replacement (the TARVA trial) and recruited his patients into both of these.

In retirement from NHS clinical practice, he has continued as Director of the Oxford Centre for Foot & Ankle Medicine, and has an ongoing interest in ankle replacement, acting as a consultant to industry on the design of implants, and acting as an expert witness in legal cases involving patents and the failure of ankle implants.

LIST OF CONTRIBUTORS

Claire Brockett, Associate Professor in Bioengineering, School of Mechanical Engineering, University of Leeds, United Kingdom.

Timothy M. Clough, Consultant Foot and Ankle Orthopaedic Surgeon, Wrightington, Wigan and Leigh NHS Foundation Trust, United Kingdom.

J. Chris Coetzee, Foot and Ankle Orthopaedic Surgeon, Minnesota Orthopedic Sports Medicine Institute (MOSMI) at Twin Cities Orthopedics in Edina, MN, USA.

Paul H. Cooke, Consultant Foot and Ankle Orthopaedic Surgeon (Ret), Oxford University Hospitals NHS Trust, United Kingdom.

Timothy R. Daniels, Associate Professor and Head of the Foot and Ankle Program at University of Toronto, and Head of Division of Orthopaedics at St. Michael's Hospital, Ontario, Canada.

James K. DeOrio, Associate Professor of Orthopaedic Surgery, Duke University, Durham, NC, USA.

Sunil Dhar, Consultant Foot and Ankle Orthopaedic Surgeon, Nottingham University Hospitals NHS Trust, United Kingdom.

H. Cornelis (Kees) Doets, Foot and Ankle Orthopaedic Surgeon (Ret), Slotervaartziekenhuis, Amsterdam, and Jan van Breemen Instituut, Amsterdam, Holland.

Brian G. Donley, Foot and Ankle Orthopaedic Surgeon and CEO of Cleveland Clinic London, United Kingdom.

Norman Espinosa, Foot and Ankle Orthopaedic Surgeon, Fussinstitut, Zurich, Switzerland.

Klammer Georg, Foot and Ankle Orthopaedic Surgeon, Fussinstitut, Zurich, Switzerland.

Sandro Giannini, Professor of Orthopaedics (Ret), Traumatology and of Physical Medicine at Bologna University and Director at the Rizzoli Institute, Italy.

Andrew J. Goldberg OBE, Consultant Orthopaedic Surgeon, The Wellington Hospital, London, and Honorary Associate Professor at the UCL Institute of Orthopaedics, Royal National Orthopaedic Hospital, London, United Kingdom.

Anders Henricson, Department of Orthopedics, Falun Central Hospital and Centre of Clinical Research, Dalarna, Falun, Sweden.

Michael T. Karski, Consultant Foot and Ankle Orthopaedic Surgeon, Wrightington, Wigan and Leigh NHS Foundation Trust, United Kingdom.

John Kirkup MBE, Consultant Foot and Ankle Orthopaedic Surgeon (Ret), Royal United Hospital Bath NHS Trust, United Kingdom.

Daniel Latt, Foot and Ankle Orthopaedic Surgeon, Tucson, Arizona, USA, and Associate Professor in Orthopaedic Surgery and Biomedical Engineering with Banner-University Medical Center South, USA.

Alberto Leardini, Director at Laboratory of Movement Analysis and Functional-Clinical Evaluation of Prosthesis, The Rizzoli Institute, Italy.

Manuel Leyes, Foot and Ankle Orthopaedic Surgeon, Clinica Cemtro, Madrid, Spain.

Haroon Majeed, Senior Fellow in Foot and Ankle Surgery, Wrightington, Wigan and Leigh NHS Foundation Trust, United Kingdom.

Ali-Asgar Najefi, Specialist Registrar in Foot and Ankle Surgery, Royal National Orthopaedic Hospitals NHS Trust, United Kingdom. **(Associate Editor)**

Ali Navi, Consultant Foot and Ankle Orthopaedic Surgeon, Hervey Bay Hospital, Queensland, Australia. **(Associate Editor)**

John J. O'Connor, Emeritus Professor of Bioengineering (Ret), Department of Engineering Science, Oxford University, Oxford, United Kingdom.

Arul Ramasamy, Honorary Clinical Senior Lecturer. The Royal British Legion Centre for Blast Injury Studies, Imperial College London, United Kingdom. **(Associate Editor)**

Pascal Rippstein, Foot and Ankle Orthopaedic Surgeon, Schulthess Clinic, Zurich, Switzerland.

Dishan Singh, Consultant Foot and Ankle Orthopaedic Surgeon (Ret), Royal National Orthopaedic Hospitals NHS Trust, United Kingdom.

Dakshinamurthy Sunderamoorthy, Consultant Foot and Ankle Orthopaedic Surgeon, Goole and Scunthorpe Hospitals, United Kingdom.

Rhys H. Thomas, Consultant Foot and Ankle Orthopaedic Surgeon, University Hospital Llandough, Cardiff, United Kingdom.

Tim Williams, Consultant Foot and Ankle Orthopaedic Surgeon, Colchester Hospital University NHS Foundation Trust, United Kingdom.

Razi Zaidi, Specialist Registrar in Foot and Ankle Surgery. Royal National Orthopaedic Hospitals NHS Trust, United Kingdom.
(Associate Editor)

ACKNOWLEDGEMENTS

To our wives and parents who are always there for us and whom have sacrificed much whilst we focused time and energy for this textbook, but never our love and devotion. To our amazing children who give us reason to teach, share knowledge and do what we do. To all the amazing contributors to this textbook who have brought their invaluable knowledge and depth of expertise despite delays, obstacles and obstructions. It would be remiss if we did not mention the four Associate Editors, Ali-Asgar Najefi, Ali Navi, Arul Ramasamy, and Razi Zaidi for their heroic efforts in pulling the project together and keeping the momentum going. And last but not least to all those read this book, and hence for giving us the reason for being.

CONTENTS

BIOMECHANICS OF THE ANKLE COMPLEX

A. Leardini, J. J. O'Connor and S. Giannini

Summary

The human ankle joint complex plays a fundamental role in gait and other activities of daily living. At the same time, it is a very complicated anatomical system where the following has not been fully described: (i) the coupled joint motion, position, and orientation of the joint axis of rotation, (ii) stress and strain in the ligaments and their role in guiding and stabilising joint motion, (iii) conformity and congruence of the articular surfaces, patterns of contact at the articular surfaces, patterns of rolling and sliding at the joint surfaces, and muscle lever arm lengths. This chapter addresses these issues, also reporting the most recent relevant findings from the literature. This is discussed for the normal and diseased ankle joint. Methods for assessment of motion, relevance of biomechanics to implant design, kinetics and kinematics effects of surgery are also discussed.

KINETICS AND KINEMATICS OF THE NORMAL ANKLE

The ankle and subtalar joints are the connecting part of the complex foot segment. During locomotion, this unit provides the rocker of the shank with respect to the foot during the three rockers of the walking cycle (Gage *et al.*, 1995). During each of these phases, the foot becomes flexible to load or becomes rigid to allow propulsion (Root *et al.*, 1977). The mechanisms have been variously called "shock absorption", "navicular drop", "windlass mechanism", "foot clearance", and "elicapodalica" (helical airscrew between the rearfoot and forefoot).

Passive stability is a measure of the limitations imposed by the anatomical structures and involves mechanical interactions between ligaments and articular surfaces. Active stability involves mechanical interactions between muscles, ligaments, and articular surfaces in response to external forces (O'Connor *et al.*, 1998).

In this chapter, we refer to the ankle (tibiotalar) and subtalar joints as "ankle complex". In real life, overall "mobility" of the foot with respect to the shank is not restricted to just these two joints but relies on a mobile foot as well. In level walking, considerable triplanar motion occurs in the ankle complex, including about 30° rotation in the sagittal plane, coupled with about 14° and 22° rotation in the frontal and transverse planes (Ingrosso *et al.*, 2009).

Kinetics is the study of motion of objects and the forces that cause those motions. In contrast, kinematics is the study of motion of objects without consideration of the forces acting on the object.

Using kinematics, ankle complex motion can be divided into that at the ankle and at the subtalar joints (Leardini *et al.*, 2000; Stagni *et al.*, 2003), though only *in vitro* studies have been able to reveal this motion separately, and almost always, in an unloaded situation. Initially, combined motion (at the ankle and subtalar joint) was considered to be a rotation about a fixed axis (Inman, 1976; Dul and Johnson, 1985). The instantaneous axis of rotation at both these joints was later shown to translate and rotate during flexion (Leardini *et al.*, 1999b, 2001b), suggesting that the original hinge joint concept was an oversimplification.

There is also an associated shift of the contact area at the ankle during flexion not only at the trochlea tali but also at the tibial mortise (Corazza *et al.*, 2005). In this joint, therefore, rolling as well as sliding occurs, consistent with multiaxial rotation. In normal joints, an isometric pattern of rotation for the calcaneofibular (CaFi) and the tibiocalcaneal (TiCa) ligaments about their origins and insertions has been reported (Leardini *et al.*, 1999b; Stagni *et al.*, 2004) (Figure 1).

From unloaded maximal dorsiflexion to maximal plantiflexion, the mean overall rotation in 20 healthy subjects using three-dimensional (3D) CT stress tests was found to be much higher at the tibiotalar (63°) than at subtalar (4°) joint *in vivo* (Tuijthof *et al.*, 2009). Smaller differences were observed in the complete and natural range from maximal combined eversion–dorsiflexion to maximal combined inversion–plantarflexion (49° vs 30°).

During the stance phase of walking, the joint rotation in the three anatomical planes were, on average, about 15°, 8°, and 8° at the tibiotalar, 7°, 10°, and 7° at the subtalar (Lundgren *et al.*, 2008). In this study, with foot bone motion tracked *in vivo* in volunteers with intracortical pins, the overall (100%) bone motion in the sagittal plane of the medial longitudinal arch was found distributed in about 38% at the tibiotalar joint, 21% at the talonavicular, 28% navicular-cuneiform, and 13% at the first metatarsal-cuneiform; these percentages were 21%, 38%, 27%, and 14% in the frontal plane, and 21%, 45%, 17%, and 17% in the transverse planes. Therefore, a false impression of good ankle movement can be retained after ankle fusion because of motion at adjacent joints.

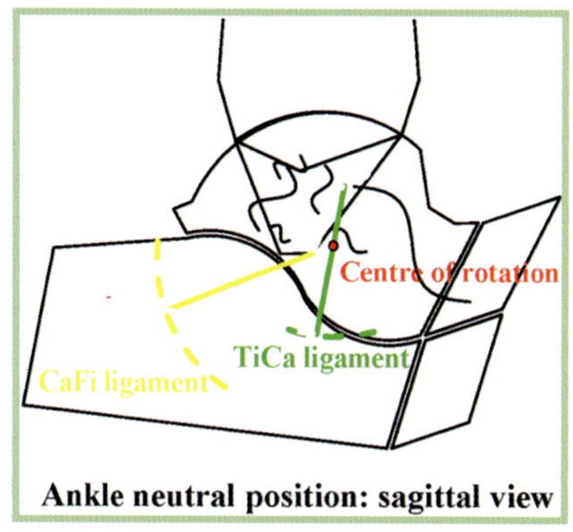

Figure 1. *Diagram for the sagittal plane model of the ankle joint (Leardini et al., 1999b), with the course of the main ligaments, including the two most isometric, the CaFi and the TiCa. The centre of instantaneous rotation at the crossing point of the two is depicted.*

KINETICS AND KINEMATICS OF THE DISEASED ANKLE

Many groups have studied the motion of the ankle complex in healthy model, both *in vitro* and *in vivo*. Our group has spent much time investigating *in vitro* the roles of the ligaments in restraining (i.e. guiding and resisting joint motion) in a healthy ankle complex. A number of studies have extended this interest in conditions simulating ankle instability, mostly by successively sacrificing ligament fibres. Very little has been reported of the changes in arthritic ankles, because access to cadaveric arthritic ankles is limited.

Pathologic gait has been studied *in vivo* in rheumatoid arthritis, posterior tibial tendon dysfunction, and hallux rigidus (Rankine *et al.*, 2008).

Access to functional analyses of pathological ankles has been provided by clinical gait analysis before and after surgery, although such studies have only considered motion of the foot as a single unit, in respect to the shank.

In unilateral, posttraumatic ankle osteoarthritis patients, smaller joint rotations in the three planes, and a weaker push-off power were observed at the ankle (Valderrabano *et al.*, 2007; Ingrosso *et al.*, 2009). In both studies, low performance may be affected by pain and difficulty in progression as suggested by low clinical scores and decreases in most of the spatiotemporal parameters. When comparing these, the alignment in varus, valgus, and neutral ankles with arthritis, there were no differences in spatial temporal mechanics, patient outcomes, or measures of physical performance (Queen *et al.*, 2011).

Patients with ankle osteoarthritis had changes in ankle and hip mechanics specifically during the push-off phase of gait. There occurred an increase in hip flexion moment and an increase in hip extension in the ankle osteoarthritis patients due to compensation for the decrease in plantarflexion moment from limited ankle motion during terminal stance (Queen, 2017).

In those with rheumatoid arthritis, the gait pattern was characterised by reduced walking speed, decreased cadence, decreased stride length, decreased ankle power, increased double limb support time, and peak plantar pressures at the forefoot. Walking velocity was reduced in psoriatic arthritis and gout with no differences in ankylosing spondylitis (Carroll *et al.*, 2015).

METHODS FOR ASSESSMENT OF MOTION OF THE ANKLE COMPLEX

Stereophotogrammetric Systems

Observation of gait is the mainstay of clinical analysis but is incapable of detecting and quantifying subtle changes. Quantitative 3D gait analysis is therefore used. There are many stereophotogrammetric systems on the market (including, BTS (BTS S.p.A., Milan, Italy); Codamotion (Charnwood Dynamics Ltd, Rothley, UK); Motion Analysis (Motion Analysis Corporation, Santa Rosa, CA); Qualysis (Qualysis, Gothenburg, Sweden); and Vicon (OMG Plc, Oxford, UK). In these systems, it is possible to track foot and ankle motion, *in vivo*. A typical gait analysis laboratory has several video cameras located around a walkway or treadmill, all connected to a central computer (Figure 2).

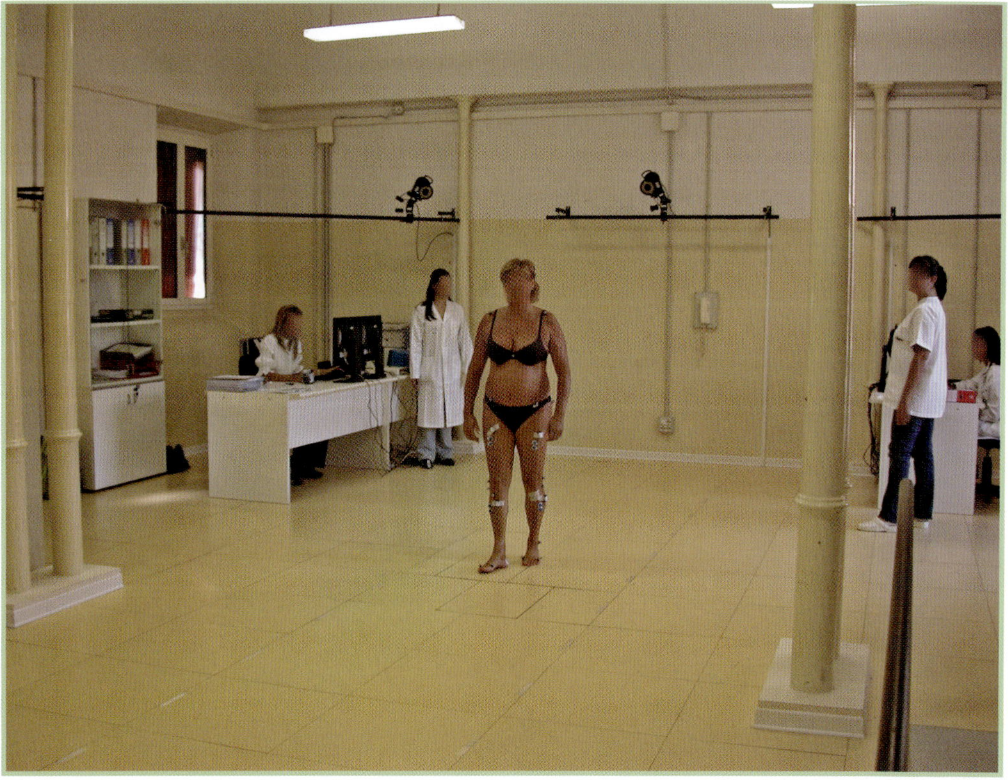

Figure 2. *Picture taken during gait analysis in a typical laboratory (courtesy of the Istituto Ortopedico Rizzoli, the Movement Analysis Laboratory); the instrumented patient is asked to walk within a field of measurements, assisted by technicians and medical doctors.*

In a conventional protocol (Davis *et al.*, 1991), surface markers are placed on the subject at various reference points such as the pelvis, condyles of the knees, medial and lateral malleoli, calcaneus, and a few metatarsal heads. Usually, the foot is considered as a single rigid segment, or even as a line segment. However, 3D segments are used in most current clinical gait analysis protocols (Figure 3). The subject is asked to walk and the position of the markers is calculated and assessed by a complex computer algorithm, which provides a breakdown of the motion at each joint.

To calculate the kinetics, the gait laboratory has various load transducers usually embedded into force platforms put into the floor to measure ground reaction forces during foot contact. Spatial distribution of pressure (vertical component of the forces in the unit area) can be measured with pedobarographic equipment such as a Novel system (Novel GmbH, Munich, Germany) or a TekScan system (TekScan Inc., Boston, MA) (Figure 4).

A computational method known as inverse dynamics is used to assess the resulting net forces and moments about various joints during each sample of the gait cycle. To assess the activity of individual muscles on motion, surface or needle electrodes are used that assess the electrical activity of the muscles electromyography (EMG). Information from deep muscles is clearly confounded by those of more superficial muscles especially when surface EMG is used.

All this information is the input for an overall complex interpretation phase to assess the subjects function. Frequently, more resolution is necessary to assess function of the foot, and this requires multisegmental foot kinematic analysis. Such protocols are available (well summarised in the reviews by Rankine *et al.* (2008), and Bishop *et al.* (2012)) and are distinguished by the number of segments tracked, types of the marker cluster (single skin markers, wands, rigid arrays of markers), 2D- or 3D-based measurements (Figure 5). Conventions for joint rotation or planar angle calculation can vary, as can the definition of the anatomical reference frames and of the neutral reference.

Initial models only analysed the rearfoot although now midfoot and forefoot segments have been modelled, probably because of the

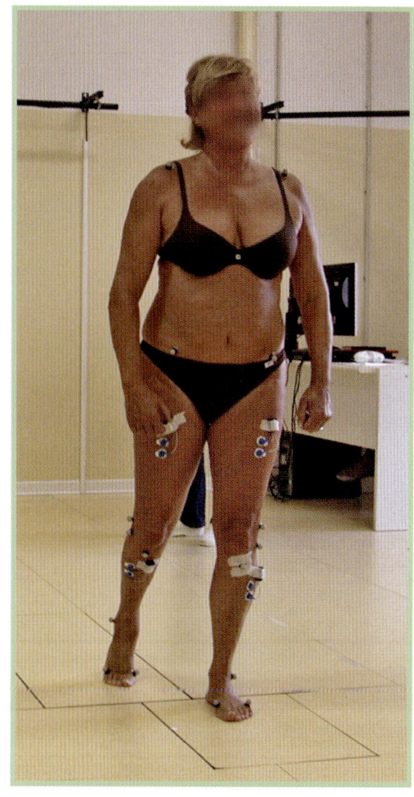

Figure 3. *Close-up of the patient (courtesy of the Istituto Ortopedico Rizzoli, the Movement Analysis Laboratory) with a typical marker set for full body kinematics analysis (Leardini et al., 2007a); with only three markers, the foot is assumed as a single rigid body.*

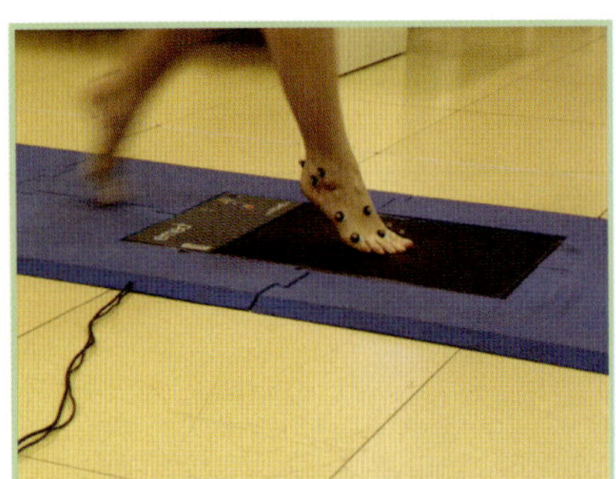

Figure 4. *Picture of one frame during landing of a foot instrumented (courtesy of the Istituto Ortopedico Rizzoli, the Movement Analysis Laboratory) with a typical marker set for multisegment foot kinematics (Leardini et al., 2007b), including the shank and the rear-, mid-, forefoot segments and the big toe. The measure is enhanced with a combined baropodometry by utilising a pressure platform.*

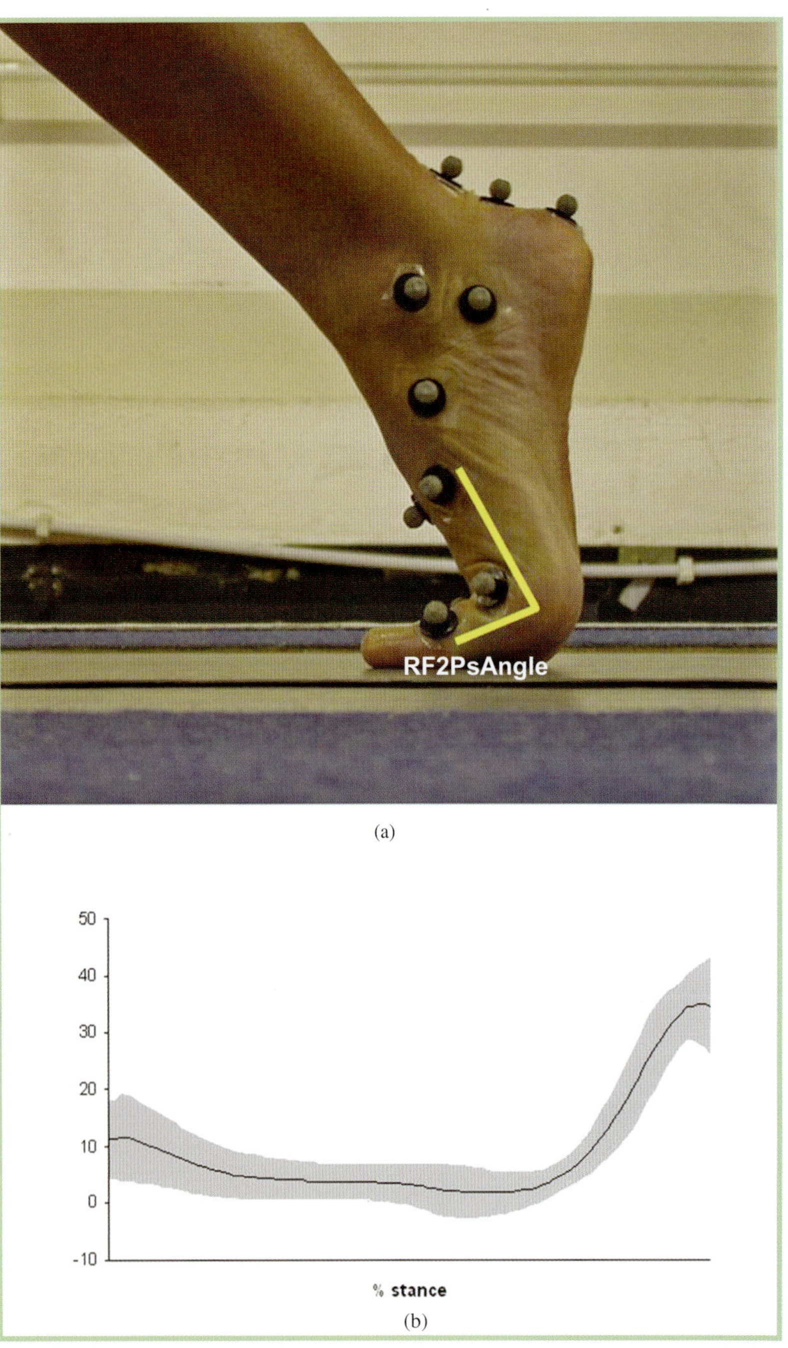

Figure 5. *One typical measure as taken from one multisegmental foot kinematic protocol (Leardini et al., 2007b). Dorsi/ plantar flexion of the first metatarsophalangeal joint, depicted in (a), and tracked throughout the stance phase of gait. (b) Mean (solid line) and standard deviation (grey) are shown.*

availability of more reliable instrumentation. The most recent studies propose 9- or even 10-segment approaches, although validation in terms of repeatability (Curtis *et al.*, 2009; Caravaggi *et al.*, 2011) and marker-to-bone association is limited (Nester *et al.*, 2010).

Limitations

Several issues still limit full acceptance and application of these techniques, including visibility, accuracy, encumbrance, and standardisation of the reports both in convention and terminology. In addition, there are technical hitches such as the markers falling off, or *in vivo* alterations of normal walking patterns (Lundgren *et al.*, 2008). The applicability of any findings in the presence of foot and leg deformities (Deschamps *et al.*, 2012), orthosis, and shoes (Bishop *et al.*, 2013) remains poorly defined.

3D Techniques

3D kinematics have also been assessed by means of electromagnetic tracking techniques, although limited to the hindfoot only (Woodburn *et al.*, 2002; Rouhani *et al.*, 2012). These systems are more practical and cheaper than the stereophotogrammetric, but cables are required and they rely once again on skin markers.

Other special techniques based on X-rays and on more modern MRI or videofluoroscopy (Figure 6) have been reported but are not routinely applied because of the invasive data acquisition, restricted field of measurement, and the intense data reduction. The field is, however, evolving at rapid pace and some preliminary studies are taking this towards a possible clinical application (Sheehan *et al.*, 2007; Fassbind *et al.*, 2011; Beimers *et al.*, 2012). A few such studies have recently addressed morphometry, explicitly to be exploited in the field of sizing in total ankle replacement (TAR) design (Fessy *et al.*, 1997; Stagni *et al.*, 2005; Kuo *et al.*, 2014), with the interesting final result that the current prostheses apparently are smaller than necessary. In these techniques, single foot bony motion can be tracked during activities of daily living.

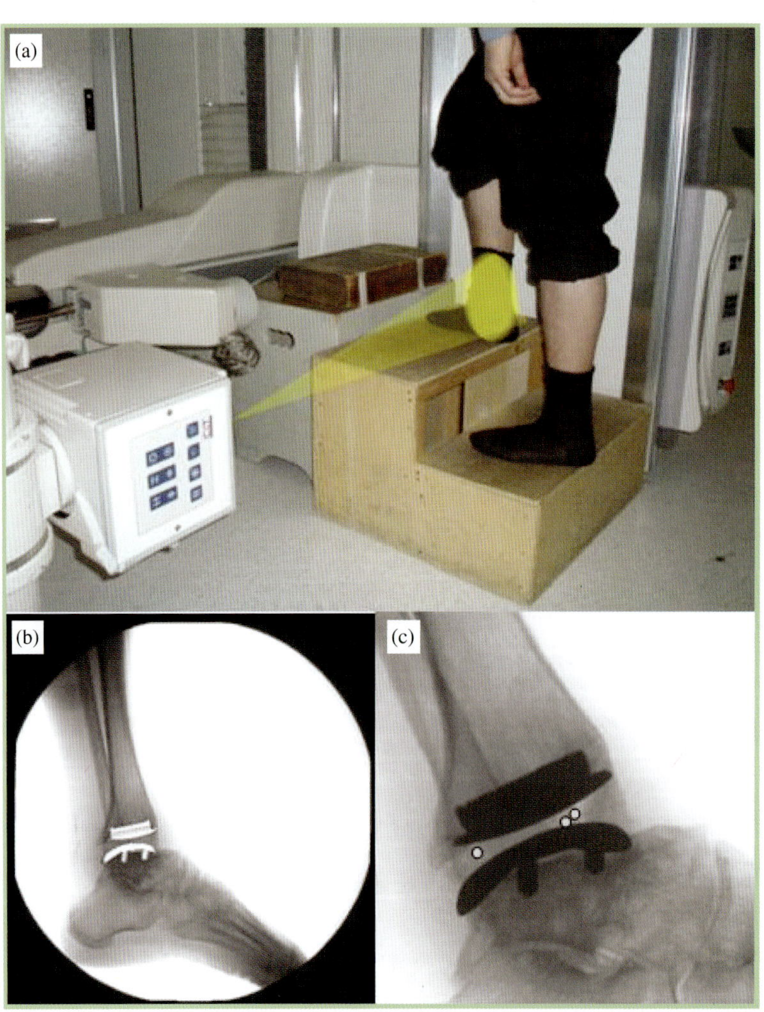

Figure 6. *Pictures from 3D videofluoroscopy (Cenni et al., 2013). From standard sagittal plane X-ray projections during execution of a motor task (a), relative position and orientation of the prosthetic components can be calculated (b), even of the polyethylene insert via tantalum beads stuck on it (c).*

Anatomical Models

In vitro tracking of foot bone motion has also been studied by gait simulators (Nester *et al.*, 2007; Whittaker *et al.*, 2011; Burg *et al.*, 2013), which are highly complicated and expensive systems using cadaveric specimens to attempt to replicate realistic kinematics and loading conditions (Figure 7). This enables access to internal

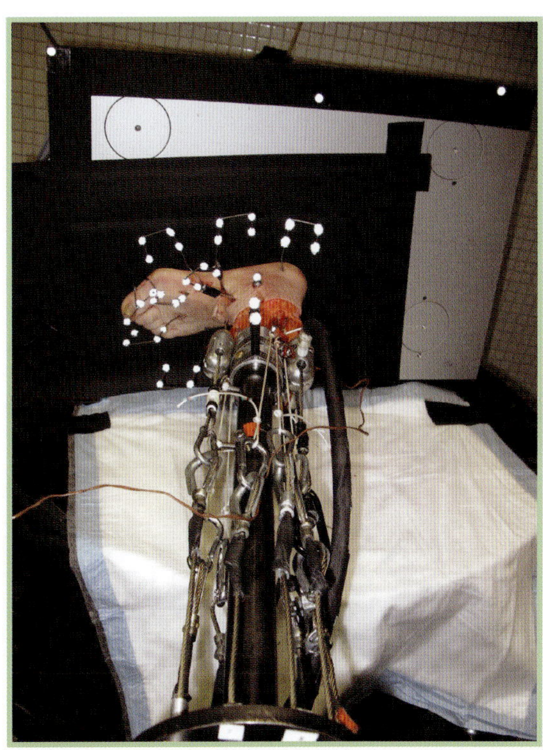

Figure 7. *The overall apparatus of the robotic gait simulator (Whittaker et al., 2011; Aubin et al., 2012). Courtesy of the VA RR&D Center of Excellence for Limb Loss Prevention and Prosthetic Engineering, VA Puget Sound Health Care System, WA, USA.*

A left foot in the robotic gait simulator, which consists of a Mikrolar R2000 parallel axis robot, a Kistler force plate, a novel pressure mat, a tibial mount, nine tendon clamps and cables, a load frame (not shown), nine linear actuators and load cells (not shown), and an eight-camera Vicon motion analysis system (not shown). Six degree of freedom kinematic data (tibia to ground) are collected from a motion analysis laboratory. In the simulator, the motion data are inverted, so that the "ground" (i.e. the force plate) moves relative to the fixed tibia to simulate gait. The vertical position of the ground and the Achilles tendon force is adjusted to insure accurate vertical ground reaction forces; the other five kinematic degrees of freedom are prescribed as are the other eight extrinsic muscle forces. Once the correct vertical ground reaction force is generated, the outputs (plantar pressure and foot bone motion) are obtained.

structures and relevant measurements, impossible *in vivo*, and a few clinical applications are now encouraging their use (Jackson *et al.*, 2011; Weber *et al.*, 2012).

In many of these models, loads and speeds have been below those in real life and the extent to which this replication is reliable has also been questioned.

In vivo skeletal tracking using percutaneous bone-anchored markers could be used to assess skeletal motion in activities of daily living (Nester *et al.*, 2007); however, the invasiveness of the procedures has limited its use to a handful of volunteers and is certainly not appropriate in routine clinical assessments (Figure 8).

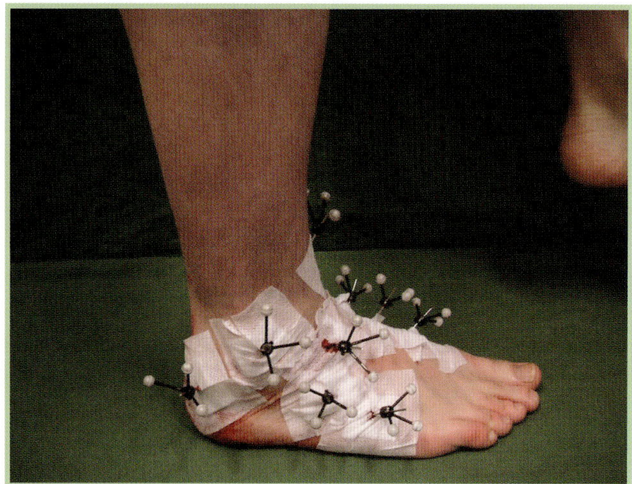

Figure 8. *Picture taken from in vivo measurement of skeletal motion by bone pins; a cluster of three markers is implanted in eight different bones (from Lundgren et al., 2008 study; original picture provided by the authors).*

Summary

Our understanding of this important topic is still based on strong mathematical assumptions, which are necessary for simplifying the huge mechanical complexity of this anatomical area.

The only measure we can rely on is the single ground reaction force applied to the single rigid foot segment. In addition, plantar pressures in a number of individual cells can be measured, and associated somehow to the bones in the foot.

Despite these limitations, the current understanding of the kinematics of the foot and of its segments during execution of standard motor tasks is reasonable, although we still know very little about the kinetics, particularly, the forces exchanged between these segments.

EFFECT OF ANKLE SURGERY ON ANKLE COMPLEX KINETICS AND KINEMATICS

After arthrodesis, either of the tibiotalar joints, tibiotalocalcaneal or a pantalar fusion, standard gait analysis with three or less markers on the foot (Bayaert *et al.*, 2004; Wu *et al.*, 2005) shows movement from the remaining unfused joints.

Some studies have attempted to distinguish between hindfoot and forefoot motion (Wu *et al.*, 2000; Thomas *et al.*, 2006). In these, rigidity of the ankle joint was compensated for by movement at the knee and foot joints. Radiographic findings at the subtalar joint have shown either a significant increase of motion (Sealey *et al.*, 2009) or stiffness and loss of motion (Thomas *et al.*, 2006). The compensatory hypermobility, particularly at the subtalar and midfoot joints, is deemed likely to contribute to subsequent adjacent joint arthritis (Bayaert *et al.*, 2004; Thomas *et al.*, 2006; Sealey *et al.*, 2009). A theoretical improvement in gait and protection of the adjacent joints are of course arguments in favour of arthroplasty (Piriou *et al.*, 2008).

Queen *et al.* demonstrated that there were no significant differences in ankle mechanics following surgery, suggesting that change was relative only to the preoperative time point. However, stride length improved by 13.9 cm, walking speed by 31 cm/s, and double-limb support time by 6%. In patients up to 5 years after surgery, most improvements were maintained through 5 years and sagittal plane ankle mechanics remained unchanged. However, some variables (walking speed, timed up and go, stride length, and stride width) declined between the 2- and 5-year time points, indicating a decline in function during this time (Queen, 2017).

In vivo, gait analysis has shown that neither arthroplasty nor arthrodesis restored fully normal walking speed or lower limb joint movements. Arthroplasty, however, allows larger motion at the ankle complex, a symmetrical gait and normal ground reaction force patterns (Piriou *et al.*, 2008; Brodsky *et al.*, 2011; Hahn *et al.*, 2012; Rouhani *et al.*, 2012). In these studies, patients with arthrodesis appeared to have faster gait and longer step length (Piriou *et al.*, 2008). Six months following ankle arthroplasty, nearly normal spatiotemporal parameters were obtained together with nearly normal patterns of ankle joint rotations and moments in all the three anatomical planes, and a good recovery of physiological muscle activity (Ingrosso *et al.*, 2009; Valderrabano *et al.*, 2007). These results were observed to be maintained at 12 months follow-up.

Increased motion at hip and knee joints and increased ankle power and flexion moment were also measured (Brodsky *et al.*, 2011). Nearly physiological motion and loading in the replaced ankle were observed also during stair climbing (Cenni *et al.*, 2013). However, deterioration of the spatio-temporal parameters and abnormal muscular activation have also been noted at longer follow-up (Benedetti *et al.*, 2008).

Fatigue and limited physical activity that is often reported in osteoarthritis patients could be associated with the decrease in energy recovery. Perhaps, gait retraining could improve walking mechanics and therefore improve energy recovery. In the TAR population, walking speed was significantly improved through the 2-year postoperative assessment; however, after controlling for walking speed, no differences in energy recovery were found (Schmitt *et al.*, 2015).

Restoration of neutral ankle alignment at the time of TAR in patients with preoperative varus or valgus tibiotalar alignment resulted in biomechanics similar to those of patients with neutral preoperative tibiotalar alignment by 24-month follow-up (Grier *et al.*, 2016).

In comparisons between ankle fusion and ankle replacement, significant improvement in foot mobility was found after replacement, whereas significant impairments remained after arthrodesis (Piriou *et al.*, 2008; Hahn *et al.*, 2012; Rouhani *et al.*, 2012; Kane *et al.*, 2017; Pedowitz *et al.*, 2016).

In summary, it appears that patients with both ankle arthrodesis and ankle replacement walk more slowly than matched controls, but gait more closely approximates normality following ankle

replacement compared to arthrodesis (Valderrabano *et al.*, 2006; Piriou *et al.*, 2008; Ingrosso *et al.*, 2009; Pedowitz *et al.*, 2016). Flavin *et al.* compared pre- and post-operative gait in patients who had ankle arthroplasty or arthrodesis. Both groups had significant improvements compared with preoperative function. However, neither group reached the function of normal control patients (Flavin, 2013). They also reported greater range of movement in the sagittal plane in those who had undergone TAR.

RELEVANCE OF BIOMECHANICS TO IMPLANT DESIGN

It is likely that the current unsatisfactory clinical results of TAR (Pyevich *et al.*, 1998; Stengel *et al.*, 2005; Chou *et al.*, 2008; Cracchiolo and Deorio, 2008; Deorio and Easley, 2008; Michael *et al.*, 2008; Saito *et al.*, 2018; and Cody *et al.*, 2019) are accounted for by limited biomechanical knowledge applied to their design.

An isometric pattern of rotation for fibres within the CaFi and the TiCa ligaments, the instantaneous axis of rotation, and the shift of the contact area at the tibial mortise during flexion imply a complex rolling and sliding combined motion at the ankle joint, as guided by the close interaction between the geometry of the ligaments and the shapes of the articular surfaces (Leardini *et al.*, 1999a, 1999b) (Figure 1).

Any design of joint replacement or ligament reconstructions should take into consideration these important findings (Leardini *et al.*, 2004) if it is to replicate the function of a normal ankle or there may be conflict between mobility and conformity (O'Connor *et al.*, 1998).

Where restoration of normal mobility is the main goal, unconforming semiconstrained designs may lead to inadequate loadbearing capacity and increased wear.

Where the main target is congruency of the artificial surfaces, full conforming articular surfaces enlarge contact areas, but may constrain motion and overload the fixation system. Most current TAR designs compromise in this respect.

The implants least susceptible to wear can be two-part completely congruent (or nearly so) or three-part (Stengel *et al.*, 2005; Younger *et al.*, 2008), i.e. with a meniscal bearing in between the two metal bone-anchored components, as in most of the current designs (Vickerstaff *et al.*, 2007). The former uses a thick layer of polyethylene associated to the tibial component. The latter employs fully congruent meniscal bearings with variable freedom to slide on each of the articular surfaces. These meniscal bearing prostheses in theory can allow translational movement and yet maintain congruence of the articular surfaces throughout the range of movements, but may require a special combination of geometry of the metal components (Leardini *et al.*, 2001a), rather than flat tibial and anatomical talar components.

The three-part implants can also accommodate limited inaccuracy in implantation, and the independent selection of an appropriate thickness of the bearing component can help restore better a normal tensioning at the retained ligaments, which seems logical.

In vitro, it has been shown that two-component prostheses restricted talar motion within the mortise much more than three-component designs, likely resulting in an increase of stress forces (Valderrabano *et al.*, 2003a, 2003b, 2003c). Queen *et al.* demonstrated improvements in ankle moment and ground reaction forces in fixed bearing implants, while the mobilebearing implant group demonstrated improvements in patient-reported pain outcome (Queen *et al.*, 2014). More recently, Queen *et al.* demonstrated that there were no statistically or clinically meaningful differences between fixed and mobilebearing implants when examining gait mechanics and pain 1 year after TAR in a randomised control trial (Queen *et al.*, 2017).

Implantability and durability are the other main objectives of TAR designs. For the former, reliability and repeatability of the operative technique is sought, with robust and accurate instrumentation to guarantee correct position of the components with minimum bone stock removal. Durability depends on good fixation of the components, with appropriate load transfer to bone and a low risk of loosening.

Current designs use a variety of fixation elements: pegs, long or short stems, fins, cylindrical or rectangular bars (Bauer *et al.*, 1996), and bone screws (Hintermann *et al.*, 2004; Vickerstaff *et al.*, 2007; Gougoulias *et al.*, 2009) (Figure 9). Apart from a few prostheses which feature ceramic on ceramic bearings, all recent two- and three-part designs have metal bone-anchored components and a polyethylene insert, either fixed or semi-constrained with the tibial, or freely movable in between (Cracchiolo and Deorio, 2008; Gougoulias *et al.*, 2009).

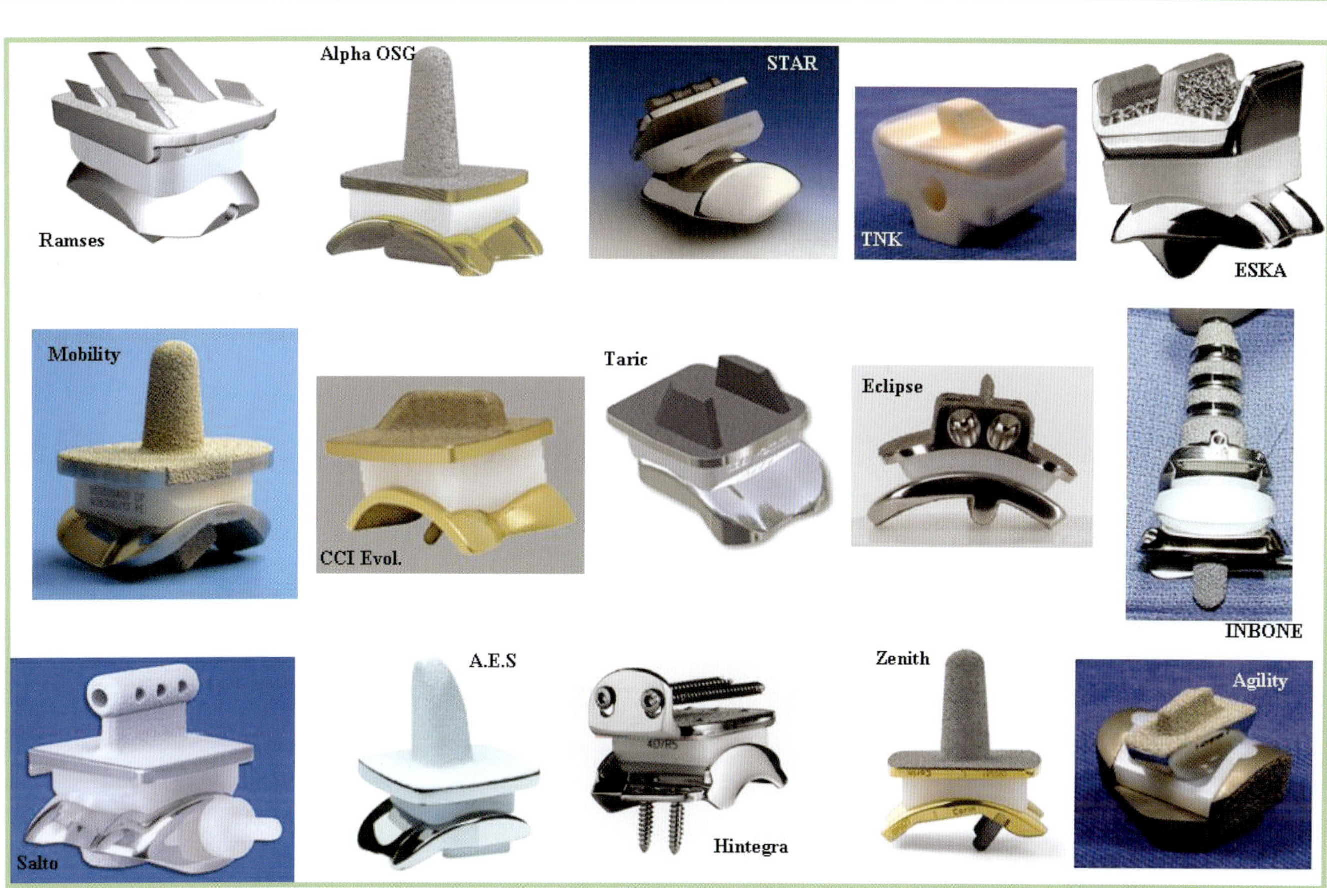

Figure 9. *Pictures from a number of current ankle prosthesis designs, showing the fixation elements in the tibial and talar components.*

CONCLUSION

We still have much to learn about the biomechanics of the ankle, particularly with reference to ankle joint replacement. However, many modern designs still do not use all available data that may lead to demonstrably improved patient outcomes.

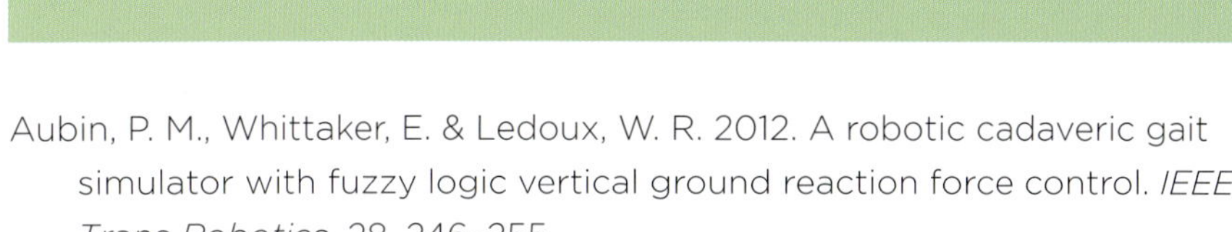

REFERENCES

Aubin, P. M., Whittaker, E. & Ledoux, W. R. 2012. A robotic cadaveric gait simulator with fuzzy logic vertical ground reaction force control. *IEEE Trans Robotics*, 28, 246–255.

Bauer, G., Eberhardt, O., Rosenbaum, D. & Claes, L. 1996. Total ankle replacement: review and critical analysis of the current status. *Foot Ankle Surg*, 2, 119–126.

Bayaert, C., Sirveaux, F., Paysant, J., Molé, D. & André, J.-M. 2004. The effect of tibio-talar arthrodesis on foot kinematics and ground reaction force progressing during walking. *Gait Posture*, 20, 84–91.

Beimers, L., Louwerens, J. W., Tuijthof, G. J., Jonges, R., Van Dijk, C. N. & Blankevoort, L. 2012. CT measurement of range of motion of ankle and subtalar joints following two lateral column lengthening procedures. *Foot Ankle Int*, 33, 386–393.

Benedetti, M. G., Leardini, A., Romagnoli, M., Berti, L., Catani, F. & Giannini, S. 2008. Functional outcome of meniscal-bearing total ankle replacement: A gait analysis study. *J Am Podiatr Med Assoc*, 98, 19–26.

Bishop, C., Paul, G. & Thewlis, D. 2012. Recommendations for the reporting of foot and ankle models. *J Biomech*, 45, 2185–2194.

Bishop, C., Paul, G. & Thewlis, D. 2013. The reliability, accuracy and minimal detectable difference of a multi-segment kinematic model of the foot-shoe complex. *Gait Posture*, 37, 552–557.

Brodsky, J. W., Polo, F. E., Coleman, S. C. & Bruck, N. 2011. Changes in gait following the Scandinavian Total Ankle Replacement. *J Bone Joint Surg Am*, 93, 1890–1896.

Burg, J., Peeters, K., Natsakis, T., Dereymaeker, G., Vander Sloten, J. & Jonkers, I. 2013. *In vitro* analysis of muscle activity illustrates mediolateral decoupling of hind and mid foot bone motion. *Gait Posture*, 38, 56–61.

Caravaggi, P., Benedetti, M. G., Berti, L. & Leardini, A. 2011. Repeatability of a multi-segment foot protocol in adult subjects. *Gait Posture*, 33, 133–135.

Carroll, M., Parmar, P., Dalbeth, N., Boocock, M. & Rome, K. 2015. Gait characteristics associated with the foot and ankle in inflammatory arthritis: A systematic review and meta-analysis. *BMC Musculoskelet Disord*, 16, 134.

Cenni, F., Leardini, A., Pieri, M., Berti, L., Belvedere, C., Romagnoli, M. & Giannini, S. 2013. Functional performance of a total ankle replacement: Thorough assessment by combining gait and fluoroscopic analyses. *Clin Biomech (Bristol, Avon)*, 28, 79–87.

Chou, L. B., Coughlin, M. T., Hansen, S., Jr., Haskell, A., Lundeen, G., Saltzman, C. L. & Mann, R. A. 2008. Osteoarthritis of the ankle: The role of arthroplasty. *J Am Acad Orthop Surg*, 16, 249–259.

Cody, E. A., Taylor, M. A., Nunley, J. A., II, Parekh S. G. & DeOrio J. K. 2019. Increased early revision rate with the INFINITY total ankle prosthesis. *Foot Ankle Int*, 40(1), 9–17. doi: 10.1177/1071100718794933. Epub 2018 Sep 3.

Corazza, F., Leardini, A., O'Connor J. J. & Parenti Castelli, V. 2005. Mechanics of the anterior drawer test at the ankle: The effects of ligament viscoelasticity. *J Biomech*, 38, 2118–2123.

Cracchiolo, A., III & Deorio, J. K. 2008. Design features of current total ankle replacements: Implants and instrumentation. *J Am Acad Orthop Surg*, 16, 530–540.

Curtis, D. J., Bencke, J., Stebbins, J. A. & Stansfield, B. 2009. Intra-rater repeatability of the Oxford foot model in healthy children in different stages of the foot roll over process during gait. *Gait Posture*, 30, 118–121.

Davis, R. B., Õunpuu, S., Tyburski, D. & Gage, J. R. 1991. A gait analysis data collection and reduction technique. *Hum Mov Sci*, 10, 575–587.

Deorio, J. K. & Easley, M. E. 2008. Total ankle arthroplasty. *Instr Course Lect*, 57, 383–413.

Deschamps, K., Staes, F., Bruyninckx, H., Busschots, E., Matricali, G. A., Spaepen, P., Meyer, C. & Desloovere, K. 2012. Repeatability of a 3D multi-segment foot model protocol in presence of foot deformities. *Gait Posture*, 36, 635–638.

Dul, J. & Johnson, G. E. 1985. A kinematic model of the human ankle. *J Biomed Eng*, 7, 137–143.

Fassbind, M. J., Rohr, E. S., Hu, Y., Haynor, D. R., Siegler, S., Sangeorzan, B. J. & Ledoux, W. R. 2011. Evaluating foot kinematics using magnetic resonance imaging: from maximum plantar flexion, inversion, and internal rotation to maximum dorsiflexion, eversion, and external rotation. *J Biomech Eng*, 133, 104502.

Fessy, M. H., Carret, J. P. & Bejui, J. 1997. Morphometry of the talocrural joint. *Surg Radiol Anat*, 19, 299–302.

Flavin, R. C. S., Tenenbaum, S. & Brodsky, J. W. 2013. Comparison of gait after total ankle arthroplasty and ankle arthrodesis. *Foot Ankle Int*, 34, 1340–1348.

Gage, J. R., Deluca, P. A. & Renshaw, T. S. 1995. Gait analysis: Principles and applications. *J Bone J Surg (Am)*, 77-A, 1607–1623.

Gougoulias, N. E., Khanna, A. & Maffulli, N. 2009. History and evolution in total ankle arthroplasty. *Br Med Bull*, 89, 111–151.

Grier, A. J., Schmitt, A. C., Adams, S. B. & Queen, R. M. 2016. The effect of tibiotalar alignment on coronal plane mechanics following total ankle replacement. *Gait Posture*, 48, 13–18.

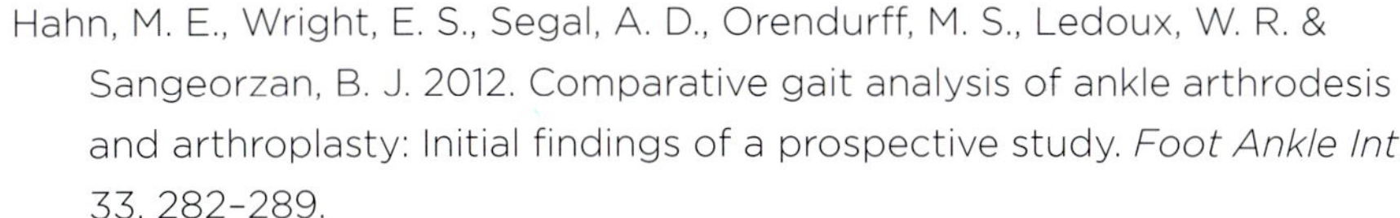

Hahn, M. E., Wright, E. S., Segal, A. D., Orendurff, M. S., Ledoux, W. R. &
   Sangeorzan, B. J. 2012. Comparative gait analysis of ankle arthrodesis
   and arthroplasty: Initial findings of a prospective study. *Foot Ankle Int*,
   33, 282–289.
Hintermann, B., Valderrabano, V., Dereymaeker, G. & Dick, W. 2004. The
   HINTEGRA ankle: Rationale and short-term results of 122 consecutive
   ankles. *Clin Orthop Relat Res*, 424, 57–68.
Ingrosso, S., Benedetti, M. G., Leardini, A., Casanelli, S., Sforza, T. & Giannini, S.
   2009. Gait analysis of a novel design of ankle replacement. *Gait Posture*,
   30, 132–137.
Inman, V. 1976. *The Joints of the Ankle*, Lipincott Williams and Wilkins,
   Balitmore, 7–73.
Jackson, L. T., Aubin, P. M., Cowley, M. S., Sangeorzan, B. J. & Ledoux, W. R.
   2011. A robotic cadaveric flatfoot analysis of stance phase. *J Biomech
   Eng*, 133, 051005.
Kane, J. M., Coleman, S. & Brodsky, J. W. 2017. Kinematics and function of total
   ankle replacements versus normal ankles. *Foot Ankle Clin*, 22, 241–249.
Kuo, C. C., Lu, H. L., Leardini, A., Lu, T. W., Kuo, M. Y. & Hsu, H. C. 2014.
   Three-dimensional computer graphics-based ankle morphometry with
   computerized tomography for total ankle replacement design and
   positioning. *Clin Anat*, 27, 659–668.
Leardini, A., O'Connor, J. J., Catani, F. & Giannini, S. 1999a. A geometric model
   of the human ankle joint. *J Biomech*, 32, 585–591.
Leardini, A., O'Connor, J. J., Catani, F. & Giannini, S. 1999b. Kinematics of the
   human ankle complex in passive flexion: A single degree of freedom
   system. *J Biomech*, 32, 111–118.
Leardini, A., O'Connor, J. J., Catani, F. & Giannini, S. 2000. The role of the
   passive structures in the mobility and stability of the human ankle joint:
   A literature review. *Foot Ankle Int*, 21, 602–615.
Leardini, A., Catani, F., Giannini, S. & O'Connor, J. J. 2001a. Computer-assisted
   design of the sagittal shapes of a ligament-compatible total ankle
   replacement. *Med Biol Eng Comput*, 39, 168–175.
Leardini, A., Stagni, R. & O'Connor, J. J. 2001b. Mobility of the subtalar joint in
   the intact ankle complex. *J Biomech*, 34, 805–809.
Leardini, A., O'Connor, J. J., Catani, F. & Giannini, S. 2004. Mobility of the
   human ankle and the design of total ankle replacement. *Clin Orthop
   Relat Res*, 39–46.
Leardini, A., Sawacha, Z., Paolini, G., Ingrosso, S., Nativo, R. & Benedetti, M. G.
   2007a. A new anatomically based protocol for gait analysis in children.
   Gait & Posture, 26(4), 560–571.

Leardini, A., Benedetti, M. G., Berti, L., Bettinelli, D., Nativo, R. & Giannini, S. 2007b. Rear-foot, mid-foot and fore-foot motion during the stance phase of gait. *Gait Posture*, 25(3): 453–462.

Lundgren, P., Nester, C., Liu, A., Arndt, A., Jones, R., Stacoff, A., Wolf, P. & Lundberg, A. 2008. Invasive *in vivo* measurement of rear-, mid- and forefoot motion during walking. *Gait Posture*, 28, 93–100.

Michael, J. M., Golshani, A., Gargac, S. & Goswami, T. 2008. Biomechanics of the ankle joint and clinical outcomes of total ankle replacement. *J Mech Behav Biomed Mater*, 1, 276–294.

Nester, C. J., Liu, A. M., Ward, E., Howard, D., Cocheba, J. & Derrick, T. 2010. Error in the description of foot kinematics due to violation of rigid body assumptions. *J Biomech*, 43, 666–672.

Nester, C. J., Liu, A. M., Ward, E., Howard, D., Cocheba, J., Derrick, T. & Patterson, P. 2007. *In vitro* study of foot kinematics using a dynamic walking cadaver model. *J Biomech*, 40, 1927–1937.

O'Connor, J. J., Lu, T. W., Wilson, D. R., Feikes, J. & Leardini, A. 1998. Review: Diarthrodial joints-kinematic pairs, mechanisms or flexible structures? *Comput Methods Biomech Biomed Engin*, 1, 123–150.

Pedowitz, D. I., Kane, J. M., Smith, G. M., Saffel, H. L., Comer, C. & Raikin, S. M. 2016. Total ankle arthroplasty versus ankle arthrodesis: A comparative analysis of arc of movement and functional outcomes. *Bone Joint J*, 98-B, 634–640.

Piriou, P., Culpan, P., Mullins, M., Cardon, J. N., Pozzi, D. & Judet, T. 2008. Ankle replacement versus arthrodesis: a comparative gait analysis study. *Foot Ankle Int*, 29, 3–9.

Pyevich, M. T., Saltzman, C. L., Callaghan, J. J. & Alvine, F. G. 1998. Total ankle arthroplasty: A unique design. Two to twelve-year follow-up. *J Bone Joint Surg Am*, 80, 1410–1420.

Queen, R. 2017. Directing clinical care using lower extremity biomechanics in patients with ankle osteoarthritis and ankle arthroplasty. *J Orthop Res*, 35, 2345–2355.

Queen, R. M., Carter, J. E., Adams, S. B., Easley, M. E., Deorio, J. K. & Nunley, J. A. 2011. Coronal plane ankle alignment, gait, and end-stage ankle osteoarthritis. *Osteoarthr Cartil*, 19, 1338–1342.

Queen, R. M., Sparling, T. L., Butler, R. J., Adams, S. B., Jr., Deorio, J. K., Easley, M. E. & Nunley, J. A. 2014. Patient-reported outcomes, function, and gait mechanics after fixed and mobile-bearing total ankle replacement. *J Bone Joint Surg Am*, 96, 987–993.

Queen, R. M., Franck, C. T., Schmitt, D. & Adams, S. B. 2017. Are there differences in gait mechanics in patients with a fixed versus mobile bearing total ankle arthroplasty? A randomized trial. *Clin Orthop Relat Res*, 475, 2599–2606.

Rankine, L., Long, J., Canseco, K. & Harris, G. F. 2008. Multisegmental foot modeling: A review. *Crit Rev Biomed Eng*, 36, 127–181.

Root, M. L., Orien, W. P. & Weed, J. H. 1977. Clinical Biomechanics: Normal and abnormal function of the foot. *Clinical Biomechanics Corps*, Los Angeles, California. 127–164.

Rouhani, H., Favre, J., Aminian, K. & Crevoisier, X. 2012. Multi-segment foot kinematics after total ankle replacement and ankle arthrodesis during relatively long-distance gait. *Gait Posture*, 36, 561–566.

Saito, G. H., Sanders, A. E., de Cesar Netto, C., O'Malley, M. J., Ellis, S. J., Demetracopoulos, C. A. 2018. Short-term complications, reoperations, and radiographic outcomes of a new fixed-bearing total ankle arthroplasty. *Foot Ankle Int*, 39(7), 787–794. doi: 10.1177/1071100718764107. Epub 2018 Mar 28.

Schmitt, D., Vap, A. & Queen, R. M. 2015. Effect of end-stage hip, knee, and ankle osteoarthritis on walking mechanics. *Gait Posture*, 42, 373–379.

Sealey, R. J., Myerson, M. S., Molloy, A., Gamba, C., Jeng, C. & Kalesan, B. 2009. Sagittal plane motion of the hindfoot following ankle arthrodesis: a prospective analysis. *Foot Ankle Int*, 30, 187–196.

Sheehan, F. T., Seisler, A. R. & Siegel, K. L. 2007. *In vivo* talocrural and subtalar kinematics: A non-invasive 3D dynamic MRI study. *Foot Ankle Int*, 28, 323–335.

Stagni, R., Leardini, A., O'Connor, J. J. & Giannini, S. 2003. Role of passive structures in the mobility and stability of the human subtalar joint: a literature review. *Foot Ankle Int*, 24, 402–409.

Stagni, R., Leardini, A. & Ensini, A. 2004. Ligament fibre recruitment at the human ankle joint complex in passive flexion. *J Biomech*, 37, 1823–1829.

Stagni, R., Leardini, A., Ensini, A. & Cappello, A. 2005. Ankle morphometry evaluated using a new semi-automated technique based on X-ray pictures. *Clin Biomech (Bristol, Avon)*, 20, 307–311.

Stengel, D., Bauwens, K., Ekkernkamp, A. & Cramer, J. 2005. Efficacy of total ankle replacement with meniscal-bearing devices: A systematic review and meta-analysis. *Arch Orthop Trauma Surg*, 125, 109–119.

Thomas, R., Daniels, T. R. & Parker, K. 2006. Gait analysis and functional outcomes following ankle arthrodesis for isolated ankle arthritis. *J Bone Joint Surg Am*, 88, 526–535.

Tuijthof, G. J., Zengerink, M., Beimers, L., Jonges, R., Maas, M., Van Dijk, C. N. & Blankevoort, L. 2009. Determination of consistent patterns of range of motion in the ankle joint with a computed tomography stress-test. *Clin Biomech (Bristol, Avon)*, 24, 517–523.

Valderrabano, V., Hintermann, B., Nigg, B. M., Stefanyshyn, D. & Stergiou, P. 2003a. Kinematic changes after fusion and total replacement of the ankle: Part 1: Range of motion. *Foot & Ankle International*, 24, 881–887.

Valderrabano, V., Hintermann, B., Nigg, B. M., Stefanyshyn, D. & Stergiou, P. 2003b. Kinematic changes after fusion and total replacement of the ankle: Part 2: Movement transfer. *Foot Ankle Int*, 24, 888–896.

Valderrabano, V., Hintermann, B., Nigg, B. M., Stefanyshyn, D. & Stergiou, P. 2003c. Kinematic changes after fusion and total replacement of the ankle: Part 3: Talar movement. *Foot Ankle Int*, 24, 897–900.

Valderrabano, V., Pagenstert, G., Horisberger, M., Knupp, M. & Hintermann, B. 2006. Sports and recreation activity of ankle arthritis patients before and after total ankle replacement. *Am J Sports Med*, 34, 993–999.

Valderrabano, V., Nigg, B. M., Von Tscharner, V., Stefanyshyn, D. J., Goepfert, B. & Hintermann, B. 2007. Gait analysis in ankle osteoarthritis and total ankle replacement. *Clin Biomech (Bristol, Avon)*, 22, 894–904.

Vickerstaff, J. A., Miles, A. W. & Cunningham, J. L. 2007. A brief history of total ankle replacement and a review of the current status. *Med Eng Phys*, 29, 1056–1064.

Weber, J. R., Aubin, P. M., Ledoux, W. R. & Sangeorzan, B. J. 2012. Second metatarsal length is positively correlated with increased pressure and medial deviation of the second toe in a robotic cadaveric simulation of gait. *Foot Ankle Int*, 33, 312–319.

Whittaker, E. C., Aubin, P. M. & Ledoux, W. R. 2011. Foot bone kinematics as measured in a cadaveric robotic gait simulator. *Gait Posture*, 33, 645–650.

Woodburn, J., Helliwell, P. S. & Barker, S. 2002. Three-dimensional kinematics at the ankle joint complex in rheumatoid arthritis patients with painful valgus deformity of the rearfoot. *Rheumatology (Oxford)*, 41, 1406–1412.

Wu, W. L., Su, F. C., Cheng, Y. M., Huang, P. J., Chou, Y. L. & Chou, C. K. 2000. Gait analysis after ankle arthrodesis. *Gait Posture*, 11, 54–61.

Wu, W. L., Huang, P. J., Lin, C. J., Chen, W. Y., Huang, K. F. & Cheng, Y. M. 2005. Lower extremity kinematics and kinetics during level walking and stair climbing in subjects with triple arthrodesis or subtalar fusion. *Gait Posture*, 21, 263–270.

Younger, A., Penner, M. & Wing, K. 2008. Mobile-bearing total ankle arthroplasty. *Foot Ankle Clin*, 13, 495–508, ix–x.

BIOMATERIALS

CHAPTER

2

27

C. Brockett

Summary

Biomaterials have played a vital contribution to the evolution of total ankle replacements (TARs). Bearing surfaces are required to produce minimal wear and have been adapted from the success of other total joint replacement designs. Limited wear studies in relation to the ankle make it difficult to determine which bearing material combination will produce the least debris long term. Fixation aims to provide stability through osseointegration between the bone and implant. The movement towards porous-coated designs with bioactive calcium phosphate finishes are preferred outside of the USA, but has yet to be proven through clinical outcome data. A lack of pre-clinical testing and long-term clinical studies make it difficult to draw conclusions about the performance of biomaterials in TAR.

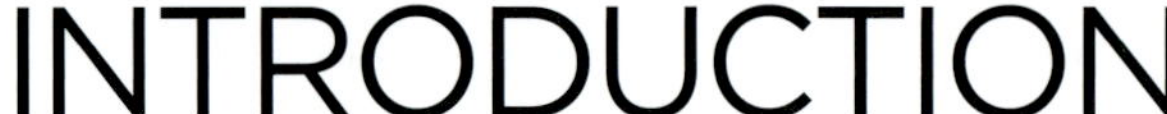

INTRODUCTION

Total ankle replacements (TARs) must function under demanding cyclic loads and within a potentially corrosive environment while maintaining mechanical and chemical integrity. The following aspects must be considered when selecting appropriate materials:

- Biocompatibility.
- Mechanical properties.
- Economically viable manufacturing modalities.

It is important to understand both the body's response to the material and the material's reaction to the bioactive environment. The ideal materials will have a high corrosion resistance, stiffness similar to that of bone, and be bioactive where necessary for fixation.

The reduced life span of TAR relative to total hip and knee replacement mean less focus has been placed on the advancement of biomaterials specific to TAR. Across the market, there are a variety of biomaterials employed but their impact on long-term performance is, to some extent, unknown.

BEARING SURFACES

Historically, metal-on-polyethylene bearings have been used extensively throughout total joint replacement. The most common combination consists of a cobalt chromium (CoCr) alloy articulating with varying grades of ultra-high molecular weight polyethylene (UHMWPE). The biomaterials are given their application due to their material properties shown in Table 1. TARs are no exception with the majority of the marketed designs opting for this material pairing as shown in Table 2.

The performance of a total joint replacement is often considered in terms of wear which can be defined as the "the removal of material from solid surfaces as a result of a mechanical action" (Rabinowicz, 1965). The wear properties of the device can be altered through biomaterial selection with joint replacements aiming to produce not only low wear volumes but also particles which cause minimal biological activity.

Table 1. Biomaterial properties compared to bone (Long and Rack, 1998; Kurtz, 2004).

Material	Ultimate tensile strength (MPa)	Yield strength (MPa)	Elastic modulus (GPa)
Cobalt chromium	600–1795	170–750	200–230
Titanium	960–970	850–900	110
UHMWPE	57	22	0.5
Alumina	300	—	380
Bone	90–140	—	10–40

Table 2. Biomaterials used in modern TAR.

Manufacturer	Brand	Bearing surfaces		Fixation surface
DePuy	Mobility	UHMWPE	Cobalt chrome	Sintered pure titanium beads
DePuy	Agility	UHMWPE	Cobalt chrome	
Stryker	STAR	UHMWPE	Cobalt chrome	Plasma sprayed titanium with electrochemical added calcium phosphate
Integra	Hintegra	UHMWPE	Cobalt chrome	Plasma sprayed titanium with HA coating (optional tibial fixation screws)
Integra	Cadence	UHMWPE	Tibia titanium allow Talus is cobalt chrome	Plasma sprayed titanium
Implantcast	TARIC	UHMWPE	Cobalt chrome	Titanium with optional HA coating
Corin	Zenith	UHMWPE	Titanium with TiN coating	Titanium with an electrochemical deposited HA coating
MatOrtho	BOX	UHMWPE	Cobalt chrome	Small cast-in metal balls with plasma sprayed HA coating
Tornier	Salto	UHMWPE	Cobalt chrome	Plasma sprayed titanium with HA coating
Tornier	Salto talaris	UHMWPE	Cobalt chrome	Plasma sprayed titanium
Wright Medical	Inbone	UHMWPE	Cobalt chrome	Plasma sprayed titanium
Wright Medical	Infinity	UHMWPE	Cobalt chrome (tibial) Titanium (talar)	Plasma sprayed titanium Trabecular metal (to be introduced in 2019)
Wright Medical	CCI	UHMWPE	Cobalt chrome with TiN coating	Plasma sprayed titanium with calcium phosphate coating

Table 2 (*Continued*)

Manufacturer	Brand	Bearing surfaces		Fixation surface
Zimmer	Trabecular metal	XPE	Cobalt chrome	Trabecular metal
Kyocera Medical	TNK	UHMWPE	Alumina ceramic	HA, cultured mesenchymal stem cells and optional fixation screw
Biomet	Rebalance	Vitamin E stabilised UHMWPE	Cobalt chrome	Unavailable
Exactech	Vantage	UHMWPE	Titanium (tibia) Cobalt chrome (Talus)	Commercially pure titanium coating
Chauveaux	Akile CLL	UHMWPE	Metal	Alumina beads with a lockable keel

Notes: UHMWPE, ultra-high molecular weight polyethylene; TiN, titanium nitride; HA, hydroxyapatite; XPE, cross-linked polyethylene.

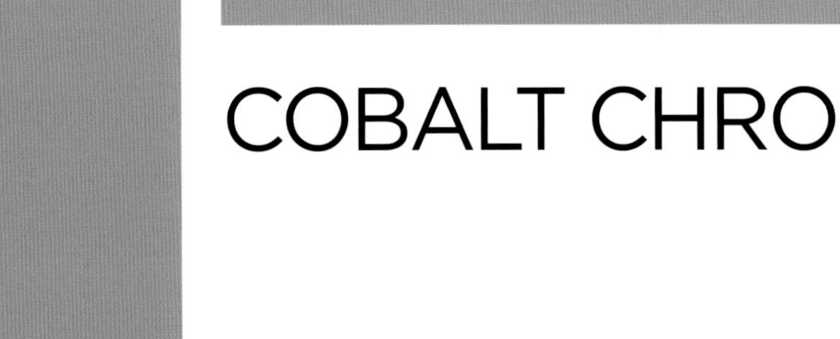

COBALT CHROMIUM

Cobalt chromium (CoCr) was first introduced to hip replacements in 1938 as an alternative to stainless steel. CoCr is renowned for its strength and resistance to corrosion and abrasive wear and is thought to strike a good balance between mechanical properties and biocompatibility. It can be manufactured via two routes: (i) cast or (ii) forged both of which have similar abrasive wear properties. This alloy has shown long-term clinical success when paired with UHMWPE. The one limitation of CoCr lies with the metal ions produced from articulation which have been associated with hypersensitivity and immune inflammatory reactions (Sonntag *et al.*, 2012).

TITANIUM NITRIDE

Ceramic-like coatings have been introduced to reduce friction and improve wear performance of bearing surfaces. These coatings may improve resistance to third-body damage and corrosion while maintaining the desired bulk properties of the metal (Lappalainen and Santavirta, 2005).

In coated ankle replacement designs, a thin film of titanium nitride (TiN) ceramic coating is applied to the titanium base (Ti-6AL-4V) by pressure vapour deposition, giving the device its identifiable gold colouring. Highly polished TiN aims to improve the wear properties by increasing the material hardness to decrease the number of biologically inert metal ions released. The oxide-protecting layer which forms should enhance the wear performance with the presence of third-body particles and due to the bulk of the material being titanium, the effects of stress shielding should be reduced as Table 1 shows that the elastic modulus is closer to that of bone. A limitation for this coating is the potential elevated rate of fretting corrosion and risk of high wear should the coating become damaged (Sonntag *et al.*, 2012). The reported results have been varied for this coating method with some *in vitro* studies indicating reduced wear compared with more conventional bearing surfaces (Pappas *et al.*, 1995). The clinical results have reported higher polyethylene wear with thin TiN layers. It has been shown experimentally that TiN coatings tend to have a higher surface roughness than a CoCr bearing, and this has previously been correlated with the level of polyethylene wear (Pappas *et al.*, 1995; Bell and Fisher, 2007; Kamali *et al.*, 2005).

CERAMIC

Ceramics are an alternative to metal. The increased material hardness and ability to be highly polished mean ceramics have been associated with reduced wear and reduced osteolysis in total hip replacement. In hip replacement, both alumina and zirconia have been employed with great success (Katti, 2004). In knee and ankle replacements, the use of ceramics has been limited to designs with less demanding loading due to the complex geometry and need for thin implant sections, which may increase fracture risk (Chevalier and Gremillard, 2009). The only ankle replacement which currently uses an alumina ceramic on polyethylene articulation is the semi-constrained TNK, primarily used in Japan with limited published long-term outcome data (Takakura, 2008).

POLYETHYLENE

UHMWPE has been used in joint replacement for decades. It consists of very long chains of ethylene which facilitate the effective transfer of load. Despite material advancements, it is still the preferred bearing material in ankle and knee replacement. The clinical and experimental performance can vary depending on design features such as thickness and conformity, which influence the level of stress transmission, and the sterilisation method. Smooth surfaces are necessary to provide optimal material properties and reduce friction. Current UHMWPE materials have good friction characteristics, when articulated with metallic bearings, good bulk biocompatibility, and good wear performance (Espinosa, 2017).

The sterilisation method of the UHMWPE has a substantial effect on its long-term properties. Until the mid-1990s, almost all UHMWPE components would undergo gamma irradiation in air as the standard sterilisation process. This method was found to be associated with oxidation which in many cases, long term, lead to delamination and fatigue failure of the UHMWPE. All modern polyethylene is sterilised in an inert atmosphere to reduce the risk of oxidative degradation (Kurtz, 2004). All TAR devices in current clinical use would be sterilised in an inert atmosphere.

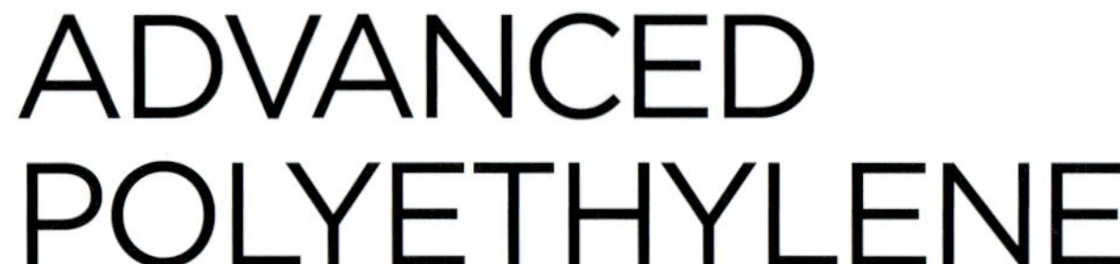

ADVANCED POLYETHYLENE

Long-term clinical failure of orthopaedic implants has frequently been associated with polyethylene wear debris-mediated osteolysis (Fisher *et al.*, 2004). Histological analysis in failed TAR showed areas of osteolysis with abundant polyethylene wear particles, present both intracellularly and extracellularly (Schipper *et al.*, 2017; Dalat *et al.*, 2013). Cross-linked polyethylene has been introduced with the aim to reduce the volume of wear debris generated. The most common method of cross-linking is irradiation of the UHMWPE material; however, chemical cross-linking may also be used. This process produces free radicals, some of which join together to create cross-links; covalent bonds between chains (Figure 1) (Kurtz, 2004).

The number of new bonds formed is proportional to the gamma dosage so the material can be cross-linked to varying degrees. As depicted in Figure 1, the higher cross-linking, the more improved wear resistance with a 73% reduction in wear under comparable conditions. Unfortunately, this improvement in wear performance comes at a cost to the mechanical properties such as toughness, fatigue, and fracture resistance, which reduce with increasing cross-linking (Figure 2).

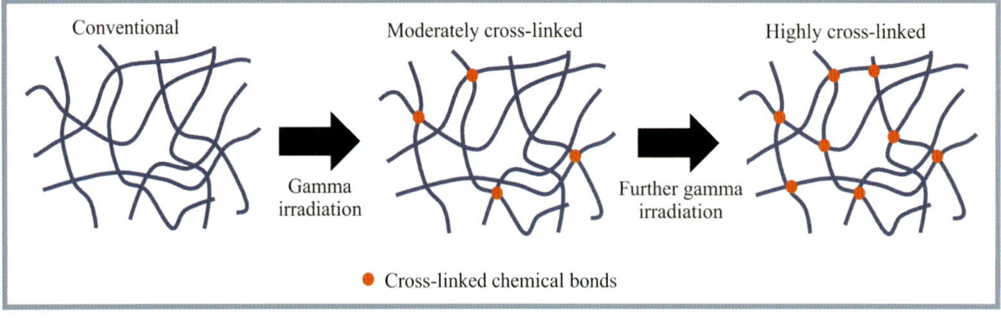

Figure 1. *Polyethylene cross-linking process.*

Highly cross-linked UHMWPE has shown significant wear benefits clinically for total hip replacement (Glyn-Jones *et al.*, 2015). Due to the trade-off between mechanical properties and wear performance, total knee replacement designs have tended towards using a moderately cross-linked polyethylene. TAR designs are typically more conforming than knee replacement but also reportedly undergo higher stresses than hip replacements. Only the recently introduced Zimmer trabecular metal implant specifies the use of highly cross-linked polyethylene and all others presently use conventional UHMWPE. More recently, studies have shown benefit of vitamin-E infused highly cross-linked polyethylene in hip arthroplasty (Rochcongar *et al.*, 2018).

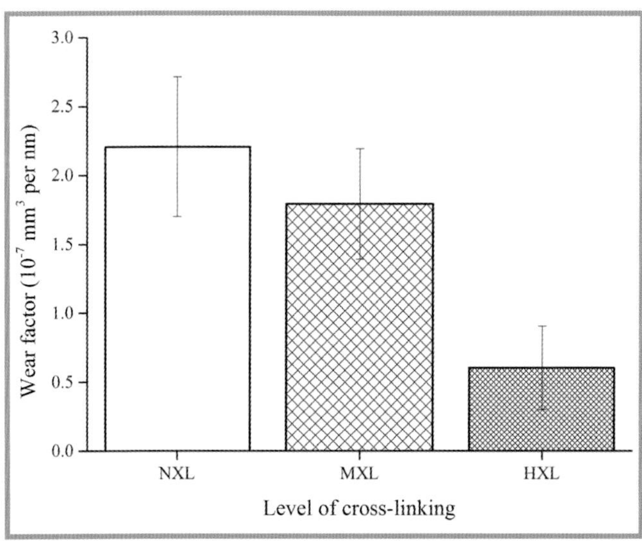

Figure 2. *Wear compared to the level of cross-linking across non-cross-linked (NXL), moderately cross-linked (MXL), and highly cross-linked (HXL) PE (Fisher et al., 2004).*

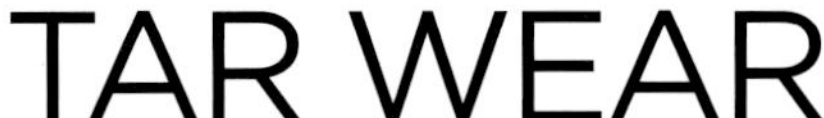

TAR WEAR

The relative merits of cross-linked UHMWPE and bearing choice in TAR are unclear as the clinical and experimental wear performance of TARs is not well documented. Experimental wear studies for TAR are limited (Table 3). Of the five designs that have been studied, the mobility and BOX comprise of a CoCr on conventional UHMWPE articulation, the Zimmer TAR used cross-linked UHMWPE, the Buechel–Pappas and the Corin Zenith are TiNi-coated devices. The Corin Zenith had a UHMWPE insert (Affatato *et al.*, 2007; Bell and Fisher, 2007; Kincaid, 2013; Smyth *et al.*, 2017).

Each study except the Corin Zenith study was run for a short period (5 million cycles or less) under different test conditions, making comparison of the implants difficult. These designs have presented wear rates of similar magnitudes despite their differing material properties. No significant difference in wear rate was found between the TiN devices compared to the CoCr. From the available information, it is impossible to draw conclusions about the "best" biomaterial for TAR. The wear rates appear similar to that of *in vitro* knee simulation which may mean, long term, similar problems such as wear debris induced osteolysis may arise for implants *in situ* beyond 10 years (Gilbert *et al.*, 2016).

Table 3. TAR wear rates from simulator studies.

	TAR design	Million cycles (Mc)	Wear rate (mm³/Mc)
Affatato *et al.* (2007)	MatOrtho BOX TAR	2	19.6 ± 12.8
Bell and Fisher (2007) (no AP)	Buechel–Pappas (BP) TAR	5	10.7 ± 11.8
	DePuy mobility TAR	5	3.3 ± 0.4
Bell and Fisher (2007) (AP)	Buechel–Pappas (BP) TAR	5	16.4 ± 17.4
	DePuy mobility TAR	5	10.4 ± 14.7
Kincaid (2013)	Zimmer trabecular metal TAR	5	3.1 ± 0.3
Smyth *et al.* (2017)	Corin zenith TAR	12	1.2 ± 0.6

FIXATION

The ultimate aim of any biomaterial used for implant fixation is to allow either bone cement (polymethyl methacrylate) or new bone growth to secure the prosthesis. The mechanical fixation of the prosthesis is important for the implant to withstand the biomechanical conditions in the ankle during activities of daily living.

Implant stability can be achieved at two time points within its lifetime. Primary stability is the initial mechanical fixation of the prosthesis attained during surgery. This can be achieved by ensuring a press fit between the implant and surrounding bone or by further mechanical restraints, such as bone cement or fixation screws. Secondary stability is the subsequent biological fixation facilitated predominantly by porous coatings and bioactive biomaterials used on the implant surface (Pegg *et al.*, 2014).

Bone cement has achieved long-term clinical success in both total hip and knee replacement. However, within the first decade of use in TAR, it was highlighted as a source of implant failure (Gougoulias *et al.*, 2009). Minimal space, low bone stock, and limited options for revision were a few of the reasons for the termination of bone cement use in TAR fixation. Cement fixation has largely stopped outside of the US market. However, it is notable that all FDA approved devices in the US are indicated for cemented use only. The alternative methods for fixation are the use of porous and/or bioactive coatings, which are specifically designed as secondary stability methods. Successful secondary stability relies on the phenomenon called osseointegration. This is the process by which lamellar bone becomes attached to the implant surface via a strong chemical bond. This may be strengthened further by enhancing the surface roughness and porosity of the fixation surface to allow mechanical fixation through bone ingrowth (Albrektsson and Johansson, 2001).

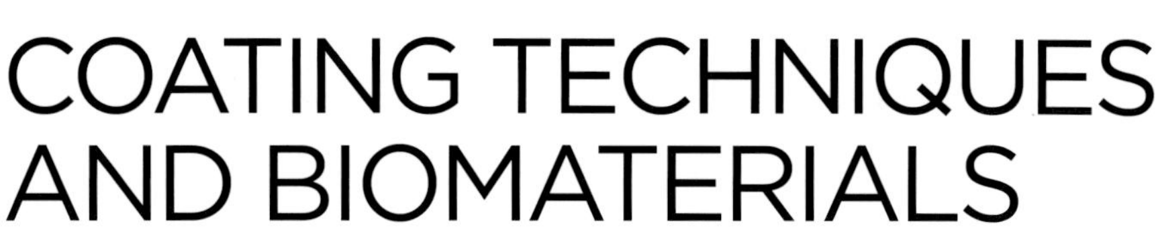

COATING TECHNIQUES AND BIOMATERIALS

The unaltered bulk material of an implant does not have the desirable properties for sustainable osseointegration. The surfaces are therefore roughened mechanically, chemically, or enhanced with a rough and/or bioactive coating in order to optimise osseointegrative potential. Two of the most commonly used biomaterials in TARs are titanium and hydroxyapatite (HA).

TITANIUM COATING

In 1952, Per-Ingvar Branemark first dubbed the term osseointegration after noticing substantial bone ingrowth in titanium implants (Branemark *et al.*, 2001). This sparked the use of titanium in orthopaedic implants which later extended to joint replacements.

Plasma spraying is a common technique used to create an interconnected open-cell porous titanium coating that promotes the anchorage of bone tissue (Massaro *et al.*, 2001). Plasma spraying consists of an extremely high temperature (20,000°C) plasma jet which collides with the injected coating powder. This forms a high speed liquid stream that impacts onto the bulk implant material with high kinetic energy (Figure 3). The characteristics of the coating can be altered by varying the spraying parameters (Ryan *et al.*, 2006). Pore sizes between 100 and 400 μm have been shown to promote high quality bone fixation (Bobyn *et al.*, 1980; Hulbert *et al.*, 1970; Itälä *et al.*, 2001), and third-generation ankle implants have a porosity within this range.

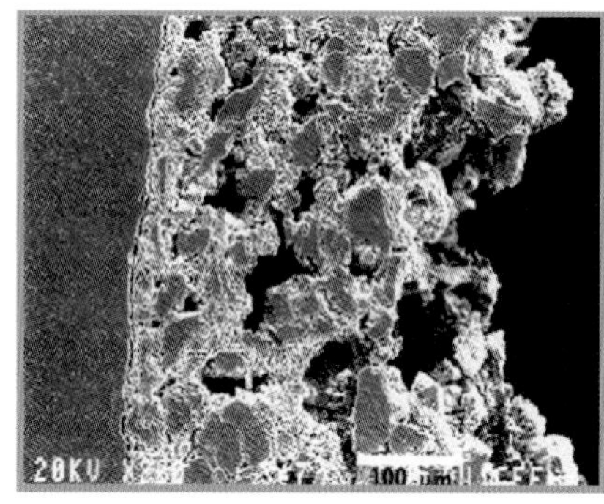

Figure 3. *Cross-section of the interface between the bulk material and coating (Ryan et al., 2006).*

The material properties of titanium when used as a coating are theoretically advantageous when compared to cobalt chrome because its mechanical properties are more similar to that of bone (Table 1). This is suggested to reduce the incidence of stress shielding with subsequent osteolysis, although a four- to five-fold mismatch in stiffness remains. To close the mismatch further, the coating technique can be modified to reduce the elastic modulus of titanium. For example, plasma-sprayed titanium creates a graduation of porosity from the solid bulk material of the implant to the highly porous outer surface of the coating. It is this graduation of porosity that creates the reduced elastic modulus and a reduced propensity to induce stress shielding (Ryan *et al.*, 2006; Otsuki *et al.*, 2006). Wood and Deakin (2003) showed that radiolucency at the bone–implant interface was 7.5 times more likely without the addition of a porous titanium coating. One potential downside to porous titanium coatings is a compromise on fatigue strength due to the stress intensification at the additional interfaces (Yue *et al.*, 1984).

Similar to uncemented total knee replacements, TARs are scarcely treated with titanium alone. A supplemental layer HA is often implemented to further augment osseointegration.

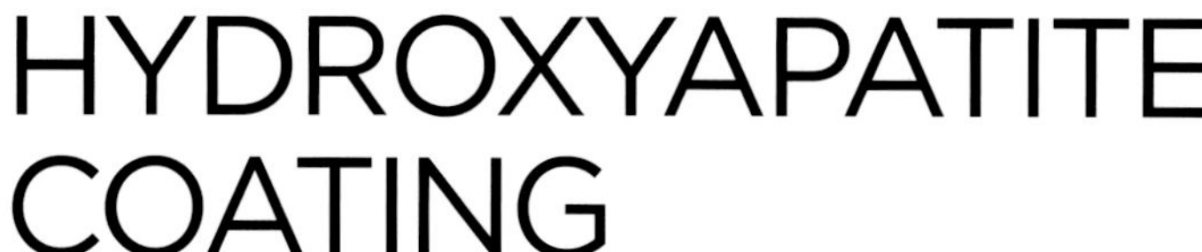

HYDROXYAPATITE COATING

For the majority of TARs sold outside of the USA, HA is applied using the plasma spray technique, similar to that mentioned for titanium coatings. However, an electrochemical-deposition method of applying HA is also being used called as Bonit's technique.

There are several benefits to HA electrochemical-deposition techniques when compared to plasma-sprayed techniques. Electrochemical-deposition HA is a non-line-of-sight method which allows complex geometries, such as those used in ankle prostheses to acquire an even coating in obscure areas. Also, electrochemical-deposition allows for substantially thinner coatings (15 μm thick) as opposed to the plasma-sprayed technique which is typically produces a coating 50 μm thick. Low thickness coatings preserve the initial porosity of the roughened surface beneath. Also, thinner coatings may reduce stresses at the HA–implant interface which could reduce the potential for coating delamination (Røkkum *et al.*, 2002). Electrochemical-deposition HA uses physiological temperatures during the manufacturing process. High temperatures such as those used in plasma spraying can alter the crystal structure of the HA which can result in heterogeneous properties across the implant surface, which may lead to accelerated interface failure (Rößler *et al.*, 2003). Both HA techniques have experimentally shown substantially greater bone apposition at both 7 and 14 days when compared to bare titanium. While both experimentally and theoretically the use of HA is promoted, the clinical evidence is not so supportive (Gandhi *et al.*, 2009; Hintermann *et al.*, 2013). It may also cause more periprosthetic bone cysts (Arcângelo, 2017). Long-term high quality studies are required to test the efficacy of HA and the different manufacturing techniques in TAR.

TRABECULAR METAL

The Zimmer Trabecular Metal TAR was released in 2013 and is the first trabecular metal fixation surface used in a commercial ankle prosthesis. Trabecular metal is plasma-spray deposited composite tantalum metal that forms a porous structure with a pore size ranging from 400 to 600 μm. The structure closely resembles the mechanical properties of cancellous bone (Bobyn *et al.*, 1999), is biologically inert, and is corrosion-resistant (Bargiotas, 2014). Short-term clinical results in trabecular metal knee replacements have been promising (O'Keefe *et al.*, 2010); however, outcomes of such ankles are awaited.

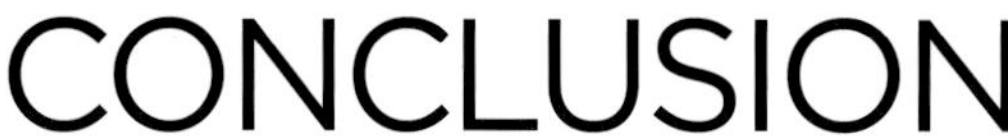

CONCLUSION

The biomaterials used for TARs are heavily reliant on the previous success reported for other total joint replacements. It is assumed that the biological and mechanical environment in the ankle is similar to that of other lower limb synovial joints. However, some difficulties identified clinically after total ankle arthroplasty, such as poor blood circulation and soft tissue imbalances, may indicate as yet unidentified biological and mechanical demands for the biomaterials used. Wear-mediated failure of TAR seems to be relatively rare compared with hip and knee replacement, potentially due to the higher rate of earlier failure. However, it would be unwise to ignore the lessons learned regarding wear debris-mediated osteolysis in these joints. At present, material selections in order to improve the stress shielding problems is certainly something which should be considered. As more knowledge is gained about the long-term performance of current generation of TARs, the best biomaterials for this application should become apparent.

REFERENCES

Affatato, S., Leardini, A., Leardini, W., Giannini, S. & Viceconti, M. 2007. Meniscal wear at a three-component total ankle prosthesis by a knee joint simulator. *J Biomech*, 40, 1871–1876.

Albrektsson, T. & Johansson, C. 2001. Osteoinduction, osteoconduction and osseointegration. *Eur Spine J*, 10(2), S96–S101.

Arcângelo, J., Guerra-Pinto, F., Pinto, A., Grenho, A., Navarro, A., & Martin Oliva, X. 2017. Peri-prosthetic bone cysts after total ankle replacement. A systematic review and meta-analysis. *Foot Ankle Surg*, S1268–7731(17), 31347–4.

Bargiotas, K. A. 2014. Trabecular metal: Bone interface in total joint arthroplasty. In: Karachalios T. (eds) *Bone-Implant Interface in Orthopedic Surgery*, 121–126 Springer, London.

Bell, C. J. & Fisher, J. 2007. Simulation of polyethylene wear in ankle joint prostheses. *J Biomed Mater Res B Appl Biomater*, 81, 162–167.

Bobyn, J. D., Pilliar, R. M., Cameron, H. U. & Weatherly, G. C. 1980. The optimum pore size for the fixation of porous-surfaced metal implants by the ingrowth of bone. *Clin Orthop Relat Res*, 150, 263–270.

Bobyn, J. D., Stackpool, G. J., Hacking, S. A., Tanzer, M. & Krygier, J. J. 1999. Characteristics of bone ingrowth and interface mechanics of a new porous tantalum biomaterial. *J Bone Joint Surg Br*, 81, 907–914.

Branemark, R., Branemark, P. I., Rydevik, B. & Myers, R. R. 2001. Osseointegration in skeletal reconstruction and rehabilitation: A review. *J Rehabil Res Dev*, 38, 175–181.

Chevalier, J. & Gremillard, L. 2009. Ceramics for medical applications: A picture for the next 20 years. *J Eur Ceramic Soc*, 29, 1245–1255.

Dalat, F., Barnoud, R., Fessy, M. H., Besse, J. L. & AFCP French Association of Foot Surgery. 2013. Histologic study of periprosthetic osteolytic lesions after AES total ankle replacement. A 22 case series. *Orthop Traumatol Surg Res*, 99, S285–S295.

Espinosa, N., Klammer, G. & Wirth, S. H. 2017. Osteolysis in total ankle replacement: How does it work? *Foot Ankle Clin*, 22, 267–275.

Fisher, J., McEwen, H. M., Tipper, J. L., Galvin, A. L., Ingram, J., Kamali, A., Stone, M. H. & Ingham, E. 2004. Wear, debris, and biologic activity of cross-linked polyethylene in the knee: Benefits and potential concerns. *Clin Orthop Relat Res*, 428, 114–119.

Gandhi, R., Davey, J. R. & Mahomed, N. N. 2009. Hydroxyapatite coated femoral stems in primary total hip arthroplasty: A meta-analysis. *J Arthroplasty*, 24, 38–42.

Gilbert, T. J., Anoushiravani, A. A., Sayeed, Z., Chambers, M. C., El-Othmani, M. M. & Saleh, K. J. 2016. Osteolysis complicating total knee arthroplasty. *JBJS Reviews*, 4(7).

Glyn-Jones, S., Thomas, G. E., Garfjeld-Roberts, P., Gundle, R., Taylor, A., McLardy-Smith, P. & Murray, D. W. 2015. The John Charnley Award: Highly crosslinked polyethylene in total hip arthroplasty decreases long-term wear: a double-blind randomized trial. *Clin Orthop Relat Res*, 473, 432–438.

Gougoulias, N. E., Khanna, A. & Maffulli, N. 2009. History and evolution in total ankle arthroplasty. *Br Med Bull*, 89, 111–151.

Hintermann, B., Zwicky, L., Knupp, M., Henninger, H. B. & Barg, A. 2013. HINTEGRA revision arthroplasty for failed total ankle prostheses. *J Bone Joint Surg Am*, 95, 1166–1174.

Hulbert, S. F., Young, F. A., Mathews, R. S., Klawitter, J. J., Talbert, C. D. & Stelling, F. H. 1970. Potential of ceramic materials as permanently implantable skeletal prostheses. *J Biomed Mat Res*, 4, 433–456.

Itälä, A. I., Ylänen, H. O., Ekholm, C., Karlsson, K. H. & Aro, H. T. 2001. Pore diameter of more than 100 μm is not requisite for bone ingrowth in rabbits. *J Biomed Mat Res*, 58, 679–683.

Kamali, A., Farrar, R., Hatto, P., Stone, M. H. & Fisher, J. 2005. Wear of ultrahigh-molecular-weight polyethylene against titanium-nitride-coated counterfaces. *Proceedings of the Institution of Mechanical Engineers, Part J: J Eng Tribol*, 219, 41–47.

Katti, K. S. 2004. Biomaterials in total joint replacement. *Colloid Surf B: Biointerfaces*, 39, 133–142.

Kincaid, B., Fryman, J. C., Gillard, D., Wentorf, F., Popoola, O. & Bischoff, J. 2013. Proceedings of the Orthopaedic Research Society Meeting, San Antonio, USA. Gravimetric wear testing of a fixed-bearing bicondylar total ankle replacement.

Kurtz, S. M. 2004. *The UHMWPE Handbook: Ultra-High Molecular Weight Polyethylene in Total Joint Replacement*, Ch 2, pp. 14–35 Elsevier Science, London.

Lappalainen, R. & Santavirta, S. S. 2005. Potential of coatings in total hip replacement. *Clin Orthop Relat Res*, 430, 72–79.

Long, M. & Rack, H. J. 1998. Titanium alloys in total joint replacement – a materials science perspective. *Biomaterials*, 19, 1621–1639.

Massaro, C., Baker, M. A., Cosentino, F., Ramires, P. A., Klose, S. & Milella, E. 2001. Surface and biological evaluation of hydroxyapatite-based coatings on titanium deposited by different techniques. *J Biomed Mater Res*, 58, 651–657.

O'Keefe, T. J., Winter, S., Lewallen, D. G., Robertson, D. D. & Poggie, R. A. 2010. Clinical and radiographic evaluation of a monoblock tibial component. *J Arthroplasty*, 25, 785–792.

Otsuki, B., Takemoto, M., Fujibayashi, S., Neo, M., Kokubo, T. & Nakamura, T. 2006. Pore throat size and connectivity determine bone and tissue ingrowth into porous implants: Three-dimensional micro-CT based structural analyses of porous bioactive titanium implants. *Biomaterials*, 27, 5892–5900.

Pappas, M. J., Makris, G. & Buechel, F. F. 1995. Titanium nitride ceramic film against polyethylene. A 48 million cycle wear test. *Clin Orthop Relat Res*, 317, 64–70.

Pegg, E. C., Mellon, S. J., Gill, H. S. 2014. Early and late mechanical stability of the cementless bone-implant interface in total joint arthroplasty. In: Karachalios T. (eds) *Bone-Implant Interface in Orthopedic Surgery*, pp. 13–26 Springer, London.

Rabinowicz, E. 1965. *Friction and Wear of Materials*, Ch 5, pp. 109–125, John Wiley & Sons, New York.

Rochcongar, G., Buia, G., Bourroux, E., Dunet, J., Chapus, V. & Hulet, C. 2018. Creep and wear in vitamin E-infused highly cross-linked polyethylene cups for total hip arthroplasty: A prospective randomized controlled trial. *J Bone Joint Surg Am*, 100, 107–114.

Røkkum, M., Reigstad, A. & Johansson, C. B. 2002. HA particles can be released from well-fixed HA-coated stems. *Acta Orthopaed*, 73, 298–306.

Rößler, S., Sewing, A., Stölzel, M., Born, R., Scharnweber, D., Dard, M. & Worch, H. 2003. Electrochemically assisted deposition of thin calcium phosphate coatings at near-physiological pH and temperature. *J Biomed Mater Res Part A*, 64, 655–663.

Ryan, G., Pandit, A. & Apatsidis, D. P. 2006. Fabrication methods of porous metals for use in orthopaedic applications. *Biomaterials*, 27, 2651–2670.

Schipper, O. N., Haddad, S. L., Pytel, P. & Zhou, Y. 2017. Histological analysis of early osteolysis in total ankle arthroplasty. *Foot Ankle Int*, 38, 351–359.

Smyth, A., Fisher, J., Suner, S. & Brockett, C. 2017. Influence of kinematics on the wear of a total ankle replacement. *J Biomech*, 53, 105–110.

Sonntag, R., Reinders, J. & Kretzer J. P. 2012. What's next? Alternative materials for articulation in total joint replacement. *Acta Biomater*, 8, 2434–2441.

Takakura, Y. 2008. Total ankle arthroplasty using TNK ankle for osteoarthritis. *Seikei-Saigaigeka*, 51, 919–924.

Wood, P. L. R. & Deakin, S. 2003. Total ankle replacements. *J Bone Joint Surg-Brit Vol*, 85, 334–341.

Yue, S., Pilliar, R. M. & Weatherly, G. C. 1984. The fatigue strength of porous-coated Ti-6%Al-4%V implant alloy. *J Biomed Mater Res*, 18, 1043–1058.

THE ANATOMY OF THE ANKLE AND HINDFOOT

CHAPTER 3

T. Williams, D. Singh and A. J. Goldberg

Summary

An appreciation of the anatomy of the ankle and hindfoot is essential before embarking on ankle arthroplasty. The ankle joint should be considered a complex in conjunction with the hindfoot and forefoot. This will ensure that when planning surgery, potential pitfalls due to distal deformity will not compromise a surgeon's results. Careful dissection through safe planes with full-thickness flaps of tissue will help protect what is a thin and often delicate soft tissue envelope. To restore anatomy is to provide a base to restoring function.

INTRODUCTION

The interrelations of the ankle and hindfoot serve to provide a stable platform for shock absorption, plantigrade stance, and propulsion with complex biomechanics. Surgical restoration of anatomy and congruent joint alignment will optimise the outcome of any implant surgery.

The bony architecture is covered by a relatively thin layer of soft tissues. This not only allows surface anatomy to be easily recognised for a surgical approach but also increases the chance of wound problems if not managed meticulously. Safe planes of dissection have been historically documented in association with ankle arthroplasty.

INNERVATION

The sciatic nerve is formed from L4 to S3 segments of the sacral plexus. In the popliteal fossa, the nerve divides into the tibial nerve and the common peroneal nerve.

In the popliteal fossa, the tibial nerve supplies the gastrocnemius and soleus as well as the knee joint, and a cutaneous branch that will join a branch of the common peroneal nerve to become the sural nerve. The tibial nerve itself continues in the deep posterior compartment deep to soleus to the back of the medial malleolus within the flexor retinaculum alongside the posterior tibial artery. In the foot, the nerve divides into medial and lateral plantar nerves.

The common peroneal nerve (L4/5, S1/2) curves around the head of the fibula where it is palpable. It divides deep to the peroneus longus into the superficial peroneal nerve and deep peroneal nerve.

The deep peroneal nerve supplies the muscles of the anterior compartment of the leg (tibialis anterior, extensor hallucis longus (EHL), extensor digitorum longus, and peroneus tertius) and the intrinsic muscles of the foot (extensor digitorum brevis and extensor hallucis brevis). The medial terminal branch of the deep peroneal accompanies the dorsalis pedis artery along the dorsum of the foot supplying branches to the first Metatarsophalangeal Joint (MTPJ) and the skin of the first web space, which is where it is clinically tested.

The superficial peroneal nerve supplies the muscles of the lateral compartment of the leg (peroneus longus and peroneus brevis) and the skin over the anterolateral aspect of the leg and the dorsum of the foot. It passes forward between the peroneal muscles and the extensor digitorum longus, and pierces the deep fascia approximately 10–12 cm above the tip of the fibula, although this position is variable and should be noted for anterolateral approaches to the ankle as well as the fixation of fibula fractures (Figure 1). Once through the deep fascia, it lies just under the skin and divides

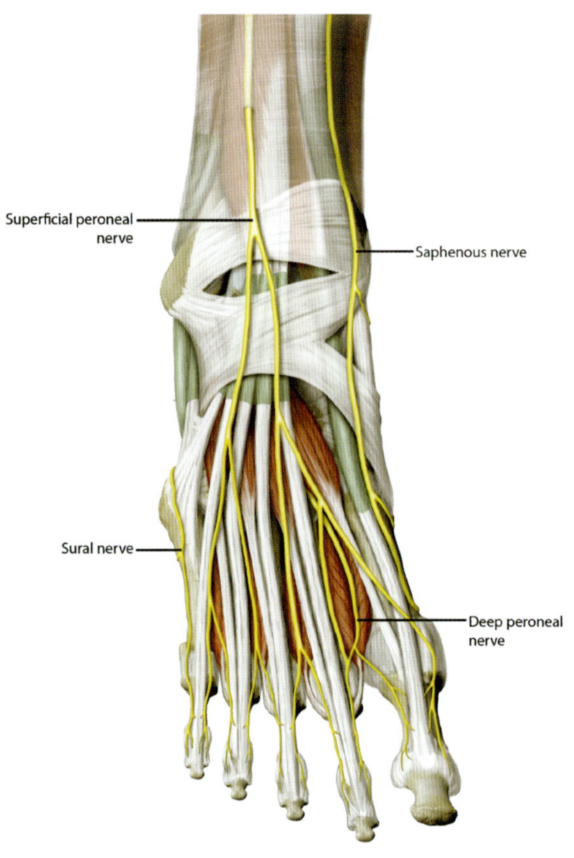

Figure 1. *Illustration of the superficial peroneal nerve. The nerve pierces the deep fascia coming from deep to superficial approximately 10–12 cm above the tip of the fibula. It then travels very superficially over the front of the ankle and is invariably encountered at the lower end of a midline anterior incision.*
Image by Catherine Sulzmann, Medical Artist.

into an intermediate dorsal cutaneous nerve (the main nerve we see) and a smaller medial dorsal cutaneous nerve (which sometimes has to be sacrificed in anterior approaches to the ankle). Figures 2(a)-(c) illustrate the sensory innervation to the lower leg.

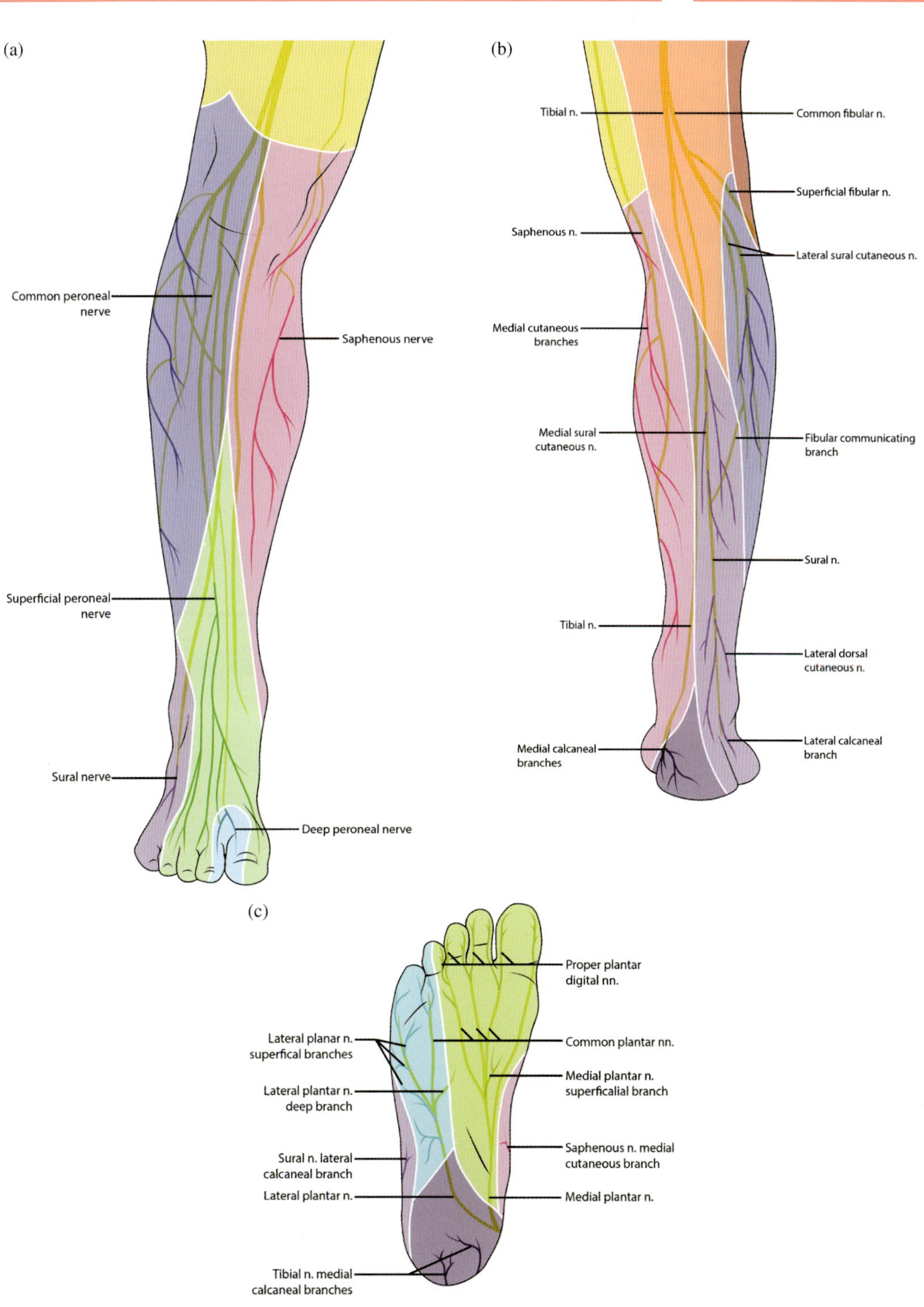

Figure 2. *Illustrations of the right leg (a) from the front, (b) from behind and (c) from under the foot, demonstrating sensory nerve supply.*
Image by Catherine Sulzmann, Medical Artist.

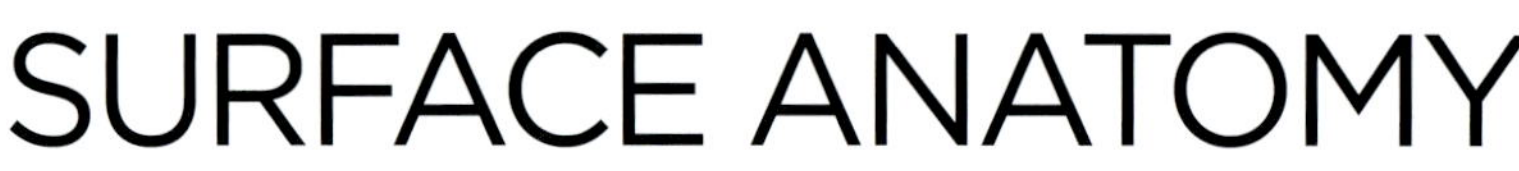

SURFACE ANATOMY

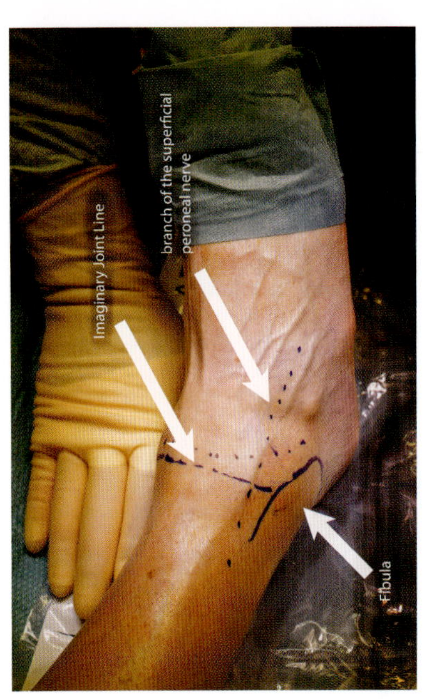

Figure 3. *A photograph of the right foot pre-operatively, with the bones marked out and the imaginary joint line illustrated approximately 1 inch above the tip of the medial malleolus.*

The ankle is a superficial joint and its bony landmarks are easily appreciated (and marked) preoperatively (Figure 3).

An imaginary line running horizontally approximately an inch above the tip of the medial malleolus indicates the level of the ankle joint. Anteriorly, the tibialis anterior tendon is identified by active dorsiflexion of the foot against resistance with the patient awake, but is large and palpable also in the anaesthetised patient. Similarly, the EHL tendon is both visibly appreciable and palpable with active or passive great toe movement.

The dorsalis pedis arterial pulse can be felt and tracked in the midline from the foot proximally, knowing that alongside this (and usually laterally) lies the deep peroneal nerve at the ankle. The lateral branch of the superficial peroneal nerve (also known as the intermediate dorsal cutaneous nerve of the foot) can be identified by the examiner pulling on the fourth toe of a relaxed, plantarflexed and inverted foot; this will tension the nerve which can be felt as a "taut fine wire" alongside the fourth toe tendon slip of the extensor digitorum longus (Figure 3). In an ankle block, the superficial peroneal is blocked at this point. The medial branch of the superficial peroneal nerve (also known as the medial dorsal cutaneous nerve of the foot) can occasionally be also palpated by pulling on the second toe. The sural nerve (lateral dorsal cutaneous nerve of the foot) is not at risk in anterior approaches but should be protected in a lateral approach; its course is variable but usually runs from about 1 cm behind the lateral malleolus to the lateral aspect of the shaft of the fifth metatarsal.

Posteriorly, the tendo-achilles is palpable right up to its insertion on the calcaneal tuberosity. Laterally, the peroneal tendons run behind the malleolus and just below the tip of the fibula is found the subtalar joint. It may be more proximal — especially, when there is severe arthritis.

Passive adduction of the ankle tensions the calcaneofibular ligament which can then be palpated.

The Ankle

The ankle is a "mortice and tenon"-like, constrained hinge joint centred under the mechanical axis of the leg in both sagittal and coronal planes. The talar dome (tenon) sits in its mortice made up of the tibial plafond and medial and lateral malleoli. The plafond primarily transmits load while the malleoli act as constraints both to sagittal translation and tilting forces (with the collateral and syndesmotic ligament complexes).

The tibial plafond has a consistent alignment in the coronal plane of 92–93° to the mechanical axis of the leg. The obliquity is from distal lateral to proximal medial. The articular surface has a subtle biconcavity with midline crista in congruence with the underlying centrally grooved talus.

In the sagittal plane, the posterior tibia extends some 3–6 mm more distal than the anterior margin. This results in an appreciable posterior downwards slope. The joint line is concave and conforms loosely to the talar dome below.

The tibiotalar hinge joint lies approximately 8° in external rotation on average, although considerable variation may occur. The talar dome is convex in the sagittal plane but not uniformly as in a section of a cylinder. It is best thought of as a frustum of a cone with its tip medially expanding laterally. This means that while the medial wall lies in the sagittal plane, the lateral wall lies in a plane that expands anterolaterally. The dome is wider anteriorly than posteriorly by some 5 mm (Pol Le Coeur, 1938). Being narrowest in ankle plantarflexion, the congruent ankle is maintained without constriction by controlled fibular excursion during dorsiflexion.

These measurements are really a guide as the actual figures vary with the size of the foot and the axes of rotation vary from individual to individual and for each individual during the gait cycle. For the purposes of implanting an arthroplasty, however, they provide a reference that will help the surgeon with prosthetic alignment.

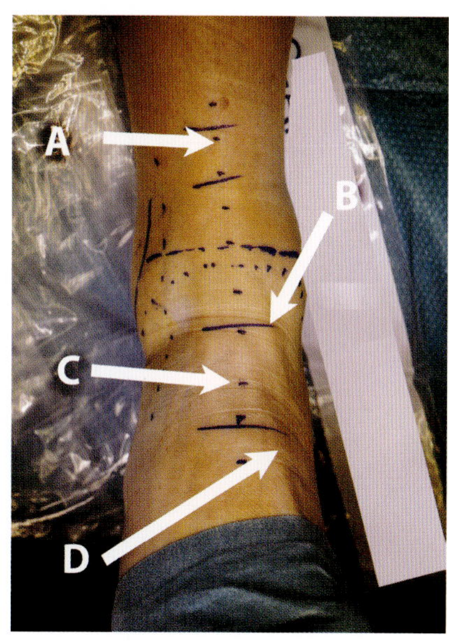

Figure 4. *A photograph of the ankle pre-operatively, demonstrating the midline incision for the anterior approach (A); the visible tibialis anterior tendon (B); the palpable dorsalis pedis (C); and the extensor hallucis longus tendon (D).*

The Syndesmosis

Just proximal to the ankle joint, the fibula has a fibrous articulation in a groove in the posterolateral tibia — known as the syndesmosis. It is stabilised by anterior, inferior, and posterior inferior tibiofibular ligaments.

Contiguous with the syndesmosis, the intraosseous membrane runs along the length of the fibula and tibia proximally before merging with the superior tibiofibular joint at the knee. This entire complex is mobile and mechanically linked to ankle movements.

As the ankle dorsiflexes, the increasing talar width causes the lateral malleolus to move away from the tibia. It retracts proximally and rotates medially about the posterior tibiofibular ligament. This is a passive process in contrast with the changes of plantarflexion, in which the fibula approximates the tibia being drawn. This also pulls the fibula distally with a slight lateral rotation. These actions ensure the mortice of the ankle is held congruent and stable throughout its range of motion.

These syndesmotic movements are subtle but must be considered in the design and positioning of any ankle prostheses. Too wide a talar component will impinge on the fibula in plantarflexion, applying excessive lateral forces with pain and potential stress risers.

Medial Supporting Structures

The medial malleolus is an extension of the tibia. It is lined with hyaline cartilage that articulates with the medial wall of the talus. Distally and medially, it serves as an origin for the deltoid ligament. Grooved posteriorly, a trochlea forms a bony boundary to the tarsal tunnel with its tendons and important neurovascular structures.

The deltoid ligament fans out from the malleolus in a deep and superficial layer.

The deep part is made up of two bands. (i) The anterior tibiotalar band runs distally and anteriorly attaching to the medial neck of the talus. (ii) Its sister posterior tibiotalar band runs distally and posteriorly and attaches under the medial articular surface of the talus along with medial tubercle of its posterior process. This posterior band is the thicker of the pair.

The superficial layer consists of a thin sheet of ligamentous strands overlying the anterior tibiotalar band. These fan out to attach distally along a line from the sustentaculum tali of the calcaneus to the tuberosity of the navicular bone. Between these two points, the complex is also adherent to the upper medial border of the plantar calcaneonavicular (spring) ligament.

Lateral Supporting Structures

The lateral malleolus is the distal end of the fibula. Its intra-articular medial wall is also lined with hyaline cartilage and articulates with the lateral talar dome. Its subcutaneous lateral and distal aspects provide origin for the lateral ligaments as well as a trochlea for the peroneal tendons.

The lateral collateral ligaments are more discrete than the deltoid. The anterior talofibular ligament (ATFL) is a broad sheet originating from the anterior tip of the lateral malleolus and inserting in the lateral talar neck. The calcaneofibular ligament (CFL) is a thicker cord that runs from the anterior tip of the fibula to the posterior tuberosity of the calcaneus. It plays an important role in subtalar stability. The posterior talofibular ligament (PTFL) runs transversely from the fibula to the posterior aspect of the talus. It gives a second tibial slip that merges with the posterior inferior tibiofibular ligament (PITFL).

The Subtalar Joint

The subtalar joint and the ankle form a link between the long bones of the leg and the perpendicular construct of the foot. Movements of the ankle require reactionary changes in the subtalar and transverse tarsal joints for effective load transmission and propulsion.

The talus acts as the loadbearing fulcrum between the ankle and subtalar joint. Its dome articulates with the ankle, its head with the navicular and its under surface with the calcaneum forming the subtalar joint. It is 60% covered in cartilage and gives rise to no muscle origin. It has a main blood supply running from anterior to posterior derived from the dorsalis pedis artery, deltoid ligament, and tarsal canal arteries.

The calcaneum is a cancellous bone that forms the bony heel with its large posterior tuberosity. The loadbearing posterior one-third of the bone is extraarticular and also acts a lever arm for its attachment of the gastrocsoleus complex. When viewed from behind in plantigrade stance, the heel sits in 10–15° of valgus with respect to the coronal axis of the leg. This alignment changes during gait.

The middle one-third is lined dorsally with hyaline articular cartilage and comprises the posterior facet of the subtalar joint. This surface has a complex oblique orientation from posterolateral to anteromedial. In this more longitudinal axis, the surface is convex, though perpendicular to this view, it is down sloping and again convex posteriorly to anterior. This shape is reflected in the under surface of talus forming a congruent subtalar joint.

The anterior one-third of the calcaneum comprises the anterior and middle facets of the subtalar joint and the sustentaculum tali.

These smaller facets are concave in an arc that is completed by the articular surface of the navicular approximating the socket of the "coxa pedis" in which sits the ball-shaped talar head. The overlying anterior talus is congruent with the calcaneum.

Short and stout interosseus talocalcaneal ligaments provide stability to this subtalar joint. They are most prominent in the sinus tarsi directly under the weightbearing axis of the leg. In addition to providing stability, they provide a semicontrolled axis of motion for the joint and in this role, they are sometimes regarded as analogous to the cruciates of the knee. Laterally and posteriorly are two thinner talocalcaneal ligaments which also play a supporting role.

Movements of the subtalar joint are complex and involve a rotatory motion of the bones. They accommodate irregularities in ground contact by unlocking the hind and midfoot during heel strike to stance phase.

Subsequently, the talar movements about the calcaneum and navicular draw the heel into varus and help supinate the foot, which creates a more rigid construct to allow propulsive power to be transmitted.

The changing talocalcaneal relationship plays a role in stabilising the ankle complex, which is sometimes seen following subtalar or triple fusion. The ankle can then be subjected to coronal forces of varus and valgus that were previously absorbed in the hindfoot. This in turn can cause eventual talar tilt and accelerated wear with uneven joint space loss.

When planning ankle arthroplasty, hindfoot alignment is important in both the fused or unfused situation to avoid consequences of instability and uneven loading.

Radiographically, this can be seen on preoperative weightbearing films of the foot and ankle and allowance made.

Kite's angle is the talocalcaneal angle in the frontal plane and represents the divergence of the respective longitudinal axes. Stance phase value of 17–21° is considered normal. On the lateral image, the calcaneal pitch is normally 20–25° from the horizontal with a talar pitch very similar. The overall lateral talocalcaneal angle is a combined value at 30–50°. Any variation outside of these values (which should also be clinically apparent) should be allowed for at the time of surgical planning.

APPROACHES TO THE ANKLE

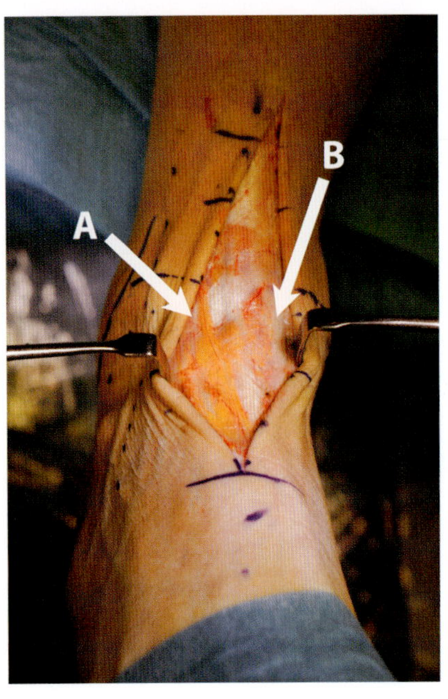

Figure 5. *Intraoperative photograph following midline incision to reveal the medial branch of the superficial peroneal nerve which crosses the lowest part of the wound (A), and tibialis anterior tendon within its sheath (B).*

Anterior Approach

The anterior approach is by far the most common approach used for ankle arthroplasty. It is largely extensile in nature through a safe tissue plane and window, but operating through such a thin layer requires meticulous care and minimal undercutting of wound edges, as well as protection of the flaps to prevent wound problems.

The patient is positioned supine with an optional bolster under the ipsilateral buttock. This will help improve the rotation of the leg, bringing the joint line into the anteroposterior plane.

A midline longitudinal incision is made over the ankle joint centred between the malleoli. This overlies the tendons of tibialis anterior and EHL. Skin and superficial fascia are incised in line and without undercutting of the skin. Careful dissection in this region may allow identification and protection of the medial branch of the superficial peroneal nerve (marked as A in Figure 5). A vascular loop can be placed around the nerve to ensure it is protected at all times (Figure 6). The tibialis anterior tendon sheath is then divided (Figure 7) to expose the tendon which can be retracted medially and the plain of dissection continues in the floor of the tendon sheath using sharp dissection onto the bone of the joint beneath. Once on bone, subperiosteal dissection, both medial and laterally, will allow exposure of the joint (Figure 8). Sufficient exposure to allow visualisation of both medial and lateral gutters requires an incision about 10–15 cm long in order that retraction does not compromise the wound edges. The wound edges may still be traumatised, especially if self-retaining retractors are used with the foot dorsiflexed and the foot is later moved into plantarflexion. We advise that self-retainers should never be used. The exposure can also be through the bed of EHL but caution is required to avoid the neurovascular structures beneath.

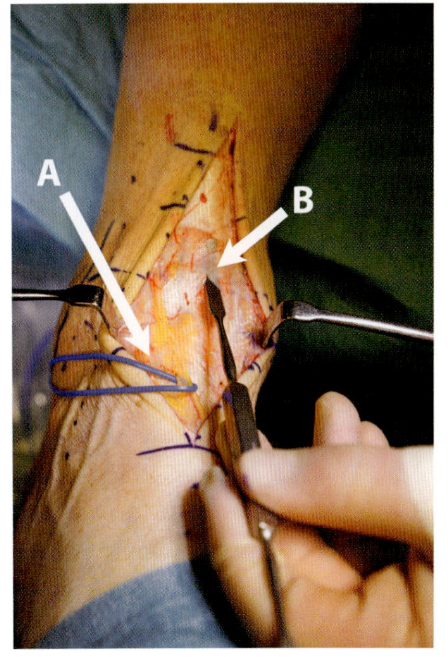

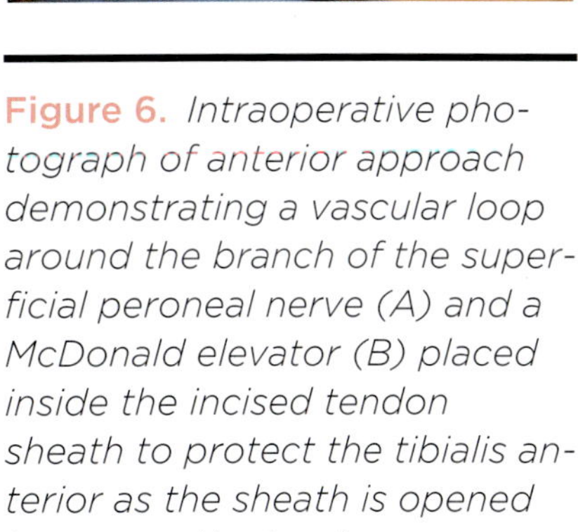

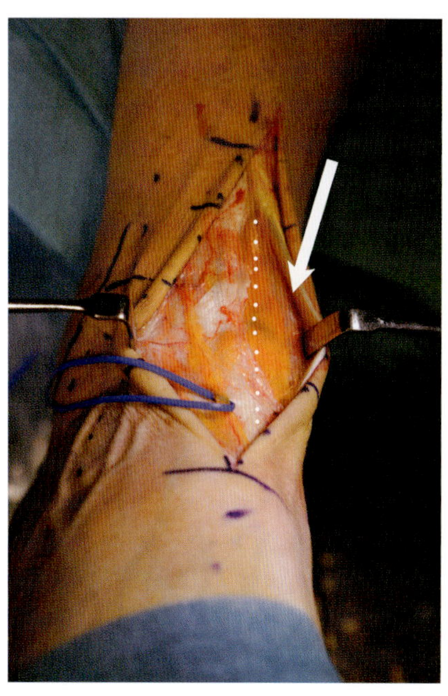

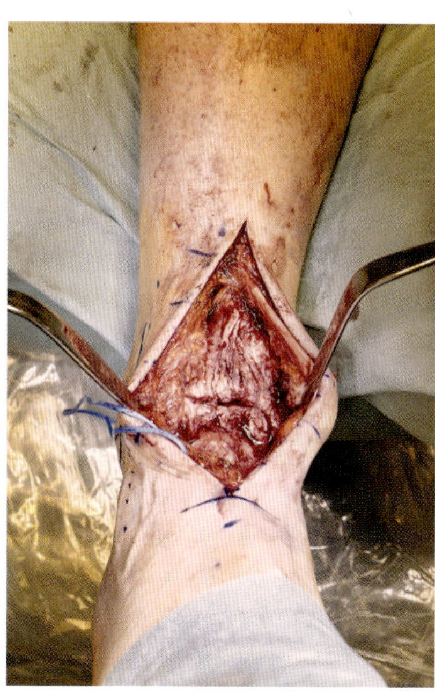

Figure 6. *Intraoperative photograph of anterior approach demonstrating a vascular loop around the branch of the superficial peroneal nerve (A) and a McDonald elevator (B) placed inside the incised tendon sheath to protect the tibialis anterior as the sheath is opened to expose the tendon.*

Figure 7. *Intraoperative photograph of anterior approach demonstrating a retracted tibialis anterior tendon (arrow) and the incision made in the bed of the tendon to expose the ankle joint (dotted line).*

Figure 8. *Intraoperative photograph of anterior approach demonstrating the exposed arthritic tibiotalar joint with two right angled retractors placed under the capsule to expose the medial and lateral gutters.*

Lateral Approach

The transfibular approach has been used to implant the ESKA© & Zimmer Trabecular Metal Ankle Total Ankle®. A direct approach is made to the superficial border of the distal fibula which is extended 1–2 cm beyond the lateral malleolus. Careful dissection will avoid damage to the superficial peroneal nerve which exits its lateral compartment approximately 10 cm above the ankle and can be found in the proximal extent of the wound. The sural nerve also lies in close proximity to the posterior aspect of the lateral malleolus and should be protected.

A transverse or chevron osteotomy is fashioned in the diaphyseal fibula and the lateral malleolus reflected distally. This allows subperiosteal dissection over the anterior tibia which should include the anterior tibiofibular ligament. The posterior tibia and talus can then be exposed subperiosteally leaving the lateral malleolus hanging distally on a calcaneofibular ligament pedicle. Following implantation of the ankle, the fibula osteotomy can be closed in compression and the ligaments repaired.

REFERENCES

Kelikian, A. S. 2012. *Sarrafian's Anatomy of the Foot & Ankle: Descriptive, Topographic, Functional,* 3rd Edition, Lippincott Williams & Wilkins, ISBN 978-0-781-79750-4.

Logan, B. & Hutchings, R. 2012. *McMinn's Colour Atlas of Foot & Ankle Anatomy*, 4th Edition, Elsevier, ISBN 978-0-323-05615-1.

Le Coeur, P. 1938. *La pince malléolaire physiologie et pathologie du péroné*, L. Arnette, Paris, p. 42.

ANKLE ARTHRITIS

CHAPTER

4

65

T. R. Daniels and R. H. Thomas

Summary

The ankle is a complex joint and appears unique when compared to the other major joints of the lower limb. Despite the ankle being subjected to high forces and being commonly injured, symptomatic ankle arthritis is only rarely seen.

Unlike the hip and knee, primary arthritis of the ankle is rare. Posttraumatic arthritis accounts for about 70% of cases, with rotational ankle fractures being the most common cause. Arthritis may develop due to changes in contact stresses and alterations in joint mechanics.

Several factors have been postulated as to why the ankle may be resistant to the development of arthritis in the absence of trauma. The ankle maintains its mechanical properties even with ageing and this may allow physiological cartilage metabolism to persist for longer. Ankle articular cartilage is uniform and thin but stiff. During weightbearing, the ankle is maximally congruent and stable. These factors may act to equalise stresses throughout the joint.

However, anatomical and biomechanical factors cannot fully explain these protective mechanisms and an increasing number of metabolic factors related to ankle cartilage are being recognised. Ankle stiffness may be related to its dense extracellular matrix due to high glycosaminoglycan (GAG) and lower water concentrations. The ankle is metabolically more active than the knee and activity varies with load.

Ankle cartilage is able to resist degeneration by producing less of a response to catabolic stimuli such as interleukin and matrix metalloproteinases (MMPs). However, it also appears to have anabolic properties to enable self-repair by increased production of matrix components.

INTRODUCTION

The pathogenesis of osteoarthritis (OA) is a complex event to which anatomic, biomechanical, and metabolic factors may all contribute. The susceptibility to OA between different joints might be explained as a balance between degeneration and repair (Poole *et al.*, 1994). Degeneration of articular cartilage may occur in all joints but the degeneration may be non-progressive or repairable in some, while progressing to symptomatic disease in other, more susceptible, joints (Figure 1).

Ankle OA is seen less commonly in clinical practice than arthritis of the hip and knee. However, symptomatic end-stage ankle OA has been shown to cause significant mental and physical disability at least as severe as that associated with end-stage hip arthritis (Glazebrook *et al.*, 2008).

The ankle is one of the most arthritis-resistant joints in the body and, unlike the hip and knee, is rarely affected by primary OA. Posttraumatic OA is the most common underlying cause of ankle arthritis. Therefore, the ankle appears to be unique amongst the major joints of the lower limb and, as such, has prompted research into the underlying mechanisms and functions of its cartilage.

This chapter aims to discuss the characteristics of the ankle that appear to afford its protection against primary arthritis but make it susceptible to arthritis following injury. These characteristics include distinctive anatomy and biomechanics though increasing focus is now being directed to the metabolism, structure, and function of the articular cartilage itself.

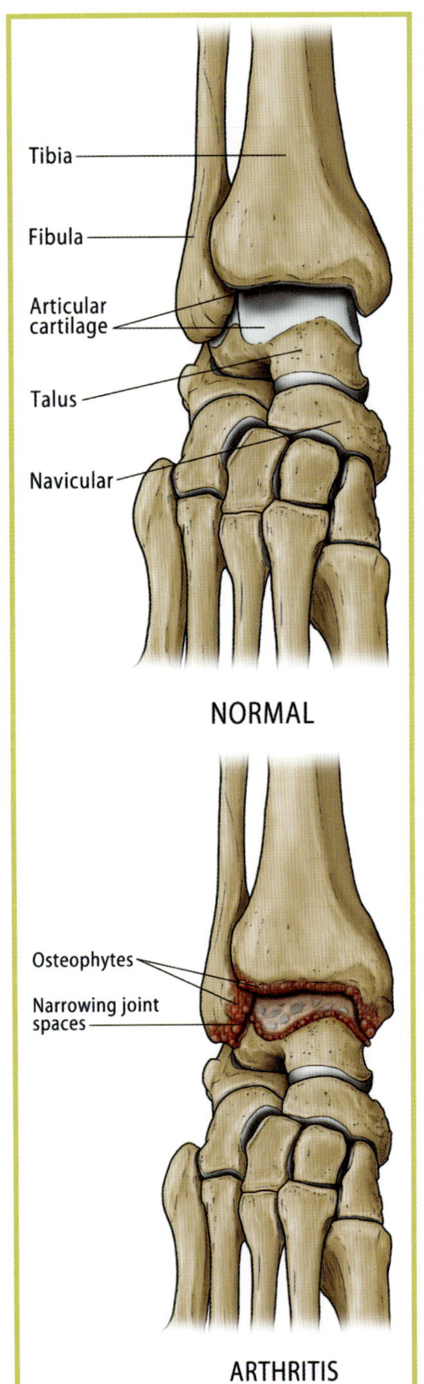

Figure 1. *Illustrations of a normal and arthritic ankle.* Image by Catherine Sulzmann, Medical Artist.

INCIDENCE

The true prevalence of ankle arthritis is difficult to determine due to the variations in correlation between degenerative change and clinical symptoms. However, cadaveric, radiographic, and clinical studies all indicate that hip and knee arthritis is more common than arthritis of the ankle (Huch *et al.*, 1997; Valderrabano *et al.*, 2009; Saltzman *et al.*, 2005; Koepp *et al.*, 1999; Cushnaghan and Dieppe, 1991; Wilson *et al.*, 1990).

Epidemiological studies have shown that 10% of the population will develop knee arthritis while symptomatic OA is rare, even in the elderly (Huch *et al.*, 1997; Wilson *et al.*, 1990; Cushnaghan and Dieppe, 1991). In clinical practice, patients with symptomatic knee pain and associated radiographic arthritis are seen up to nine times more commonly than those with symptomatic ankle arthritis. Hip arthritis is observed three times more often (Saltzman *et al.*, 2005).

The demand incidence of symptomatic ankle OA has been estimated to be 47.7 per 100,000 in the United Kingdom (Zaidi *et al.*, 2013).

It is estimated that knee replacement is performed about 23 times more frequently, and hip replacement about 18 times more frequently, than either arthrodesis or arthroplasty for end-stage ankle arthritis (Green, 2016).

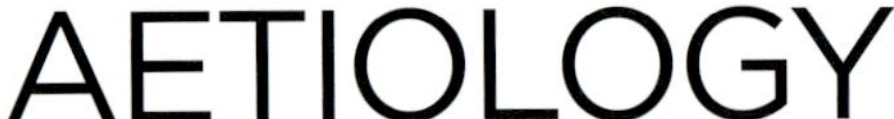

AETIOLOGY

Posttraumatic OA is the most common cause of degenerative change in the ankle (Weatherall *et al.*, 2013; Barp *et al.*, 2017).

Two recent studies have evaluated this in more detail by looking at a cohort of patients presenting to a tertiary referral centre with symptomatic end-stage arthritis. The Iowa group (Saltzman *et al.*, 2005) reviewed 639 ankles and the Swiss group reviewed 406 ankles (Valderrabano *et al.*, 2009). Both groups identified a history of previous trauma in at least 70% of ankles (Table 1). Only 7% of ankles had no identifiable underlying cause and were labelled as "primary" arthritis. This compared with a diagnosis of primary arthritis in 82% of knees and 65% of hips.

Malleolar ankle fractures were shown to be the initiating factor in 40% of those ankles with posttraumatic arthritis (Table 2).

Several factors have been identified as potential predictors of arthritis following a rotational ankle fracture including the severity of the initial injury, reflected in damage to the articular cartilage.

Table 1. Aetiology of ankle OA.

	Iowa (%)	Swiss (%)
Posttraumatic arthritis	70	78
Secondary arthritis	23	13
Primary	7	9

Table 2. Aetiology of posttraumatic arthritis.

	Iowa (%)	Swiss (%)
Malleolar fracture	37	49
Ligamentous	28	20
Plafond	9	18
Tibia	12	6
Talus	8	3

Lindsjo reported a series of more than 300 ankle fractures treated with operative internal fixation. The overall prevalence of ankle arthritis was 14% (Lindsjo, 1985). Prevalence was directly correlated to the fracture pattern, with arthritis seen in 4% Weber A fractures, 12% Weber B, and 33% Weber C. The presence of a posterior malleolar fracture, however small, indicates a more severe injury, with an increased incidence of posttraumatic arthritis (McDaniel and Wilson, 1977).

Lindjso's study also suggested that adequacy of reduction may influence outcome. Radiographic changes of OA were seen in a greater proportion of patients with a non-anatomic reduction compared with those stabilised anatomically. This study only included fractures treated operatively and it is unknown if there is any difference in outcome between anatomically reduced ankle fractures that maintained using closed treatment as opposed to open methods.

Radiographic changes of arthritis tended to occur within two years of injury; however, such changes may not progress (Lindsjo, 1985).

Ligamentous ankle injury is the second most common identifiable cause of posttraumatic arthritis. This occurs in approximately 15% of cases of posttraumatic arthritis. Instability of the ankle following chronic lateral ligament laxity may lead to the development of arthritis on the medial side of the talocrural joint through recurrent cartilage degeneration (Harrington, 1979). It is also postulated that a single episode of instability may lead to arthritis, where the force is sufficient to create osteochondral injury to the talus. OA has been reported in 20–50% of patients who have sustained osteochondral fractures and is related to the size and location of the lesion, the patients weight, and the presence of ongoing ligamentous laxity (Sanders, 2007). Several series reporting on aetiology did not create a specific category to cover ligament injury and it is probable that these groups included chronic instability within their primary osteoarthritis category (Haddad *et al.*, 2007; Wood *et al.*, 2008).

Tibial plafond fractures are the result of high-energy forces. They are associated with a high rate of posttraumatic OA, secondary to initial cartilage damage to the plafond or talus, and avascular necrosis of fracture fragments (Marsh *et al.*, 2002). It is thought that the immediate severity of injury to the articular cartilage is the major determinant of the development of OA. This would explain why AO fracture types C1 and C2 fractures have better outcomes than the more complex C3 fractures, regardless of treatment (Harris *et al.*, 2006). Some studies have demonstrated a correlation between quality of reduction and functional outcome (Rüedi, 1974) while others have shown no direct link (DeCoster *et al.*, 1999).

Rheumatoid arthritis is the commonest cause of secondary ankle arthritis not related to trauma. Other causes are secondary to neuroarthropathy, haemophilia, avascular necrosis, septic arthritis, and haemochromatosis (Valderrabano *et al.*, 2009).

DEFORMITY

Varus is the dominant malalignment seen throughout all groups of ankle OA: posttraumatic, secondary, and primary (Saltzman *et al.*, 2005; Valderrabano *et al.*, 2009).

Malaligned fractures of the ankle, tibial plafond, and tibial shaft may all result in varus deformity. Chronic lateral ligament laxity is recognised as causing alterations in joint kinematics. Ankles with lateral ligament laxity abnormally pronate and externally rotate at heel strike and supinate and internally rotate during acceleration (Hashimoto and Inokuchi, 1997). Caputo *et al.* studied *in vivo* kinematics in (Anterior Talo-Fibular Ligament) ATFL-deficient ankles compared to intact ankles (Caputo *et al.*, 2009). Physiological loading was studied using 3D magnetic resonance model and fluoroscopy. They observed that deficiency of the ATFL increased anterior translation, internal rotation, and superior translation of the talus. No significant difference in inversion was seen between normal and injured ankles. Furthermore, this group studied the change in strain with lateral ankle instability. They confirmed that peak cartilage strain is increased in the injured ankle and the location of this strain is translated anteriorly by 15.5 ± 7.1 mm and medially by 12.9 ± 4.3 mm relative to the intact ankle. These changes correspond to the region of clinically observed OA that appears at the anteromedial aspect on the ankle (Bischof *et al.*, 2010). It is suggested that anterior translation might increase wear on the tibiotalar joint. Internal rotation of the talus may lead to increased cartilage loading on the medial side of the talus due to the curvature of the cartilage on the medial malleolus and also due to increased shear stresses. The observed increase in superior translation is reflected in the increase in peak strain seen in this area.

Injuries to the lateral ligaments of the ankle are far more common than those of the medial side. This would go some way to explain why varus malalignment is seen more frequently than valgus. However, following fracture both varus and valgus are seen.

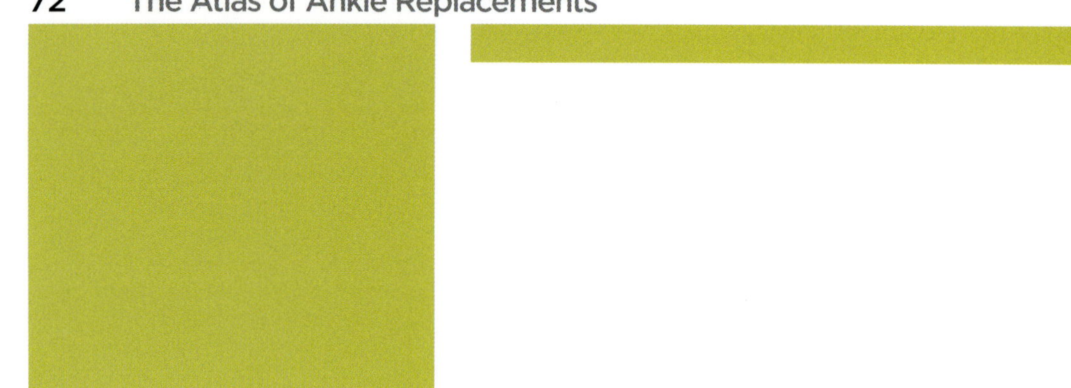

It is, as yet, unknown whether the ankle is more susceptible to developing arthritis on the medial surface as compared to the lateral.

- The normal ankle joint is highly congruent and stable.
- In contrast to hips and knees, primary OA is rare.
- The commonest cause of ankle OA is posttraumatic.
- Rotational ankle fractures and acute or chronic ligament instability are risk factors.
- The commonest malalignment is varus.

MECHANICAL PROPERTIES

OA in the hip and knee increases with age, while primary OA of the ankle is rare even in the elderly. This is despite the ankle joint being the first major articulation responsible for transfer of ground reaction forces to the remainder of the body. All joints of the lower limb are subjected to similar loads during weightbearing (Unsworth, 1991); however, the ankle is subjected to the highest forces per unit area and is the joint most commonly injured.

In the knee, cartilage degeneration with fibrillation and full thickness articular changes are believed to precede OA. Similar changes may be seen in the ankle but may not progress in the same manner. Random autopsy studies of knees and ankles found full-thickness cartilage defects in 44% of knees and only 2% of ankles (Meachim, 1975; Meachim and Emery, 1974).

Cole *et al.*, analysed 2142 joints from donors with no preceding history of joint disease (Cole *et al.*, 2003). They found at least macroscopic grade 2 disease (deep fibrillation and fissuring) in 24% of tali compared to 46% of distal femurs. Approximately, 50% of the ankles had macroscopically normal (grade 0) articular surfaces compared with only 30% of knees. The degree of degeneration in ankle cartilage is similar in both limbs in almost 80% of cases (Kuettner and Cole, 2005).

If all degeneration deteriorated with age, then, given these figures, one would expect the frequency of significant osteoarthritic changes in the ankle to be much higher than clinically observed. Koepp and colleagues found that although the frequency of degenerative changes in donors increased with age, a proportion of knee and ankle joints were found to have no detectable degeneration, even in those over 60 years (38% of the ankle, 4% of the knee) (Koepp *et al.*, 1999). In ankles where degenerative change was seen, disease of at least equal severity or worse was observed in the knee. This may suggest that joint degeneration is not as common a part of normal ageing as previously thought and that changes described as pre-osteoarthritic (or early degeneration) may not progress in the same manner between the knee and ankle joints.

It is postulated that the cartilage in the hip and knee becomes weaker with the ageing process, while the ankle retains its mechanical properties.

A number of studies have compared the biomechanical properties of ankle articular cartilage with that of the hip and knee. Kempson investigated the effect of ageing on the mechanical properties of cartilage of the hip and ankle joints by testing the tensile properties of normal, intact cartilage from postmortem subjects. The tensile fracture stress of cartilage from both the superficial and mid zones of the femoral head decreased significantly with age, while that of the talus did not. It was felt that the decline in tensile properties is related to the disruption of the normal collagen fibril network by progressive fatigue. However, even in the eighth or ninth decades, talar cartilage is likely to be strong enough to resist normal physiological stresses (Kempson, 1991).

Cyclical loading affects chondrocytes metabolism (Palmoski and Brandt, 1984). As talar cartilage is less affected by the physiological stresses of ageing, chondrocytes may continue to synthesise the main constituents of cartilage. This inherent characteristic may help prevent primary osteoarthritic change in the ankle. Higher stresses that occur in the ankle following trauma may lead to a change in chondrocytes metabolism, deterioration in collagen, and the potential to develop OA.

Swann and Seedhom found ankle cartilage to be stiffer than that of the knee. A relationship is suggested whereby areas that regularly experience high stress adapt by increasing stiffness and those areas that are only occasionally exposed to high stresses may develop arthritic changes (Swann and Seedhom, 1993). Topographic studies have shown cartilage properties to be more uniform in the ankle than in the hip and knee (Athanasiou *et al.*, 1995).

- Primary OA joint changes are usually bilateral.
- Macroscopic changes more severe in knee than the ankle.
- Changes may not be progressive.
- Ageing ankle cartilage maintains tensile strength.

ARTICULAR CARTILAGE THICKNESS

The thickness of articular cartilage will influence stresses and strains within the cartilage matrix. The thickness and uniformity of cartilage have been shown to differ amongst the joints of the lower limb (Adam *et al.*, 1998; Shepherd and Seedhom, 1999). In cadaveric lower limb joints, the ankle was found to have the thinnest cartilage, whereas the knee always had the thickest. In the same study, an inverse relationship was found between cartilage thickness and its compressive modulus. That is, thin ankle cartilage has a high compressive modulus.

Ankle cartilage is relatively uniform in thickness, generally ranging between 1.0 to 1.7 mm. Knee cartilage has a wide variation in thickness, from 1.0 to 1.6 mm. The major difference between the two joints appears to be in the thickness of the middle and deep cartilage layers (Oegema Jr *et al.*, 2003).

- Thin cartilage: high compressive modulus.
- Ankle cartilage: 1.0–1.7 mm.
- Knee cartilage: 1.0–1.6 mm.

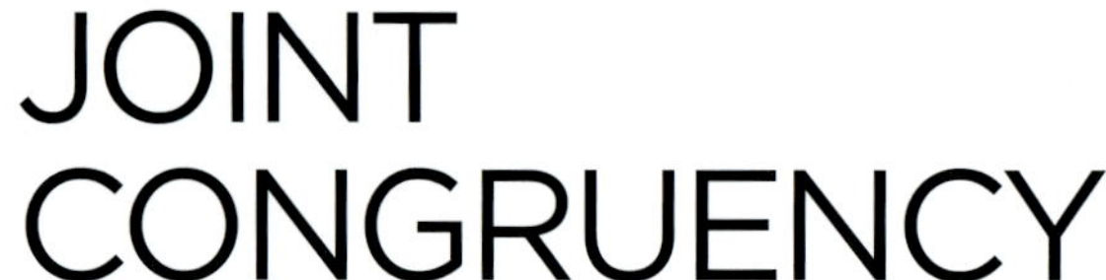

JOINT CONGRUENCY

Simon suggested that the thickness of articular cartilage is related to the congruency of the joint, with thinnest cartilage being found in the most congruent joints and thickest cartilage in incongruent joints (Simon, 1971). This correlation between cartilage thickness and congruence was suggested to act to equalise stresses within joints. Congruent joints with thin cartilage, such as the ankle, would only deform a small amount, yet, because of their congruence, the area of contact is large enough to distribute the load and maintain an acceptable level of stress. With incongruent joints like the knee, deformation of the thick cartilage increases the contact area between the joint surfaces sufficiently to decrease the stress to an acceptable level (Simon *et al.*, 1973).

This concept was extrapolated into a mathematical model, which demonstrated a change in congruency in the ankle with a change in load (Wynarsky and Greenwald, 1983). The area of stress changes from two localised areas to one continuous large area of stress distribution as loads are increased during the stance phase of walking, thus transforming the joint from incongruent to congruent. Wan *et al.* studied the contact area of the ankle using fluoroscopy and MRI-generated 3D models (Wan *et al.*, 2006). They found that the contact area of the ankle was significantly larger at mid-stance (417 mm^2) than at heel strike (273 mm^2) or toe-off (336 mm^2). As well as dissipating load, such a change may have a beneficial effect upon joint lubrication and nutrition, therefore adding a further contribution to protection from primary arthritis.

- A congruent joints act to dissipate load.
- The contact area changes with gait cycle.
- Largest contact area at mid-stance.

ARTICULAR CONTACT AREA

The potential articular surface area of the ankle is actually not too dissimilar to that of the hip and knee. With loading, however, the actual articular surface area reduces. At 500 N load, the ankle has a contact area of 350 mm^2, compared with 1100 mm^2 for the hip and 1120 mm^2 for the knee (Brown and Shaw, 1983; Wan *et al.*, 2006; Ihn *et al.*, 1993).

Changes in contact stress and contact area may occur following trauma. A decrease in contact area gives an increase in force per unit area. Such changes may increase the probability of fatigue fracture of the articular cartilage and bone of the distal tibia resulting in posttraumatic arthritis. Ramsey and Hamilton undertook a classic biomechanical study in order to investigate the change in ankle contact area caused by talar displacement and showed that 1 mm of lateral displacement decreased the tibiotalar contact area by 42% (Ramsey and Hamilton, 1976). These results are often quoted to reinforce the importance of anatomic reduction following ankle fractures.

It is important to note that their study does not represent a physiological state because a static cadaveric model void of all soft tissues was used. Other non-physiological studies have reproduced similar results (Lloyd *et al.*, 2006; Moody *et al.*, 1992).

Further studies have evaluated more dynamic/unconstrained models and have stressed the importance of the medial structures as primary stabilisers of the ankle. Curtis *et al.* placed unconstrained ankles through 20 degrees of motion and measured contact areas with both fibular displacement and deltoid division (Curtis *et al.*, 1992). There was greater than 30% decrease in tibiotalar contact with both fibular shortening and external rotation, and this reduction in contact area was accentuated further when the deltoid was divided. Clarke *et al.* also developed a dynamic weightbearing cadaveric model to assess tibiotalar stability in ankle fractures and reported that 6 mm of distal fibula displacement alone without soft tissue disruption caused no change in contact area, but that additional

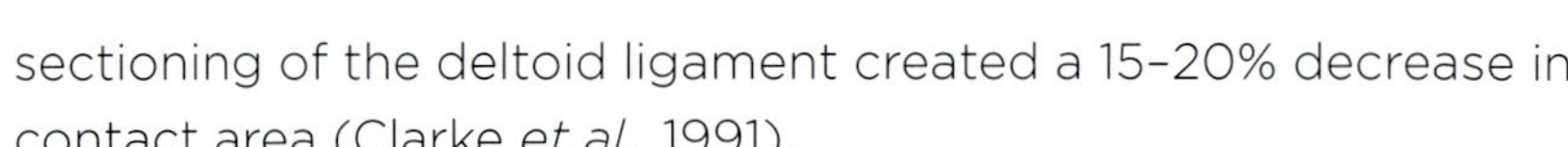

sectioning of the deltoid ligament created a 15–20% decrease in contact area (Clarke *et al.*, 1991).

To assess the value of the medial stabilisers in preventing displacement, Van den Bekerom *et al.* reviewed supination-external rotation (SER) II fractures (intact deltoid) with apparent displacement of 2 mm or more at the lateral malleolus (van den Bekerom and van Dijk, 2010). They found that the fracture displacement consists mainly of medial displacement of the proximal fibula with little displacement of the distal fracture. In view of this, they recommended conservative treatment of the majority of these fractures. However, they reinforced that these recommendations are not applicable for SER fractures with deltoid ligament injury (SER IV). Thus, physiological studies seem to demonstrate the importance of the medial structures as primary stabilisers of the ankle, and that with a displaced fibular fracture the talus tends not to follow the distal fibular displacement maximally unless there is insufficiency of the deltoid.

It is also important to consider the effect of weightbearing on the ankle joint. During normal level walking, the ankle carries loads of up to 5 times body weight (Stauffer *et al.*, 1977). The differences in findings in these studies may result from the fact that during loading, the ankle tends to adopt a stable position, and that loading leads to increased joint congruity.

• Trauma may decrease articular contact area. • The medial structures are primary stabilisers. • The ankle carries up to 5X bodyweight. • The ankle is more stable with weightbearing.

ANKLE JOINT METABOLISM

The anatomic and biomechanical differences already highlighted may go some way to explaining the differences in susceptibility to arthritis between the ankle, hip, and knee. However, the importance of metabolic differences is becoming increasingly recognised. It would appear that ankle cartilage not only has an inherent resistance to joint degeneration but may also be able to repair early degeneration once it occurs.

Articular cartilage acts as a shock absorber to the more rigid underlying bone. This task is achieved by providing elasticity and resistance to compressive forces, mainly via tissue water and the extracellular matrix, which makes up approximately 95% of the tissue volume. Collagens and proteoglycans (PGs) form the major constituents of the extracellular matrix. The major PG in cartilage is aggrecan, which provides much of the equilibrium compressive stiffness of the tissue due to electrostatic repulsion between the highly charged and closely packed GAG chains. The extracellular matrix is controlled and maintained by chondrocytes, which react to the biophysical modulation of the tissue. Articular cartilage has no blood vessels or nerve supply and derives its nutrition from the synovial fluid.

There appears to be significant differences in the biochemical and biomechanical properties of the knee and ankle (Treppo *et al.*, 2000). In the ankle, the extracellular matrix is denser, while the collagen content is similar, the sulphated GAG content is higher, and the water content is significantly lower. Together, these findings are consistent with the higher dynamic stiffness and lower hydraulic permeability seen in the ankle. These properties could increase ankle cartilage stiffness, thus protecting the cartilage from the harmful effects of higher compressive forces. This hypothesis was investigated by applying injurious compression to knee and ankle explants (Patwari *et al.*, 2007). Using a protocol that damaged nearly 50% of knee cartilage samples, it was observed that in ankle cartilage, the same level of insult caused little visible damage and had no significant effect on PG loss.

The higher concentration of sulphated GAG within the ankle is a result of a higher rate of synthesis by chondrocytes. Ankle cartilage also has a reduced half-life for PGs, implying that the ankle is metabolically more active in both synthesising and breaking down PGs. It is likely that aggrecan is the PG principally responsible for these changes (Kuettner and Cole, 2005).

Ankle versus knee hyaline cartilage

- Ankle has denser extracellular matrix.
  - GAG higher than knee, water content is lower.
- Ankle has higher dynamic stiffness.
- Ankle has lower hydraulic permeability.
- Ankle has increased stiffness.

Synthesis of PGs, collagens, and other proteins varies under load. With compression, knee chondrocytes will produce increased levels of protein similar to those seen in the unloaded ankle. Dynamic loading will cause an increase in protein synthesis, thus confirming the need for regular loading to maintain articular cartilage. In the ankle, dynamic compression also appears to cause an increase in collagen synthesis but not PGs. With static compression, collagen synthesis is suppressed at a lower level of compression than synthesis of protein or PG.

Interestingly, the extracellular matrix appears to play an important regulatory role in this mechanism rather than it being genetically programmed into the chondrocytes themselves (Kerin *et al.*, 2002; Kuettner and Cole, 2005).

If the original matrix is stripped and a new one synthesised, then the response to loading by both ankle and knee chondrocytes stops being significantly different. In addition, there are no longer differences neither in GAG synthesis nor in half-lives. Finally, no differences were observed in response to the catabolic cytokine, interleukin-1beta (IL-1β).

Anti-Catabolic Properties

Ankle cartilage is further protected by the ability of ankle chondrocytes to resist catabolic stimulation. Interleukin-1 is a pro-inflammatory catabolic cytokine that acts on chondrocytes. At low concentrations, it suppresses the synthesis of matrix components and thus decreases potential cartilage repair. At higher concentrations, IL-1 stimulates the production of proteolytic enzymes that increase matrix degradation. Ankle chondrocytes demonstrate a reduced catabolic response to stimulation with IL-1β as compared to the knee, and continue to produce GAG in a dose-dependent manner. Once a high concentration of IL-1 is reached, both knee and ankle respond in a similar manner. The greater inhibitory response seen in the knee appears to be related to the numbers or type of receptors present on the chondrocytes. The effect of IL-1 receptor antagonist was overcome more effectively in the ankle than in the knee.

As the extracellular matrix starts to degenerate, fragments of matrix components, such as fibronectin, can activate both anti-anabolic and catabolic pathways. Kang and colleagues demonstrated that knee chondrocytes showed greater PG loss and increased aggrecanase activity when stimulated by fibronectin fragments (Kang *et al.*, 1998). Ankle cartilage was much more refractory to damage than knee cartilage from the same donor.

Matrix metalloproteinases (MMPs) are a family of substances that are proteolytic to cartilage matrix components and can lead to development of OA. Chubinskaya and colleagues demonstrated that expression for MMP-8 was detected in normal knee joint cartilage, but not in normal ankle cartilage (Chubinskaya *et al.*, 1996). MMP-8 expression was seen following the action of the catabolic cytokine IL-1β on normal ankle cartilage. It is suggested that some MMPs may play a role in normal cartilage homeostasis, with only the expression of some members (MMP-3, MMP-8) being related to articular cartilage damage (Chubinskaya *et al.*, 1999).

Further studies are identifying factors, such as tissue inhibitor of metalloproteinase-3 [TIMP-3], associated with protection of articular cartilage degeneration (Morris *et al.*, 2010).

> - Less response to IL-1.
> - Less response to matrix degradation products.
> - Normally, no expression for MMP.
> - Inhibitors to MMPs.

Anabolic Properties

As well as being more resistant to cartilage breakdown, ankle cartilage may also be better able to repair early damage. Ankle chondrocytes show a heightened response to anabolic agents, such as osteogenic protein-1, by elevated PG synthesis.

Similar conclusions were made when *in vivo* studies were performed on joints with evidence of early cartilage lesions (Aurich *et al.*, 2006). Ankle cartilage demonstrated upregulation of matrix turnover with an increase in collagen synthesis and aggrecan turnover. This response was absent in the knee, which demonstrated an increase in type II collagen cleavage. These differences continue to support the notion of repair in early cartilage lesions in the ankle and degradation in the knee. There is evidence that this upregulation of matrix turnover in ankles with degenerative lesions may indicate a physiological response of the entire articular surface to repair the damaged matrix, and are not just restricted to the site of the lesion.

In OA of the hip and knee, cartilage changes are accompanied by an increase in the density of the underlying subchondral bone. However, even in ankles with moderate cartilage degeneration, a decrease in subchondral bone density is observed (Muehleman *et al.*, 2002). This may support the theory that bony involvement may need to occur before arthritis can progress.

> - Increased PG & collagen synthesis.
> - Increased aggrecan turnover.
> - No increase in bone density.

CONCLUSIONS

Differences in the incidence and aetiology of OA suggest that the ankle is more resistant to primary OA by its metabolic properties, tensile characteristics, uniformity, congruency, and restrained movement. However, such characteristics may also place it at risk for degeneration following trauma. The thinness of ankle articular cartilage and the high peak contact stresses to which it is submitted may make it less adaptable to the incongruity, decreased stability, or increased stresses that may follow a traumatic event.

Ankle OA may cause severe symptoms, and, given its post-traumatic nature, is more likely to affect a younger, working population than those with OA of the hip and knee. With this in mind, it is important to obtain an indepth understanding of the mechanisms of resistance to and development of posttraumatic ankle OA. Potential benefits of protective agents such as anti-apoptotic agents are currently being explored. Such research will not only have a possible benefit in the treatment and prevention of ankle OA but may also be extrapolated to other joints.

Increasing investigation is now concentrating on the ankle joint to determine why it demonstrates resistance to primary degeneration, with the potential that such an insight may lead to novel mechanisms and treatments that may be applied to less resistant joints such as the hip and knee.

REFERENCES

Adam, C., Eckstein, F., Milz, S. & Putz, R. 1998. The distribution of cartilage thickness within the joints of the lower limb of elderly individuals. *J Anat,* 193, 203–214.

Athanasiou, K. A., Niederauer, G. G. & Schenck, R. C., Jr. 1995. Biomechanical topography of human ankle cartilage. *Ann Biomed Eng*, 23, 697–704.

Aurich, M., Mwale, F., Reiner, A., Mollenhauer, J. A., Anders, J. O., Fuhrmann, R. A., Kuettner, K. E., Poole, A. R. & Cole, A. A. 2006. Collagen and proteoglycan turnover in focally damaged human ankle cartilage: evidence for a generalized response and active matrix remodeling across the entire joint surface. *Arthritis Rheum*, 54, 244–252.

Barp, E. A., Erickson, J. G. & Hall, J. L. 2017. Arthroscopic treatment of ankle arthritis. *Clin Podiatr Med Surg*, 34, 433–444.

Bischof, J. E., Spritzer, C. E., Caputo, A. M., Easley, M. E., Deorio, J. K., Nunley, J. A., II & Defrate, L. E. 2010. *In vivo* cartilage contact strains in patients with lateral ankle instability. *J Biomech*, 43, 2561–2566.

Brown, T. D. & Shaw, D. T. 1983. *In vitro* contact stress distributions in the natural human hip. *J Biomech*, 16, 373–384.

Caputo, A. M., Lee, J. Y., Spritzer, C. E., Easley, M. E., Deorio, J. K., Nunley, J. A., II & Defrate, L. E. 2009. *In vivo* kinematics of the tibiotalar joint after lateral ankle instability. *Am J Sports Med*, 37, 2241–2248.

Chubinskaya, S., Huch, K., Mikecz, K., Cs-Szabo, G., Hasty, K. A., Kuettner, K. E. & Cole, A. A. 1996. Chondrocyte matrix metalloproteinase-8: Up-regulation of neutrophil collagenase by interleukin-1 beta in human cartilage from knee and ankle joints. *Lab Invest*, 74, 232–240.

Chubinskaya, S., Kuettner, K. E. & Cole, A. A. 1999. Expression of matrix metalloproteinases in normal and damaged articular cartilage from human knee and ankle joints. *Lab Invest*, 79, 1669–1677.

Clarke, H. J., Michelson, J. D., Cox, Q. G. & Jinnah, R. H. 1991. Tibio-talar stability in bimalleolar ankle fractures: A dynamic in vitro contact area study. *Foot Ankle*, 11, 222–227.

Cole, A. A., Margulis, A. & Kuettner, K. E. 2003. Distinguishing ankle and knee articular cartilage. *Foot Ankle Clin*, 8, 305–316, x.

Curtis, M. J., Michelson, J. D., Urquhart, M. W., Byank, R. P. & Jinnah, R. H. 1992. Tibiotalar contact and fibular malunion in ankle fractures. A cadaver study. *Acta Orthop Scand*, 63, 326–329.

Cushnaghan, J. & Dieppe, P. 1991. Study of 500 patients with limb joint osteoarthritis. I. Analysis by age, sex, and distribution of symptomatic joint sites. *Ann Rheum Dis*, 50, 8–13.

Decoster, T. A., Willis, M. C., Marsh, J. L., Williams, T. M., Nepola, J. V., Dirschl, D. R. & Hurwitz, S. R. 1999. Rank order analysis of tibial plafond

fractures: does injury or reduction predict outcome? *Foot Ankle Int*, 20, 44–49.

Glazebrook, M., Daniels, T., Younger, A., Foote, C. J., Penner, M., Wing, K., Lau, J., Leighton, R. & Dunbar, M. 2008. Comparison of health-related quality of life between patients with end-stage ankle and hip arthrosis. *J Bone J Surg (Am)*, 90, 499–505.

Green, M., Howard, P., Porter, M., Price, A., Wilkinson, M., Wishart, N. 2016. 13th Annual Report. *Natl Jt Regist*.

Harrington, K. D. 1979. Degenerative arthritis of the ankle secondary to long-standing lateral ligament instability. *J Bone Joint Surg Am*, 61, 354–361.

Harris, A. M., Patterson, B. M., Sontich, J. K. & Vallier, H. A. 2006. Results and outcomes after operative treatment of high-energy tibial plafond fractures. *Foot Ankle Int,* 27, 256–265.

Hashimoto, T. & Inokuchi, S. 1997. A kinematic study of ankle joint instability due to rupture of the lateral ligaments. *Foot Ankle Int*, 18, 729–734.

Huch, K., Kuettner, K. E. & Dieppe, P. 1997. Osteoarthritis in ankle and knee joints. *Semin Arthritis Rheum*, 26(4), 667–674.

Ihn, J. C., Kim, S. J. & Park, I. H. 1993. *In vitro* study of contact area and pressure distribution in the human knee after partial and total meniscectomy. *Int Orthop*, 17, 214–218.

Kang, Y. *et al.* 1998. *J Orthop Res*, 16(5), 551–556.

Kempson, G. E. 1991. Age-related changes in the tensile properties of human articular cartilage: a comparative study between the femoral head of the hip joint and the talus of the ankle joint. *Biochim Biophy Acta (BBA) — General Subjects*, 1075, 223–230.

Kerin, A., Patwari, P., Kuettner, K., Cole, A. & Grodzinsky, A. 2002. Molecular basis of osteoarthritis: Biomechanical aspects. *Cell Mol Life Sci*, 59, 27–35.

Koepp, H., Eger, W., Muehleman, C., Valdellon, A., Buckwalter, J. A., Kuettner, K. E. & Cole, A. A. 1999. Prevalence of articular cartilage degeneration in the ankle and knee joints of human organ donors. *J Orthop Sci*, 4, 407–412.

Kuettner, K. E. & Cole, A. A. 2005. Cartilage degeneration in different human joints. *Osteoarthritis Cartilage*, 13, 93–103.

Lindsjo, U. 1985. Operative treatment of ankle fracture-dislocations. A follow-up study of 306/321 consecutive cases. *Clin Orthop Relat Res*, 199, 28–38.

Lloyd, J., Elsayed, S., Hariharan, K. & Tanaka, H. 2006. Revisiting the concept of talar shift in ankle fractures. *Foot Ankle Int*, 27, 793–796.

Marsh, J. L., Buckwalter, J. A., Gelberman, R., Dirschl, D. R., Olson, S., Brown, T. D. & Llinias, A. 2002. Articular fractures: Does an anatomic reduction really change the result?. *J Bone J Surg (Am)*, 84, 1259–1271.

Mcdaniel, W. J. & Wilson, F. C. 1977. Trimalleolar fractures of the ankle. An end result study. *Clin Orthop Relat Res*, 122, 37–45.

Meachim, G. 1975. Cartilage fibrillation at the ankle joint in Liverpool necropsies. *J Anat*, 119, 601–610.

Meachim, G. & Emery, I. H. 1974. Quantitative aspects of patello-femoral cartilage fibrillation in Liverpool necropsies. *Ann Rheum Dis*, 33, 39–47.

Moody, M. L., Koeneman, J., Hettinger, E. & Karpman, R. R. 1992. The effects of fibular and talar displacement on joint contact areas about the ankle. *Orthop Rev*, 21, 741–744.

Morris, K. J., Cs-Szabo, G. & Cole, A. A. 2010. Characterization of TIMP-3 in human articular talar cartilage. *Connect Tissue Res*, 51, 478–490.

Muehleman, C., Berzins, A., Koepp, H., Eger, W., Cole, A. A., Kuettner, K. E. & Sumner, D. R. 2002. Bone density of the human talus does not increase with the cartilage degeneration score. *Anatomic Record*, 266, 81–86.

Oegema, T. R., Jr., Carlson, C. S. & Cole, A. A. 2003. Histological analysis of cartilage conditions. *Handbook of Histology Methods for Bone and Cartilage*, Chapter 31. pp. 423–439. Springer Science+Business Media New York, ISBN 978-1-61737-277-3.

Palmoski, M. J. & Brandt, K. D. 1984. Effects of static and cyclic compressive loading on articular cartilage plugs *in vitro*. *Arthritis Rheum*, 27, 675–681.

Patwari, P., Cheng, D. M., Cole, A. A., Kuettner, K. E. & Grodzinsky, A. J. 2007. Analysis of the relationship between peak stress and proteoglycan loss following injurious compression of human post-mortem knee and ankle cartilage. *Biomech Model Mechanobiol*, 6, 83–89.

Poole, A. R., Ionescu, M., Swan, A. & Dieppe, P. A. 1994. Changes in cartilage metabolism in arthritis are reflected by altered serum and synovial fluid levels of the cartilage proteoglycan aggrecan. Implications for pathogenesis. *J Clin Invest*, 94, 25–33.

Ramsey, P. L. & Hamilton, W. 1976. Changes in tibiotalar area of contact caused by lateral talar shift. *J Bone Joint Surg Am*, 58, 356–357.

Rüedi, T. 1974. Fractures of the lower end of the tibia into the ankle joint: results 9 years after open reduction and internal fixation. *Injury*, 5, 130–134.

Saltzman, C. L., Salamon, M. L., Blanchard, G. M., Huff, T., Hayes, A., Buckwalter, J. A. & Amendola, A. 2005. Epidemiology of ankle arthritis: Report of a consecutive series of 639 patients from a tertiary orthopaedic center. *Iowa Orthop J*, 25, 44–46.

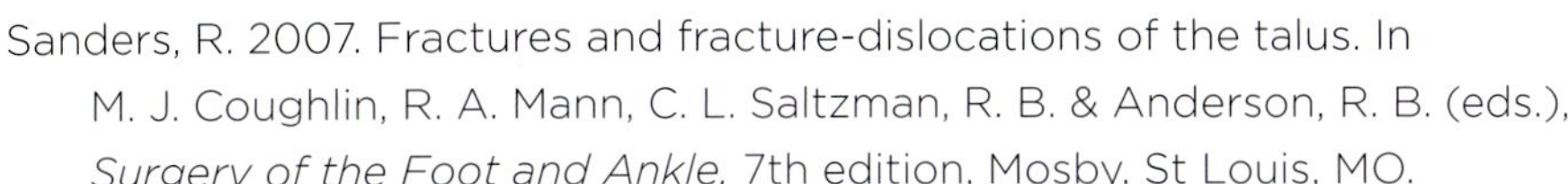

Sanders, R. 2007. Fractures and fracture-dislocations of the talus. In M. J. Coughlin, R. A. Mann, C. L. Saltzman, R. B. & Anderson, R. B. (eds.), *Surgery of the Foot and Ankle,* 7th edition, Mosby, St Louis, MO.

Shepherd, D. E. & Seedhom, B. B. 1999. Thickness of human articular cartilage in joints of the lower limb. *Ann Rheum Dis*, 58, 27–34.

Simon, W. H. 1971. Scale effects in animal joints. II. Thickness and elasticity in the deformability of articular cartilage. *Arthritis Rheum*, 14, 493–502.

Simon, W. H., Friedenberg, S. & Richardson, S. 1973. Joint congruence: a correlation of joint congruence and thickness of articular cartilage in dogs. *J Bone J Surg (Am)*, 55, 1614–1620.

Stauffer, R. N., Chao, E. Y. & Brewster, R. C. 1977. Force and motion analysis of the normal, diseased, and prosthetic ankle joint. *Clin Orthop Relat Res*, 127, 189–196.

Swann, A. C. & Seedhom, B. B. 1993. The stiffness of normal articular cartilage and the predominant acting stress levels: Implications for the aetiology of osteoarthrosis. *Rheumatology*, 32, 16–25.

Treppo, S., Koepp, H., Quan, E. C., Cole, A. A., Kuettner, K. E. & Grodzinsky, A. J. 2000. Comparison of biomechanical and biochemical properties of cartilage from human knee and ankle pairs. *J Orthop Res*, 18, 739–748.

Unsworth, A. 1991. Tribology of human and artificial joints. *Proc Inst Mech Eng, Part H: J Eng Med*, 205, 163–172.

Valderrabano, V., Horisberger, M., Russell, I., Dougall, H. & Hintermann, B. 2009. Etiology of ankle osteoarthritis. *Clin Orthop Relat Res*, 467, 1800–1806.

Van Den Bekerom, M. P. J. & Van Dijk, C. N. 2010. Is fibular fracture displacement consistent with tibiotalar displacement? *Clin Orthop Rel Res,* 468, 969–974.

Wan, L., De Asla, R. J., Rubash, H. E. & Li, G. 2006. Determination of *in-vivo* articular cartilage contact areas of human talocrural joint under weightbearing conditions. *Osteoarthr Cartil*, 14, 1294–1301.

Weatherall, J. M., Mroczek, K., Mclaurin, T., Ding, B. & Tejwani, N. 2013. Post-traumatic ankle arthritis. *Bull Hosp Jt Dis (2013)*, 71, 104–112.

Wilson, *et al.* 1990. Idiopathic symptomatic osteoarthritis of the hip and knee: A population-based incidence study. *Mayo Clin Proc*, 65(9), 1214–1221.

Wynarsky, G. T. & Greenwald, S. A. 1983. Mathematical model of the human ankle joint. *J Biomech*, 16, 241–251.

Zaidi, R., Cro, S., Gurusamy, K., Siva, N., Macgregor, A., Henricson, A. & Goldberg, A. 2013. The outcome of total ankle replacement: A systematic review and meta-analysis. *Bone Joint J*, 95-b, 1500–1507.

INDICATIONS AND CONTRAINDICATIONS FOR TOTAL ANKLE REPLACEMENT

H. Cornelis (Kees) Doets

Summary

Ankle arthritis differs from arthritis of the hip and knee as there is a low rate of degenerative arthritis and a predominance of posttraumatic arthritis and inflammatory joint disease (IJD). Posttraumatic arthritis can develop secondary to intra-articular ankle fractures, to lower leg fractures or to ligament injury. End-stage ankle arthritis occurs often at a younger age and is known to have an important negative influence on the quality of life and on the ability of patients to perform their occupational and recreational activities.

If conservative treatment fails, surgical reconstruction is often necessary. Then the choice has to be made between ankle fusion and total ankle replacement (TAR). Although ankle fusion usually gives a satisfactory clinical result, gait remains disturbed and with longer follow-up, there is probably an increased risk of secondary hindfoot arthritis.

Over the last few years, good, medium to long-term results with third-generation mobile bearing implants have been reported. Therefore, interest in TAR has grown considerably. This is reflected by the increasing number of TARs performed and also by an increase in scientific publications on TAR.

Since the pathology of the arthritic ankle may differ substantially between individual cases and between different aetiologies, TAR should not be considered as a standard procedure like endoprosthetic replacement of the hip or the knee. The ideal indication for TAR is end-stage arthritis with little or no deformity, with a normal foot, good bone stock, and a good range of motion. This situation occurs most closely in postfracture ankles and in primary degenerative arthritis. Bilateral ankle arthritis and IJD can also be regarded good indications for TAR. Deformity, stiff ankles, and younger age are among the controversial indications, although in experienced hands, good results can be expected. Contraindications are high-demand and non-compliant patients, neurovascular disease, periarticular bone loss, severe deformity, and infection.

INTRODUCTION

In contrast to the hip and the knee, primary osteoarthritis of the ankle has a relatively low prevalence. Posttraumatic arthritis is the most frequent condition leading to deterioration of the ankle joint (Saltzman *et al.*, 2005; Valderrabano *et al.*, 2009; Rebecca A Nieuwe Weme, 2015; Weatherall *et al.*, 2013). Posttraumatic ankle arthritis can occur as sequelae of fractures either around the ankle or at a distance (lower leg or hindfoot): "postfracture arthritis". Furthermore, posttraumatic arthritis can develop secondary to severe sprains or chronic ligament laxity with recurrent sprains (Valderrabano *et al.*, 2009; Verhagen *et al.*, 1995), a condition that the author prefers to describe as "instability arthritis", analogous to posttraumatic arthritis seen in the cruciate-deficient knee. Inflammatory joint disease (IJD), usually rheumatoid arthritis (RA), can also lead to destruction of either the joints of the hindfoot, the ankle, or both (Lehtinen *et al.*, 1996; Spiegel and Spiegel, 1982). Kuper *et al.* (1997), in their cross-sectional study, found an 11% incidence of RA affecting the ankle 6 years after onset of the disease: in 7% unilateral and in 4% bilateral. Within this context, Scott (2004) noted that rheumatoid factor positive RA (Rf+RA) is known to produce more radiographic destruction than rheumatoid factor negative RA (Rf − RA). Other, infrequent causes of secondary ankle arthritis include haemochromatosis, talar osteonecrosis, osteochondritis of the talar dome, haemophilia, crystal arthropathy, clubfoot, and infection (Preis *et al.*, 2017; Athanasiou *et al.*, 1995; Saltzman *et al.*, 2005; Huch *et al.*, 1997).

Ankle arthritis, giving rise to mild or moderate clinical symptoms, is relatively common in an adult patient population due to the high incidence of sport-related injuries. However, ankle arthritis may often not develop into end-stage ankle arthritis requiring surgical reconstruction. However, if symptomatic end-stage ankle arthritis

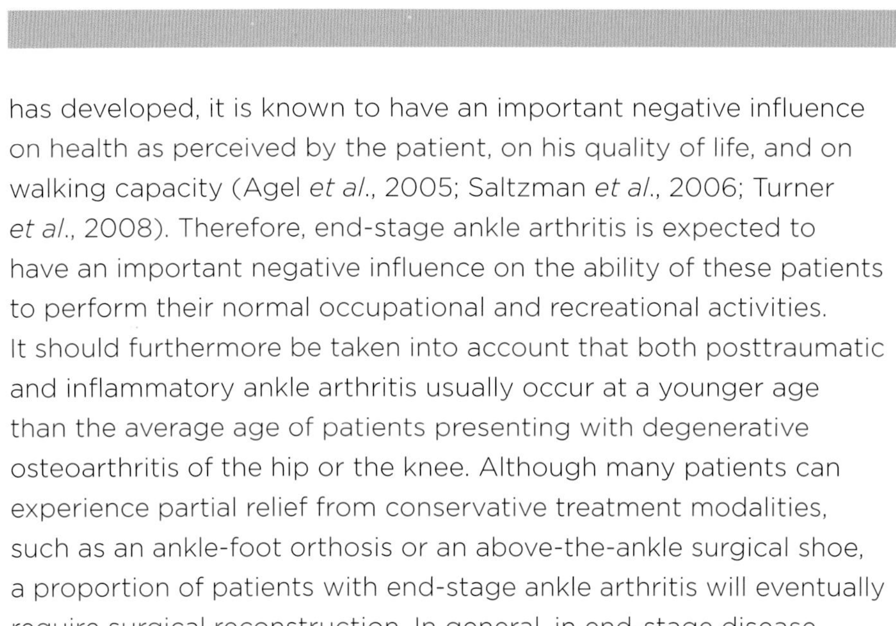

has developed, it is known to have an important negative influence on health as perceived by the patient, on his quality of life, and on walking capacity (Agel *et al.*, 2005; Saltzman *et al.*, 2006; Turner *et al.*, 2008). Therefore, end-stage ankle arthritis is expected to have an important negative influence on the ability of these patients to perform their normal occupational and recreational activities. It should furthermore be taken into account that both posttraumatic and inflammatory ankle arthritis usually occur at a younger age than the average age of patients presenting with degenerative osteoarthritis of the hip or the knee. Although many patients can experience partial relief from conservative treatment modalities, such as an ankle-foot orthosis or an above-the-ankle surgical shoe, a proportion of patients with end-stage ankle arthritis will eventually require surgical reconstruction. In general, in end-stage disease, the choice has to be made between ankle fusion and total ankle replacement (TAR), as there is mostly little place for other surgical modalities such as debridement or corrective osteotomy.

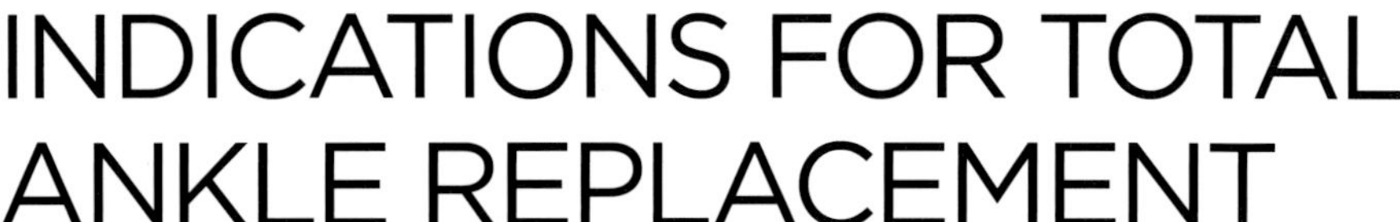

INDICATIONS FOR TOTAL ANKLE REPLACEMENT

Prosthetic replacement of the ankle joint with such devices has been shown to give good medium to long-term results, up to a level comparable to or may be even better than ankle fusion (Buechel Sr *et al.*, 2004; Doets *et al.*, 2006; Gougoulias, 2009; Haddad *et al.*, 2007; Knecht *et al.*, 2004; Saltzman *et al.*, 2009; Stengel *et al.*, 2005; Wood *et al.*, 2008; Pedowitz *et al.*, 2016; Rodriguez-Merchan, 2015; Dauty *et al.*, 2015; Daniels *et al.*, 2014; Kofoed, 2014). However, currently, the choice between ankle fusion and TAR is not only made on clear clinical arguments but also frequently depends upon the experience and the preference of the surgeon and, to some extent, on the preference of the patient. This is mainly due to the fact that there remains some uncertainty about the long-term outcome of TAR as only a few long-term studies on the outcome of TAR have been published (Bonnin *et al.*, 2011; Buechel Sr *et al.*, 2004; Doets *et al.*, 2006; Henricson *et al.*, 2011; Knecht *et al.*, 2004; Wood *et al.*, 2008; Zaidi *et al.*, 2013; Kraal *et al.*, 2013; Koivu *et al.*, 2017a, 2017b; Giannini *et al.*, 2017; Eckers *et al.*, 2017; Kerkhoff *et al.*, 2016; Jastifer and Coughlin, 2015). The first short-term non-randomised study was published by Saltzman *et al.*, which compared the outcome of ankle fusion versus TAR (Saltzman *et al.*, 2009). This study showed that patients treated by mobile-bearing TAR had a somewhat better function and equivalent pain relief compared to a control group of patients treated by ankle fusion. Haddad *et al.* (2007), in a systematic review of the literature, found similar clinical results and revision rates between the two procedures at 5 to 10 years. Their only strong clinical argument in favour of TAR was the lower below-knee amputation rate: 1% for TAR versus 5% for ankle fusion. This lower amputation rate after TAR compared to ankle fusion has also been reported by Saltzman *et al.* (2009) and SooHoo *et al.* (2007), although the influence of comorbidities is not always clear. For instance, diabetic patients with deforming arthritis and higher risk of amputation were maybe more likely to be over-represented in the fusion group. More recent studies have demonstrated a greater range of movement and better pain relief after TAR compared with arthrodesis (Pedowitz *et al.*, 2016; Hahn *et al.*, 2012).

Furthermore, gait studies have shown that ankle fusion leads to an altered gait with abnormal tarsal kinematics, an altered activity pattern of the lower leg muscles, and also changes in the ground reaction forces (Bayaert *et al.*, 2004; Thomas *et al.*, 2006; Wu *et al.*, 2000). Investigations on gait after successful TAR have shown a more normal gait, with tarsal kinematics, muscle activity patterns, and ground reaction forces usually similar to normal (Doets *et al.*, 2007; Dyrby *et al.*, 2004; Flavin, 2013). A gait pattern similar to normal can be seen as a functional argument in favour of TAR.

Another clinical argument in favour of TAR is generally thought to be the presence of a concurrent stiff or arthritic ipsilateral hindfoot. In such a condition, an ankle fusion would lead to an increased risk of hindfoot symptoms when the hindfoot joints are not ankylosed and to an even more abnormal gait pattern compared to gait after tibiotalar fusion when the hindfoot is fully stiff (tibiotalocalcaneal fusion). It is the author's experience that non-symptomatic arthritic tarsal joints without an important deformity of the hindfoot will usually remain asymptomatic after TAR, both in posttraumatic and in rheumatoid ankles and that arthritic hindfeet will not need to be fused routinely after TAR (Figure 1).

The three major causes of end-stage ankle arthritis are postfracture arthritis (including instability arthritis), inflammatory arthritis (including RA), followed by primary osteoarthritis. There is no reason of course why a patient cannot have dual pathology. For example, a patient with RA can also have postfracture arthritis, so this must be borne in mind when assessing papers. Saltzman *et al.* (2005), in a consecutive cohort of 639 patients with endstage ankle arthritis, found that 70% were of posttraumatic origin, 12% were rheumatoid ankles, 7% were idiopathic, and 11% were miscellaneous. Valderrabano *et al.* (2009) found a quite similar aetiological distribution in their cohort, with 62% postfracture arthritis, 16% secondary to ligament injury, 5% RA, 9% idiopathic, and 8% miscellaneous. In the prospective study on 200 TARs described by Wood *et al.* (2008), the distribution was 60% IJD and 40%

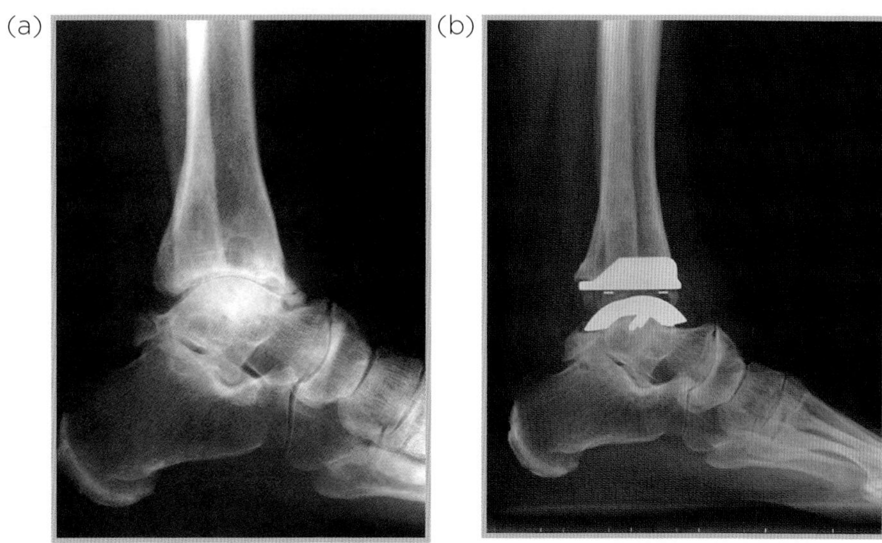

Figure 1. *Lateral weightbearing radiographs of a 49-year-old woman with end-stage ankle arthritis secondary to a malleolar fracture. The ankle joint was symptomatic but no pain could be provoked during clinical examination at the level of the tarsal joints. (a) Preoperative view showing arthritic changes both at the ankle joint, the subtalar joint, and the talonavicular joint. (b) At the 5-year follow-up interval after successful TAR with use of a CCI Evolution prosthesis, the tarsal joints showed no progression of the arthritic changes. Motion at the hindfoot was only minimally restricted and the patient was fully painfree.*

osteoarthritis (12.5% postfracture). In the review study by Haddad *et al.* (2007), comparing the outcome of TAR with ankle fusion, the patient characteristics were different between the TAR group and the fusion group: a higher incidence of RA in the TAR group (38.9% vs 12.9%) and patients in the TAR group also had a higher mean age at surgery (58 years vs 50 years). Both Haddad *et al.* (2007) and Wood *et al.* (2008) did not identify ligament injury as a separate cause for ankle arthritis and they probably grouped this aetiologic factor under non-specific or primary osteoarthritis.

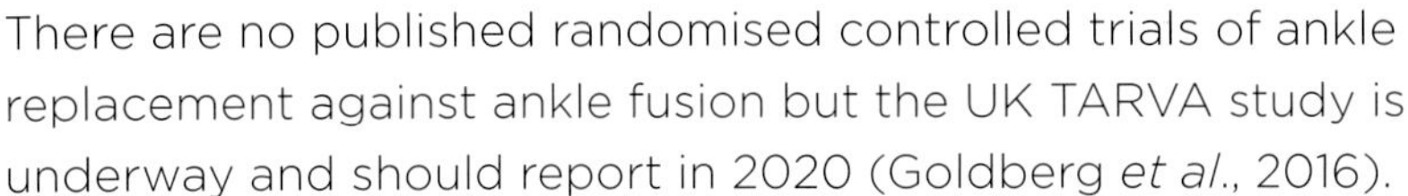

There are no published randomised controlled trials of ankle replacement against ankle fusion but the UK TARVA study is underway and should report in 2020 (Goldberg *et al.*, 2016).

The patient characteristics of the TAR population implanted from 1988 to 2011 at Slotervaartziekenhuis, Amsterdam, the institution where the author worked until 2012, are summarised in Table 1. As this institution is a reference centre for RA surgery, it explains the relatively high rate of rheumatoid ankles. Comparing our first 100 TARs (implanted between 1988 and 2002) with our last 100 TARs (implanted between 2009 and 2011), the rate of IJD decreased from 85% to 17%. This change in aetiology has mostly been the result of changes in medication for IJD and a wider awareness that TAR can be used for post-trauma OA.

Without any doubt, a learning curve will exist for surgeons on starting to perform TAR and it can be expected that this learning curve might not always be very steep. Results improve with gained experience, being expressed by a significant reduction in complications and reoperations (Henricson *et al.*, 2007;

Table 1. Indications for TAR at Slotervaartziekenhuis from 1988 to 2011.

Diagnosis	Ankles (pts)	Percentage	M/F	Age at surgery mean (range)
RA	145 (120)	40.4	25/120	58.0 (29–81)
IJD (non-RA)	21 (16)	5.9	2/19	48.1 (24–73)
Postfracture	79 (79)	22.1	41/38	56.0 (25–75)
Instability arthritis	78 (72)	21.7	56/22	60.4 (32–82)
Primary osteoarthritis	25 (24)	7	12/13	66.2 (49–84)
Haemochromatosis	6 (5)	1.7	6/—	57.9 (44–74)
Clubfoot (post-triple)	3 (2)	0.8	3/0	59.9 (58–62)
Talar osteonecrosis	2 (2)	0.6	2/—	42.2 (39–46)
Total	359 (320)		145/214	58.0 (24–84)

Saltzman *et al.*, 2009; SooHoo *et al.*, 2007) and by better survival. In experienced hands, a level can be reached that TAR might become the procedure of choice for most ankles with end-stage arthritis. Nowadays, both at the above-mentioned institution and at several other centres with long-term experience, TAR has become the procedure of choice for the surgical reconstruction of end-stage ankle arthritis and ankle fusion is mainly performed when contraindications for TAR are present.

Although the literature is unclear if patient-related risk factors for failure play an important role for the long-term outcome, gender does not influence implant survival significantly, but preoperative deformity is a risk factor (Doets *et al.*, 2006; Haskell and Mann, 2004; Henricson and Ågren, 2007; Henricson *et al.*, 2007; Wood *et al.*, 2008; Zaidi *et al.*, 2013; Hanselman *et al.*, 2015; de Asla *et al.*, 2014; Barg *et al.*, 2012). An overview of both generally accepted and undecided indications for TAR is presented in Table 2.

Among the undecided indications for TAR, younger age is one of the most important issues. Average age at surgery for TAR in published series was between 49 years of age (Buechel Sr, 2003) and 60 years of age (Wood and Deakin, 2003). However, in all series,

Table 2. Overview of indications for TAR.

Accepted indications	Undecided indications
IJD	Stiff ankles
Postfracture arthritis	Younger age (<50 years)
Instability arthritis without deformity	Instability arthritis with deformity
Degenerative arthritis	Obese patients
Ankylosed or arthritic ipsilateral hindfoot	Talar osteonecrosis
Haemochromatosis	Haemophiliac arthropathy
Contralateral ankle fusion	Conversion of ankle fusion to TAR

the range is usually quite wide. In the series published by Wood and Deakin (2003), the youngest patient was 18 years of age at the time of surgery while the oldest patient was 83 years of age, and both these patients were suffering from RA, the youngest probably from juvenile chronic arthritis (JCA). As with endoprosthetic joint replacement of other joints, the question can be raised if young age is a contraindication for TAR or not. In total hip and total knee replacement, younger age has been identified as a risk factor for failure (Havelin *et al.*, 2009; W-Dahl *et al.*, 2010). In both these register studies, an approximately 5% lower 10-year survival was found between patients younger and older than 55–60 years of age. For TAR, Henricson *et al.* (2011), in their Swedish register-based study, described an increased risk of failure in women below the age of 60 with osteoarthritis. The other register studies that have been published, from Norway (Fevang *et al.*, 2007), Finland (Skytta *et al.*, 2010), and New Zealand (Hosman *et al.*, 2007), found no influence of lower age on survival. Also in our two-centre study on TAR in IJD (Doets *et al.*, 2006), younger age could not be identified as a risk factor for failure. It can therefore be concluded that there is no substantial evidence that for TAR, younger age is a risk factor for failure in inflammatory disease. However, the surgeon and the patient should take into account that a reoperation (implant revision or conversion to arthrodesis) might become necessary. Conversion to arthrodesis of a failed TAR, although demanding, has been shown to give good clinical and radiographic results if a proper technique has been applied (Anderson *et al.*, 2005; Culpan *et al.*, 2007; Doets and Zürcher, 2010; Hopgood *et al.*, 2006; Gross *et al.*, 2016; Gross *et al.*, 2015). As only case reports have been published on revision of TAR, the result of implant exchange has yet to be defined (Kamrad *et al.*, 2015). The author's personal experience is that ankle implant exchange is well feasible in the event of either malposition or instability, and sometimes also for aseptic loosening.

CONTRAINDICATIONS FOR TOTAL ANKLE REPLACEMENT

Contraindications for TAR can be subdivided into contraindications for any reconstructive surgery and to prosthetic replacement-specific contraindications. Contraindications for both ankle fusion and TAR are an active infection, substantial bone loss, a compromised perfusion of the lower leg, (heavy) smokers, the non-compliant patient, and the patient with severe comorbidity. To evaluate any potentially existing contraindication, a thorough clinical and radiographic evaluation should be done prior to TAR. An overview of the contraindications for TAR with their specific entities, pathology, and recommendations is given in Table 3. In the end, the surgeon has to make the final decision if TAR can reasonably be performed for the individual patient or whether another treatment modality, either conservative treatment or ankle fusion, should be preferred.

Table 3. Contraindications for TAR.

Contraindications	Specific conditions and recommendations
Severe deformity	Severe deformity in the frontal or sagittal plane (equinus; anterior subluxation; supramalleolar deformity)
	Severe foot deformity; severe hip or knee deformity
Substantial bone loss	Talar osteonecrosis
	Posttraumatic or iatrogenic periarticular bone loss; charcot osteoarthropathy
Severe osteopenia	Severe generalised or local osteopenia
Peripheral vascular disease	Arteriosclerosis of the lower leg
	Microvascular disease (diabetes; smokers; hypertension)
Neuropathy	Sensory loss (both skin and proprioception); hereditary motor and sensory neuropathy (HMSN); loss of motor control of the lower leg
Active infection	Deep or superficial infection, either locally or at distance; venous lower leg ulcers
History of active or latent infection	Biopsy recommended
High-demand patients	Abandon high-impact activities
Non-compliant patients	Alcohol abuse; drug abuse: smokers

DISEASE-SPECIFIC CHARACTERISTICS AND RECOMMENDATIONS

The main indications for reconstructive surgery are posttraumatic arthritis (either postfracture or instability arthritis) and IJD. Each of these indications has its disease-specific characteristics that should be taken into account when TAR is considered. Furthermore, indications for additional surgery in combination with TAR, either as a one-stage or a two-stage procedure, such as Achilles tendon lengthening, hindfoot fusion, or hindfoot osteotomy are common.

Patients with postfracture arthritis frequently have undergone previous surgery, resulting in the presence of scars and often a reduced range of motion. If the fracture has healed with malunion, this could influence the alignment of the ankle–hindfoot complex. Some shortening of the lateral malleolus can be acceptable and should not be regarded as a contraindication for arthroplasty.

Gross malalignment should be corrected as a first step by, for example, a supramalleolar osteotomy before TAR is carried out. A widening of the ankle mortise due to injury to the tibiofibular syndesmosis should be corrected by performing a synostosis between fibula and tibia at the time of arthroplasty. In general, after an ankle fracture, the local bone stock has remained intact, so that implantation of the prosthetic components can be done without severe difficulty. As patients with postfracture arthritis more frequently have limited dorsiflexion, Achilles tendon lengthening or gastrocnemius recession may be necessary in order to obtain an adequate dorsiflexion (Queen *et al.*, 2014).

Instability arthritis is caused by chronic lateral ligament laxity. Due to this instability, the talus has a tendency to tilt into varus and/or to develop an anterior displacement with respect to the vertical axis of the lower leg (Figures 2 and 3). This persistent instability creates a problem when arthroplasty is considered, as neutral alignment in both the frontal and the sagittal plane is a prerequisite for a good result. Restoration of alignment can be done by correct component positioning and restoration of stability by either a lateral ligament reconstruction or a medial ligament release (Brigido *et al.*, 2017; Hanselman *et al.*, 2015; Barg *et al.*, 2012). As an alternative to medial

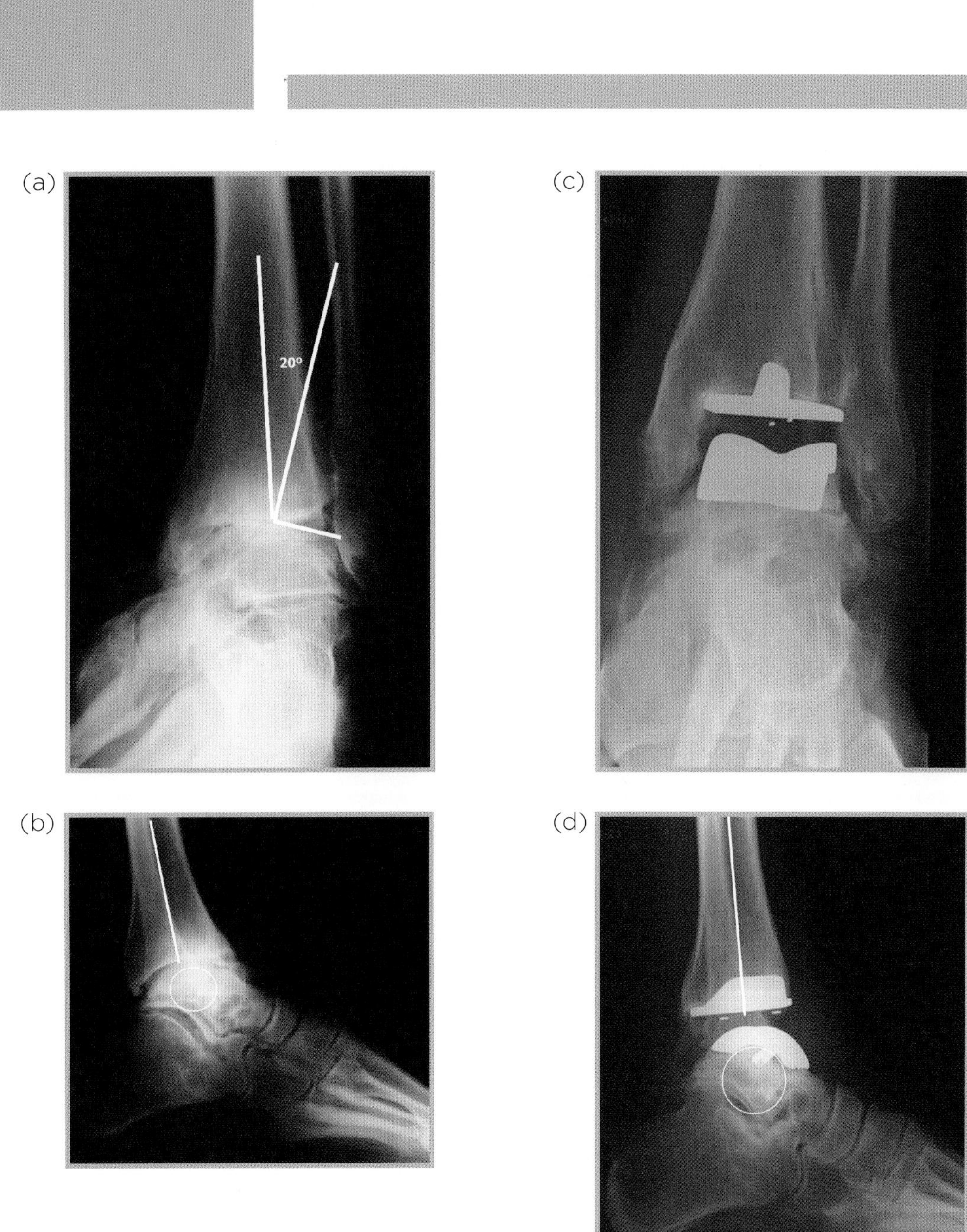

Figure 2. *Weightbearing radiographs both preoperative and 1-year postoperative after TAR with use of a CCI Evolution prosthesis in a 53-year-old man with end-stage instability arthritis. Correction of the varus deformity was done by a lengthening osteotomy of the medial malleolus. (a) Preoperative antero-posterior view showing a 20° varus deformity of the talus in the ankle mortise. (b) Preoperative lateral view showing a slight anterior displacement of the talus with respect to the vertical axis of the lower leg. (c) and (d) The 1-year postoperative views show a restored alignment of the talus in the ankle mortise, both in the frontal and the sagittal plane.*

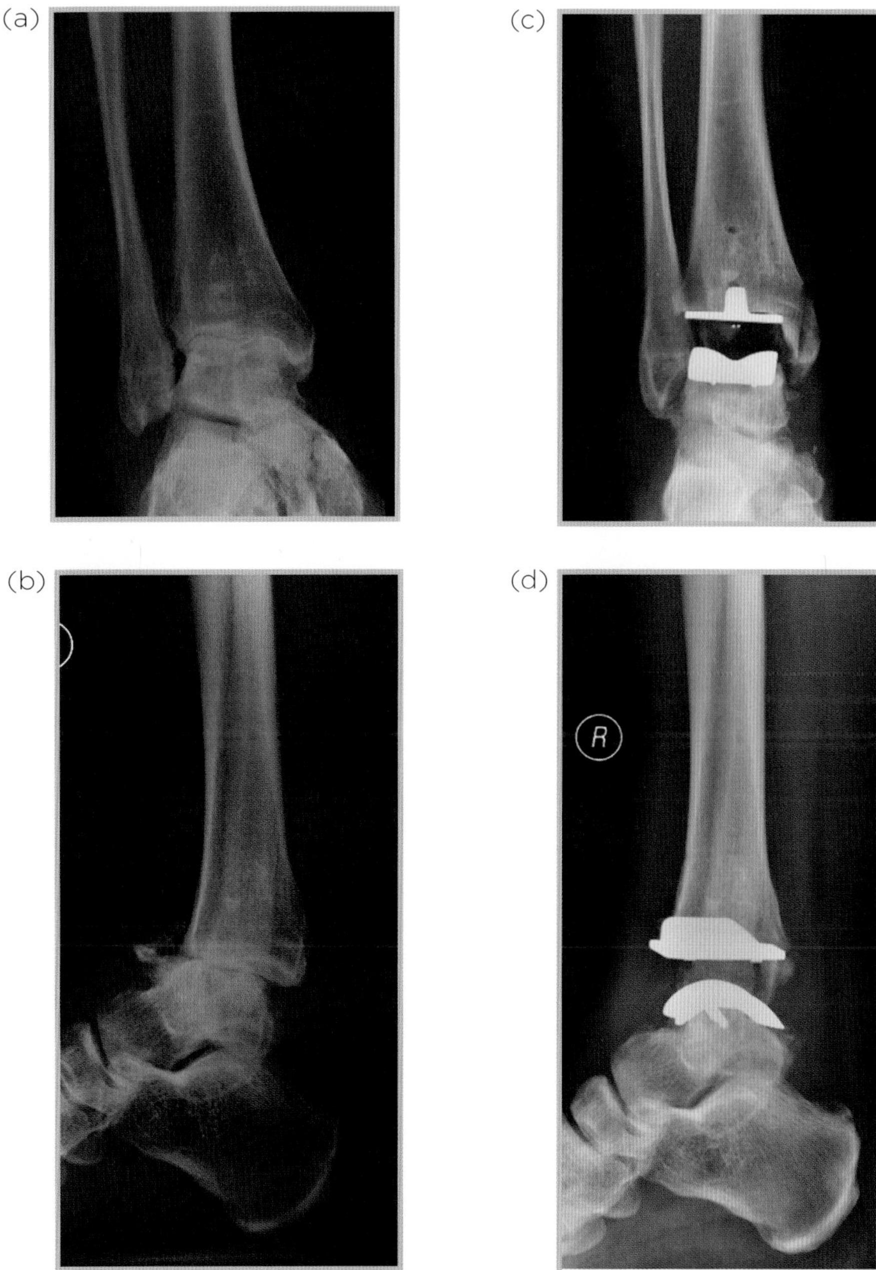

Figure 3. *Radiographs of a 45-year-old man with non-specific oligoarthritis and symptoms of his left ankle for 3 years. (a) The preoperative anteroposterior weightbearing view shows a complete obliteration of the joint space. (b) The preoperative weightbearing lateral view shows a significant anterior displacement of the talus with respect to the lower leg. (c) and (d) Early postoperative views after TAR with use of a CCI Evolution prosthesis and balancing of the ankle by a medial malleolar lengthening osteotomy. There is a full restoration of the anterior subluxation of the talus.*

ligament release, a medial malleolar lengthening osteotomy for the restoration of neutral alignment has been developed. Mid-term results with this medial malleolar lengthening technique are encouraging, although widespread use did not follow (Doets *et al.*, 2008).

IJD (mostly RA) that has resulted in end-stage ankle arthritis is usually considered an excellent indication for TAR. Frequently, in rheumatoid ankles, the joints of the hindfoot and forefoot are also involved. Arthritis of the hindfoot may lead to arthritic changes or to spontaneous ankylosis of the tarsal joints with or without concurrent deformity. In longstanding RA, planovalgus deformity is the most frequently encountered entity, resulting from a combination of tarsal joint arthritis, ligament destruction, and tibialis posterior insufficiency (Cracchiolo III, 1997). But already early after the onset of RA, disturbances in tarsal kinematics and loading of the foot have been demonstrated by Woodburn *et al.* (2002). They found an excessive eversion at the hindfoot during walking, both barefooted and shod, in a subset of RA patients with a painful hindfoot valgus at an average disease duration of 3 years. Valgus deformity at the hindfoot will not only lead to a disturbed gait but also to an eccentric loading of the ankle joint and to asymmetric joint space narrowing. As valgus deformity at the ankle joint has been identified as a risk factor for failure after TAR (Doets *et al.*, 2006; Wood *et al.*, 2008; Brigido *et al.*, 2017; Dodd and Daniels, 2017), correction of such a deformity both at the level of the hindfoot and the ankle is considered mandatory for a good long-term result. Flexible hindfoot deformity can probably best be corrected as a one-stage procedure together with TAR by an additional subtalar and/or talonavicular fusion (Figure 4). As a fixed hindfoot deformity is usually more difficult to correct, such a deformity is best corrected prior to TAR, with a minimum interval between the two procedures of 4–6 weeks.

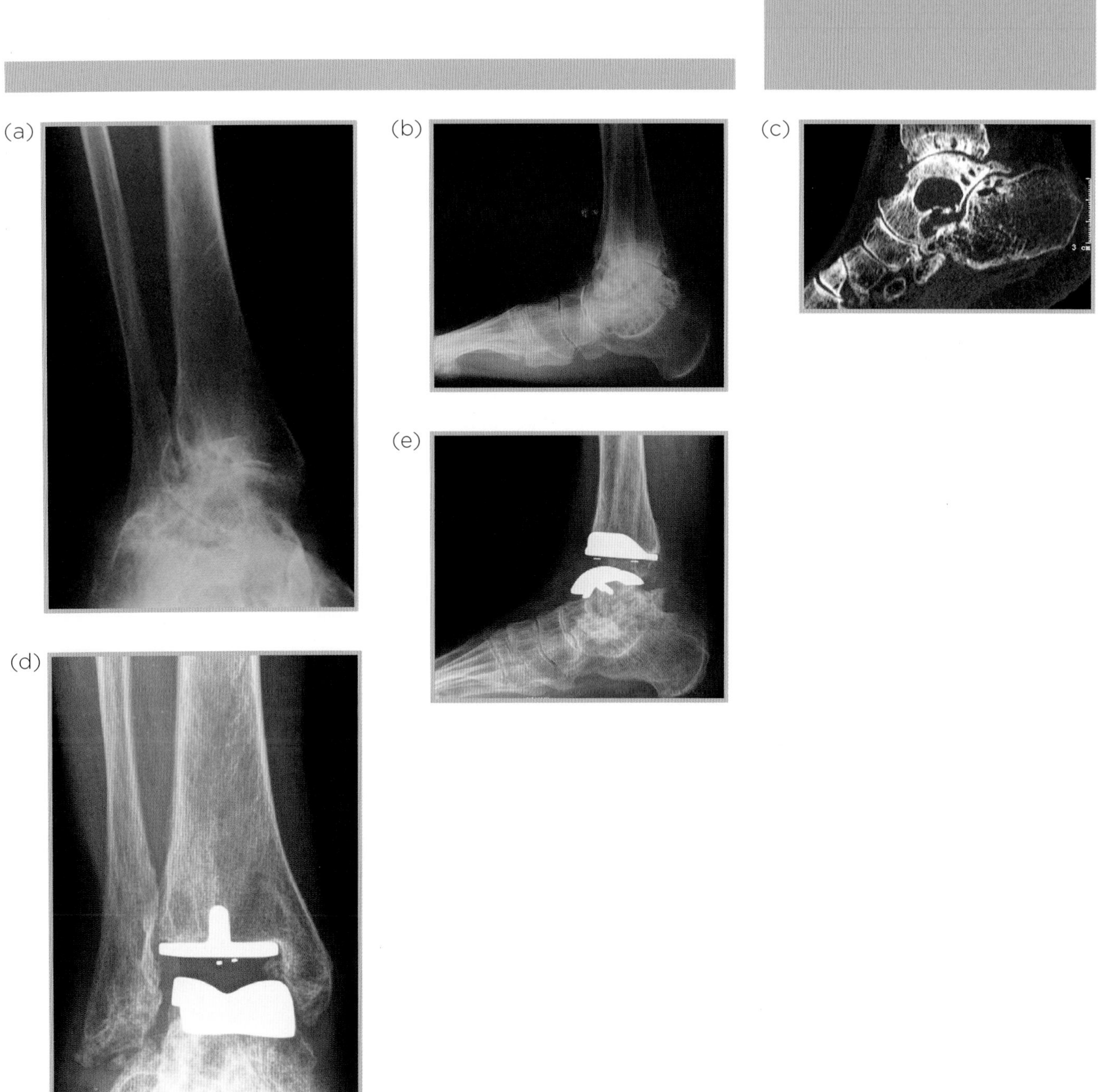

Figure 4. *Radiographs of a 68-year-old woman with longstanding RA and ankle symptoms for 7 years. (a) and (b) Preoperative anteroposterior and lateral weightbearing views show severe arthritic changes of the ankle and the subtalar joint with concurrent valgus deformity. (c) Preoperative CT scan of the ankle and hindfoot showing a large cyst in the talar body and juxta-articular cysts in the ankle and subtalar joint. (d) and (e) 1-year postoperative views after TAR with use of the CCI Evolution prosthesis and simultaneous subtalar fusion. Height of the hindfoot has been restored and the valgus deformity has significantly improved.*

PATIENT SELECTION

A good result of TAR starts with proper patient selection and an adequate preoperative workup. Many inferior results experience with TAR could, at least in part, be attributed to improper patient selection and insufficient preoperative evaluation. Therefore, a complete medical history and physical examination, followed by an adequate preoperative imaging and planning are of paramount importance in order to obtain a good result. Any adverse phenomenon, such as a comorbidity influencing the neurovascular function (e.g. smoking, diabetes mellitus) of the lower leg, a history of wound healing disturbance, or a history of latent or overt infection should be recorded and thoroughly evaluated. A systematic assessment of the functional capacities should be done, preferably by filling out a commonly used ankle score like the LCS ankle score (Buechel *et al.*, 1988), the American Orthopaedic Foot and Ankle Society score (Kitaoka *et al.*, 1994), or the Kofoed Ankle Score (Kofoed and Stürup, 1994). For research purposes, preferably self-assessment instruments like a Visual Analog Scale (VAS), the Foot Function Index (Budiman-Mak *et al.*, 1991) or the Ankle Osteoarthritis Scale instrument derived Ankle Osteoarthritis Scale (Domsic and Saltzman, 1998) should be used in addition to the physician-based scoring systems. The MOXFQ score is a more recently derived validated score of PROM (patient recorded outcome measure) which is increasingly used, especially in the UK (Dawson *et al.*, 2012, Morley *et al.*, 2013).

Physical examination should start with an assessment of the alignment of both legs, with specific attention for the alignment of the ankle and hindfoot, followed by an evaluation of all the joints of lower leg. The active motion of the ankle and hindfoot should be recorded and the stability of the ankle joint should be tested. The skin condition should be evaluated, including scars from any previous surgery. Finally, the neurovascular status should be assessed, and in the event of abnormalities, evaluation by a neurologist and/or vascular surgeon is indicated.

After completion of the physical examination, adequate imaging is an essential next step. For preoperative imaging, standard anteroposterior and lateral weightbearing radiographs of the ankle and the whole foot are recommended, as only with such views, a reliable assessment of the radiographic alignment of the ankle and foot can be made. In the event of suspected or apparent bone loss, a computer tomography (CT) scan with high-quality image reconstructions in the frontal and sagittal plane should be done, as only by this technique can a full assessment of the bony anatomy be made. In the event of suspected or apparent tendon and/or muscular abnormalities, a magnetic resonance imaging (MRI) scan should be done for a systematic assessment of these structures.

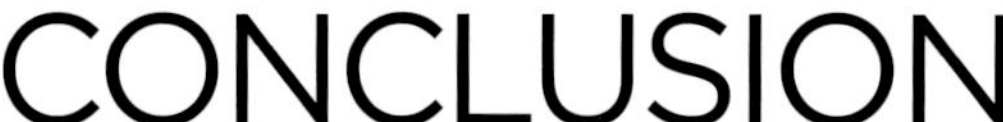

CONCLUSION

The aetiology of ankle arthritis has a predominance of posttraumatic and inflammatory disorders, different from the aetiology of arthritis of the hip and knee. The best indications for TAR are ankles that have a diagnosis of postfracture arthritis or RA, without a significant deformity and with a good range of motion. In the event of a deformity in either the frontal or the sagittal plane, the surgeon should be able to correct this deformity at the time of surgery, as stability in neutral alignment after TAR is mandatory for a lasting result. In experienced hands, indications for TAR can also include more complex conditions such as malunited fractures, instability arthritis with significant deformity, and finally even conversion to TAR of a fused ankle in patients with symptomatic hindfoot arthritis.

REFERENCES

Agel, J., Coetzee, J. C., Sangeorzan, B. J., Roberts, M. M. & Hansen, S. T., Jr. 2005. Functional limitations of patients with end-stage ankle arthrosis. *Foot Ankle Int*, 26, 537–539.

Anderson, T., Maxander, P., Rydholm, U., Besjakov, J. & Carlsson, A. 2005. Ankle arthrodesis by compression screws in rheumatoid arthritis: Primary nonunion in 9/35 patients. *Acta Orthop*, 76, 884–890.

Athanasiou, K. A., Niederauer, G. G. & Schenck, R. C., Jr. 1995. Biomechanical topography of human ankle cartilage. *Ann Biomed Eng*, 23, 697–704.

Barg, A., Pagenstert, G. I., Leumann, A. G., Muller, A. M., Henninger, H. B. & Valderrabano, V. 2012. Treatment of the arthritic valgus ankle. *Foot Ankle Clin*, 17, 647–663.

Bayaert, C., Sirveaux, F., Paysant, J., Molé, D. & André, J.-M. 2004. The effect of tibio-talar arthrodesis on foot kinematics and ground reaction force progressing during walking. *Gait Posture*, 20, 84–91.

Benich, M. R., Ledoux, W. R., Orendurff, M. S., Shofer, J. B., Hansen, S. T., Davitt, J., *et al.* 2017. Comparison of treatment outcomes of arthrodesis and two generations of ankle replacement implants. *J Bone Joint Surg Am* [Internet], 99(21): 1792–1800.

Bonnin, M., Gaudot, F., Laurent, J. R., Ellis, S., Colombier, J. A. & Judet, T. 2011. The Salto total ankle arthroplasty: Survivorship and analysis of failures at 7 to 11 years. *Clin Orthop Relat Res*, 469, 225–236.

Brigido, S. A., Carrington, S. C. & Protzman, N. M. 2017. Complex total ankle arthroplasty. *Clin Podiatr Med Surg*, 34, 529–539.

Budiman-Mak, E., Conrad, K. J. & Roach, K. E. 1991. The foot function index: A measure of foot pain and disability. *J Clin Epidemiol*, 44, 561–570.

Buechel, F. F., Pappas, M. J. & Lorio, L. J. 1988. New Jersey low contact stress total ankle replacement: Biomechanical rationale and review of 23 cementless cases. *Foot Ankle*, 8, 279–290.

Buechel Sr, F. F., Buechel Jr, F. F. & Pappas, M. J. 2003. Ten-year evaluation of cementless Buechel–Pappas meniscal bearing total ankle replacement. *Foot Ankle Int*, 24, 462–472.

Buechel Sr, F. F., Buechel Jr, F. F. & Pappas, M. J. 2004. Twenty-year evaluation of cementless mobile-bearing total ankle replacements. *Clin Orthop Rel Res*, 424, 19–26.

Cracchiolo III, A. 1997. Rheumatoid arthritis: Hindfoot disease. *Clinical Orthop Rel Res*, 340, 58–68.

Culpan, P., Le Strat, V., Piriou, P. & Judet, T. 2007. Arthrodesis after failed total ankle replacement. *J Bone Joint Surg Br*, 89, 1178–1183.

Daniels, T. R., Younger, A. S., Penner, M., Wing, K., Dryden, P. J., Wong, H. & Glazebrook, M. 2014. Intermediate-term results of total ankle

replacement and ankle arthrodesis: A COFAS multicenter study. *J Bone Joint Surg Am*, 96, 135–142.

Dauty, M., Gross, R., Leboeuf, F. & Trossaert, M. 2015. Comparison of total ankle replacement and ankle arthrodesis in patients with haemophilia using gait analysis: Two case reports. *BMC Res Notes*, 8, 768.

Dawson, J., Boller, I., Doll, H., Lavis, G., Sharp, R., Cooke, P. & Jenkinson, C. 2012. Responsiveness of the Manchester-Oxford Foot Questionnaire (MOXFQ) compared with AOFAS, SF-36 and EQ-5D assessments following foot or ankle surgery. *J Bone Joint Surg Br*, 94, 215–221.

De Asla, R. J., Ellis, S., Overley, B., Parekh, S. & Brigido, S. 2014. Total ankle arthroplasty in the setting of valgus deformity. *Foot Ankle Spec*, 7, 398–402.

Dodd, A. & Daniels, T. R. 2017. Total ankle replacement in the presence of talar varus or valgus deformities. *Foot Ankle Clin*, 22, 277–300.

Doets, H. C., Brand, R. & Nelissen, R. G. 2006. Total ankle arthroplasty in inflammatory joint disease with use of two mobile-bearing designs. *J Bone Joint Surg Am*, 88, 1272–1284.

Doets, H. C., Van Middelkoop, M., Houdijk, H., Nelissen, R. G. H. H. & Veeger, H. E. J. 2007. Gait analysis after mobile bearing total ankle arthroplasty. A comparative study with a normal control group. *Foot Ankle Int*, 28, 313–322.

Doets, H. C., Van Der Plaat, L. W. & Klein, J.-P. 2008. Medial malleolar osteotomy for the correction of varus deformity during total ankle arthroplasty. Results in 15 ankles. *Foot Ankle Int*, 29, 171–177.

Doets, H. C. & Zürcher, A. W. 2010. Salvage arthrodesis for failed total ankle arthroplasty. Clinical outcome and influence of method of fixation on union rate in 18 ankles followed for 3–12 years. *Acta Orthop*, 81, 142–147.

Domsic, R. T. & Saltzman, C. L. 1998. Ankle osteoarthritis scale. *Foot Ankle Int*, 19, 466–471.

Dyrby, C., Chou, L. B., Andriacchi, T. P. & Mann, R. A. 2004. Functional evaluation of the Scandinavian Total Ankle Replacement. *Foot Ankle Int*, 25, 377–381.

Eckers, F., Bauer, D.E., Hingsammer, A., Sutter, R., Brand, B., Viehöfer, A., Wirth, S. H. 2018. Mid- to long-term results of total ankle replacement in patients with haemophilic arthropathy: A 10-year follow-up. *Haemophilia*. 24(2): 307–315. doi: 10.1111/hae.13386. Epub 2017 Dec 22.

Fevang, B. T., Lie, S. A., Havelin, L. I., Brun, J. G., Skredderstuen, A. & Furnes, O. 2007. 257 ankle arthroplasties performed in Norway between 1994 and 2005. *Acta Orthop*, 78, 575–583.

Flavin, R. C. S., Tenenbaum, S. & Brodsky, J. W. 2013. Comparison of gait after total ankle arthroplasty and ankle arthrodesis. *Foot Ankle Int*, 34, 1340–1348.

Giannini, S., Romagnoli, M., Barbadoro, P., Marcheggiani Muccioli, G. M., Cadossi, M., Grassi, A. & Zaffagnini, S. 2017. Results at a minimum follow-up of 5 years of a ligaments-compatible total ankle replacement design. *Foot Ankle Surg*, 23, 116–121.

Goldberg, A., Zaidi Thomson, C., Doré, C., Skene, S., Cro, S., Round, J., Molloy, A., Davies, M., Karski, M., Kim, L., Cooke, P. 2016. Total ankle replacement versus arthrodesis (TARVA): Protocol for a multicentre randomised controlled trial. *BMJ Open*, 6(9): e012716. doi: 10.1136/bmjopen-2016-012716 PMCID: PMC5020669.

Gougoulias, N. E., Khanna, A. & Maffulli, N. 2009. How successful are current ankle replacements? A systematic review of the literature. *Clinl Orthop Rel Res*, 468, 199–208.

Gross, C., Erickson, B. J., Adams, S. B. & Parekh, S. G. 2015. Ankle arthrodesis after failed total ankle replacement: A systematic review of the literature. *Foot Ankle Spec*, 8, 143–151.

Gross, C. E., Lewis, J. S., Adams, S. B., Easley, M., Deorio, J. K. & Nunley, J. A., II 2016. Secondary arthrodesis after total ankle arthroplasty. *Foot Ankle Int*, 37, 709–714.

Haddad, S. L., Coetzee, J. C., Estok, R., Fahrbach, K., Banel, D. & Nalysnyk, L. 2007. Intermediate and long-term outcomes of total ankle arthroplasty and ankle arthrodesis. A systematic review of the literature. *J Bone Joint Surg Am*, 89, 1899–1905.

Hahn, M. E., Wright, E. S., Segal, A. D., Orendurff, M. S., Ledoux, W. R. & Sangeorzan, B. J. 2012. Comparative gait analysis of ankle arthrodesis and arthroplasty: Initial findings of a prospective study. *Foot Ankle Int*, 33, 282–289.

Hanselman, A. E., Powell, B. D. & Santrock, R. D. 2015. Total ankle arthroplasty with severe preoperative varus deformity. *Orthopedics*, 38, e343–e346.

Haskell, A. & Mann, R. A. 2004. Ankle arthroplasty with preoperative coronal plane deformity: Short-term results. *Clin Orthop Relat Res*, 424, 98–103.

Havelin, L. I., Fenstad, A. M., Salomonsson, R., Mehnert, F., Furnes, O., Overgaard, S., Pedersen, A. B., Herberts, P., Karrholm, J. & Garellick, G. 2009. The Nordic Arthroplasty Register Association: A unique collaboration between 3 national hip arthroplasty registries with 280,201 THRs. *Acta Orthop*, 80, 393–401.

Henricson, A. & Ågren, P.-H. 2007. Secondary surgery after total ankle replacement: The influence of preoperative hindfoot alignment. *Foot Ankle Surg*, 13, 41–44.

Henricson, A., Skoog, A. & Carlsson, A. 2007. The Swedish ankle arthroplasty register: An analysis of 531 arthroplasties between 1993 and 2005. *Acta Orthop*, 78, 569–574.

Henricson, A., Nilsson, J. A. & Carlsson, A. 2011. 10-year survival of total ankle arthroplasties: A report on 780 cases from the Swedish Ankle Register. *Acta Orthop*, 82, 655–659.

Henricson, A., Frediksson, M. 2016. CA. Total ankle replacement and contralateral ankle arthrodesis in 16 patients from the Swedish Ankle Registry: Self-reported function and satisfaction. *Foot Ankle Surg*, 22(1): 32–34.

Hintermann, B., Barg, A., Knupp, M. & Valderrabano, V. 2009. Conversion of painful ankle arthrodesis to total ankle arthroplasty. *J Bone Joint Surg Am*, 91, 850–858.

Hobson, S. A., Karantana, A. & Dhar, S. 2009. Total ankle replacement in patients with significant pre-operative deformity of the hindfoot. *J Bone Joint Surg Br*, 91, 481–486.

Hopgood, P., Kumar, R. & Wood, P. L. 2006. Ankle arthrodesis for failed total ankle replacement. *J Bone Joint Surg Br*, 88, 1032–1038.

Hosman, A. H., Mason, R. B., Hobbs, T. & Rothwell, A. G. 2007. A New Zealand national joint registry review of 202 total ankle replacements followed for up to 6 years. *Acta Orthop*, 78, 584–591.

Huch, K., Kuettner, K. E. & Dieppe, P. 1997. Osteoarthritis in ankle and knee joints. *Seminars in Arthritis and Rheumatism*. Elsevier, pp. 667–674.

Jastifer, J. R. & Coughlin, M. J. 2015. Long-term follow-up of mobile bearing total ankle arthroplasty in the United States. *Foot Ankle Int*, 36, 143–150.

Kamrad, I., Henricsson, A., Karlsson, M. K., Magnusson, H., Nilsson, J. A., Carlsson, A. & Rosengren, B. E. 2015. Poor prosthesis survival and function after component exchange of total ankle prostheses. *Acta Orthop*, 86, 407–411.

Kerkhoff, Y. R., Kosse, N. M., Metsaars, W. P. & Louwerens, J. W. 2016. Long-term functional and radiographic outcome of a mobile bearing ankle prosthesis. *Foot Ankle Int*, 37, 1292–1302.

Kim, B. S., Choi, W. J., Kim, Y. S. & Lee, J. W. 2009. Total ankle replacement in moderate to severe varus deformity of the ankle. *J Bone Joint Surg Br*, 91, 1183–1190.

Kitaoka, H. B., Alexander, I. J., Adelaar, R. S., Nunley, J. A., Myerson, M. S. & Sanders, M. 1994. Clinical rating systems for the ankle-hindfoot, midfoot, hallux, and lesser toes. *Foot Ankle Int*, 15, 349–353.

Knecht, S. I., Estin, M., Callaghan, J. J., Zimmerman, M. B., Alliman, K. J., Alvine, F. G. & Saltzman, C. L. 2004. The agility total ankle arthroplasty. Seven to sixteen-year follow-up. *J Bone Joint Surg Am*, 86-a, 1161–1171.

Kofoed, H. & Stürup, J. 1994. Comparison of ankle arthroplasty and arthrodesis. *The Foot*, 4, 6–9.

Kofoed, H. 2014. Is ankle arthrodesis or total ankle replacement the better treatment for end stage arthrosis? *Foot Ankle Surg*, 20, 1.

Koivu, H., Kohonen, I., Mattila, K., Loyttyniemi, E. & Tiusanen, H. 2017a. Long-term results of Scandinavian total ankle replacement. *Foot Ankle Int*, 38, 723–731.

Koivu, H., Kohonen, I., Mattila, K., Loyttyniemi, E. & Tiusanen, H. 2017b. Medium to long-term results of 130 Ankle Evolutive System total ankle replacements-Inferior survival due to peri-implant osteolysis. *Foot Ankle Surg*, 23, 108–115.

Kraal, T., Van Der Heide, H. J., Van Poppel, B. J., Fiocco, M., Nelissen, R. G. & Doets, H. C. 2013. Long-term follow-up of mobile-bearing total ankle replacement in patients with inflammatory joint disease. *Bone Joint J*, 95-b, 1656–1661.

Kuper, H. H., Van Leeuwen, M. A., Van Riel, P. L., Prevoo, M. L., Houtman, P. M., Lolkema, W. F. & Van Rijswijk, M. H. 1997. Radiographic damage in large joints in early rheumatoid arthritis: Relationship with radiographic damage in hands and feet, disease activity, and physical disability. *Br J Rheumatol*, 36, 855–860.

Lehtinen, A., Paimela, L., Kreula, J., Leirisalo-Repo, M. & Taavitsainen, M. 1996. Painful ankle region in rheumatoid arthritis. Analysis of soft-tissue changes with ultrasonography and MR imaging. *Acta Radiol*, 37, 572–577.

Morley, D., Jenkinson, C., Doll, H., Lavis, G., Sharp, R., Cooke, P. & Dawson, J. 2013. The Manchester–Oxford Foot Questionnaire (MOXFQ): Development and validation of a summary index score. *Bone Joint Res.* 2(4): 66–69.

Nieuwe Weme, R. A., van Solinge, G., Doornberg, J. N. Sierevelt, I., Haverkamp, D. & Cornelis Doets, H. 2015. Total ankle replacement for posttraumatic arthritis. Similar outcome in postfracture and instability arthritis: A comparison of 90 ankles. *Acta Orthop.* 86(4): 401–406. doi: 10.3109/17453674.2015.1029842. Epub 2015 Mar 14.

Pedowitz, D. I., Kane, J. M., Smith, G. M., Saffel, H. L., Comer, C. & Raikin, S. M. 2016. Total ankle arthroplasty versus ankle arthrodesis: A comparative analysis of arc of movement and functional outcomes. *Bone Joint J*, 98-B, 634–640.

Preis, M., Bailey, T., Jacxsens, M. & Barg, A. 2017. Total ankle replacement in patients with haemophilic arthropathy: Primary arthroplasty and conversion of painful ankle arthrodesis to arthroplasty. *Haemophilia*, 23, e301–e309.

Queen, R. M., Grier, A. J., Butler, R. J., Nunley, J. A., Easley, M. E., Adams, S. B., Jr. & Deorio, J. K. 2014. The influence of concomitant triceps surae lengthening at the time of total ankle arthroplasty on postoperative outcomes. *Foot Ankle Int*, 35, 863–870.

Rodriguez-Merchan, E. C. 2015. Total ankle replacement or ankle fusion in painful advanced hemophilic arthropathy of the ankle. *Expert Rev Hematol*, 8, 727–731.

Saltzman, C. L., Salamon, M. L., Blanchard, G. M., Huff, T., Hayes, A., Buckwalter, J. A. & Amendola, A. 2005. Epidemiology of ankle arthritis: Report of a consecutive series of 639 patients from a tertiary orthopaedic center. *Iowa Orthop J*, 25, 44–46.

Saltzman, C. L., Zimmerman, M. B., O'rourke, M., Brown, T. D., Buckwalter, J. A. & Johnston, R. 2006. Impact of comorbidities on the measurement of health in patients with ankle osteoarthritis. *J Bone Joint Surg Am*, 88, 2366–2372.

Saltzman, C. L., Mann, R. A., Ahrens, J. E., Amendola, A., Anderson, R. B., Berlet, G. C., Brodsky, J. W., Chou, L. B., Clanton, T. O., Deland, J. T., Deorio, J. K., Horton, G. A., Lee, T. H., Mann, J. A., Nunley, J. A., Thordarson, D. B., Walling, A. K., Wapner, K. L. & Coughlin, M. J. 2009. Prospective controlled trial of STAR total ankle replacement versus ankle fusion: Initial results. *Foot Ankle Int*, 30, 579–596.

Scott, D. L. 2004. Radiological progression in established rheumatoid arthritis. *J Rheumatol Suppl*, 69, 55–65.

Segal, A. D., Cyr, K. M., Stender, C. J., Whittaker, E. C., Hahn, M. E., Orendurff, M. S., *et al.* 2018. A three-year prospective comparative gait study between patients with ankle arthrodesis and arthroplasty. *Clin Biomech* [Internet], 54, 42–53.

Skytta, E. T., Koivu, H., Eskelinen, A., Ikavalko, M., Paavolainen, P. & Remes, V. 2010. Total ankle replacement: A population-based study of 515 cases from the Finnish Arthroplasty Register. *Acta Orthop*, 81, 114–118.

SooHoo, N. F., Zingmond, D. S. & Ko, C. Y. 2007. Comparison of reoperation rates following ankle arthrodesis and total ankle arthroplasty. *J Bone Joint Surg Am*, 89, 2143–2149.

Spiegel, T. M. & Spiegel, J. S. 1982. Rheumatoid arthritis in the foot and ankle — diagnosis, pathology, and treatment. The relationship between foot and ankle deformity and disease duration in 50 patients. *Foot Ankle*, 2, 318–324.

Stengel, D., Bauwens, K., Ekkernkamp, A. & Cramer, J. 2005. Efficacy of total ankle replacement with meniscal-bearing devices: A systematic review and meta-analysis. *Arch Orthop Trauma Surg*, 125, 109–119.

Thomas, R., Daniels, T. R. & Parker, K. 2006. Gait analysis and functional outcomes following ankle arthrodesis for isolated ankle arthritis. *J Bone Joint Surg Am*, 88, 526–535.

Turner, D. E., Helliwell, P. S., Siegel, K. L. & Woodburn, J. 2008. Biomechanics of the foot in rheumatoid arthritis: Identifying abnormal function and the factors associated with localised disease "impact". *Clin Biomech (Bristol, Avon)*, 23, 93–100.

Valderrabano, V., Horisberger, M., Russell, I., Dougall, H. & Hintermann, B. 2009. Etiology of ankle osteoarthritis. *Clin Orthop Relat Res*, 467, 1800–1806.

Verhagen, R. A., De Keizer, G. & Van Dijk, C. N. 1995. Long-term follow-up of inversion trauma of the ankle. *Arch Orthop Trauma Surg*, 114, 92–96.

W-Dahl, A., Robertsson, O. & Lidgren, L. 2010. Surgery for knee osteoarthritis in younger patients. *Acta Orthop*, 81, 161–164.

Weatherall, J. M., Mroczek, K., Mclaurin, T., Ding, B. & Tejwani, N. 2013. Post-traumatic ankle arthritis. *Bull Hosp Jt Dis (2013)*, 71, 104–112.

Wood, P. L. & Deakin, S. 2003. Total ankle replacement. The results in 200 ankles. *J Bone Joint Surg Br*, 85, 334–341.

Wood, P. L., Prem, H. & Sutton, C. 2008. Total ankle replacement: Medium-term results in 200 Scandinavian total ankle replacements. *J Bone Joint Surg Br*, 90, 605–609.

Woodburn, J., Helliwell, P. S. & Barker, S. 2002. Three-dimensional kinematics at the ankle joint complex in rheumatoid arthritis patients with painful valgus deformity of the rearfoot. *Rheumatology (Oxford)*, 41, 1406–1412.

Wu, W. L., Su, F. C., Cheng, Y. M., Huang, P. J., Chou, Y. L. & Chou, C. K. 2000. Gait analysis after ankle arthrodesis. *Gait Posture*, 11, 54–61.

Zaidi, R., Cro, S., Gurusamy, K., Siva, N., Macgregor, A., Henricson, A. & Goldberg, A. 2013. The outcome of total ankle replacement: A systematic review and meta-analysis. *Bone Joint J*, 95-b, 1500–1507.

ALTERNATIVE TREATMENTS FOR ANKLE ARTHRITIS

CHAPTER

6

B. G. Donley and M. Leyes

Summary

In this chapter, we review the surgical alternatives to total ankle replacement in the management of ankle arthritis, including arthroscopic debridement, arthrodiastasis, ankle osteotomy, and ankle fusion. We pay particular attention to the indications, surgical technique, results, and complications of the different treatment options.

Arthroscopic ankle debridement with removal of loose bodies, drilling of osteochondral lesions, and removal of anterior osteophytes can be useful in the early stages of arthritis.

Ankle arthrodiastasis is a viable alternative to ankle arthrodesis or ankle replacement in selected cases, particularly, in young patients with moderate ankle arthritis and an arc of at least 30° of motion.

Despite being a technically demanding surgical procedure, supramalleolar osteotomy is an effective joint preserving procedure with few complications. Besides, ankle fusion or total ankle replacement, if necessary, can be performed more easily and with better results after ankle osteotomy, if deformity has been corrected.

Ankle fusion is a relatively simple procedure with a high success rate that provides early relief of symptoms. It is a viable option when total ankle replacement is contraindicated, allows correction of large deformities, and is a potential lifelong definitive treatment. On the other hand, ankle fusion may cause arthritis in adjacent joints that may eventually require fusion. Patients who undergo ankle fusion may have biomechanical and functional impairment and may develop complications such as pain, non-union, and instability or arthritis of adjacent joints.

INTRODUCTION

The treatment of posttraumatic ankle arthritis is one of the most controversial aspects in orthopaedic surgery. There are some biomechanical and anatomical data that should be considered.

Second only to the 1st metatarsophalangeal joint, the ankle is the joint that withstands the highest loads, reaching between 5 and 7 times body weight in the final phase of the walking cycle (Felson, 1990). These are great loads when compared with the 3–4 times body weight applied at the knee and the 2–3 times at the hip. However, the prevalence of degenerative changes in the ankle is approximately nine times lower than in the knee or hip due to its biomechanical and anatomical characteristics (Marco Sanz, 2003).

The area of the ankle articular surface is similar to those of the knee and hip, but the contact area during weightbearing is only one-third of them (350 mm^2 compared to 1100 mm^2).

The ankle is a relatively congruent joint covered by a thin layer of cartilage. The average thickness of the ankle articular cartilage is 1.6 mm compared to 6–8 mm in the knee (Tochigi *et al.*, 2006; Kimizuka *et al.*, 1980).

In this chapter, we review the surgical alternatives to total ankle replacement, including arthroscopic debridement, arthrodiastasis, ankle osteotomy, and ankle fusion.

ANKLE DEBRIDEMENT

The role of arthroscopy for degenerative joint disease of the ankle remains controversial (Cheng and Ferkel, 1998). Arthroscopic ankle debridement can be useful in the early stages of arthritis. Unfortunately, patients with advanced arthritis and loss of joint space do not respond well to arthroscopic debridement: removal of anterior osteophytes, removal of loose bodies, debridement, and drilling of osteochondral lesions. In fact, there is a chance of significant symptomatic worsening after debriding an arthritic ankle.

Operative arthroscopy for ankle arthritis can provide an interim alternative to arthrodesis in early arthritis with preserved range of motion (Cheng and Ferkel, 1998; Barp et al., 2017). Ogilvie-Harris and Sekyi-Otu (1995) reviewed 27 patients who had arthroscopic debridement for osteoarthritis of the ankle. At an average follow-up of 45 months, they found a statistically significant improvement in pain, swelling, stiffness, limp, and activity level in 17 of 27 patients, although only 2 ankles were restored to normal function. The authors concluded that arthroscopic debridement of the ankle can offer relief to approximately two-thirds of patients, but it is important to stress to patients that the degree of improvement is limited. In Hassouna's (2007) series, 28% of osteoarthritic patients progressed to major ankle surgery within 5 years of ankle arthroscopic debridement. Age did not appear to affect the prognosis in this osteoarthritic group. Osti et al. demonstrated that anterior ankle arthroscopy for management of mild to moderate ankle arthritis is safe, effective, and allows former athletes to safely return to ordinary daily activities and recreational sport activities (Osti et al., 2016).

ARTHRODIASTASIS

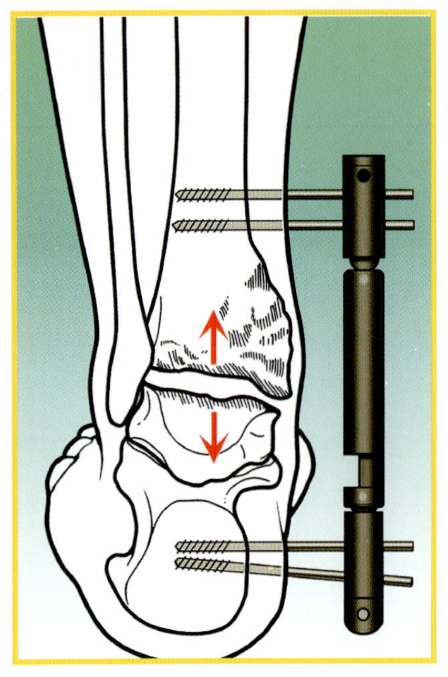

Figure 1. *Arthrodiastasis of the ankle (from Giannini et al., 2007).*

Ankle joint distraction with a hinged external fixator is another viable alternative to ankle arthrodesis or ankle replacement in selected cases, particularly in young patients with moderate ankle arthritis and an arc of at least 30° of sagittal motion (Marijnissen *et al.*, 2002) (Figure 1).

Joint distraction is based on the concept that osteoarthritic cartilage has some reparative power when there is release of mechanical stress on the cartilage, while intra-articular intermittent fluid pressure is maintained (Lafeber *et al.*, 1992).

A hinged external fixator frame is applied across the ankle and 5–10 mm gradual distraction of the joint is achieved. The fixator is left in place for 6–12 weeks and weightbearing and ankle motion as tolerated are encouraged (van Roermund *et al.*, 2002; Inda *et al.*, 2003).

A congruent, painful, mobile, and arthritic ankle joint that is treated with this technique can achieve good to excellent results both clinically and radiographically at intermediate-term follow-up (Marijnissen *et al.*, 2003). Paley *et al.* (2005) reviewed 32 patients who underwent ankle arthrodiastasis and found that 78% of patients had maintained their ankle range of motion and had no pain or only occasional moderate pain that could generally be managed with non-steroidal anti-inflammatory drugs alone. Zhao *et al.* found a failure rate of 21.7% at a mean 42.8 months, despite early improved functional outcomes. The failure rate was especially high for those obese patients and patients with varus or valgus deformity (Zhao *et al.*, 2017).

Combining adjunct procedures such as anterior blocking osteophyte resection, ankle realignment procedures, and equinus contracture release improves the results (Paley *et al.*, 2008; Badahdah and Zgonis, 2017). Tellisi *et al.* (2009) reviewed 25 patients who had undergone ankle distraction and were followed for 30 months after frame removal (range, 12–60 months).

Adjuvant procedures included, Achilles tendon lengthening ($n = 5$), ankle arthroscopy ($n = 4$), open arthrotomy ($n = 1$), and supramalleolar tibial and distal fibular osteotomy to correct deformity ($n = 6$). Ninety one per cent of patients reported improved pain, and the average AOFAS score improved from 55 preoperatively to 74 postoperatively. Only two patients (8%) had been fused at the latest follow up.

In addition, ankle arthrodiastasis does not seem to burn bridges for a possible future need for arthrodesis or ankle replacement, provided nerve injury is avoided and meticulous pin site care is used to prevent infection.

ANKLE OSTEOTOMY

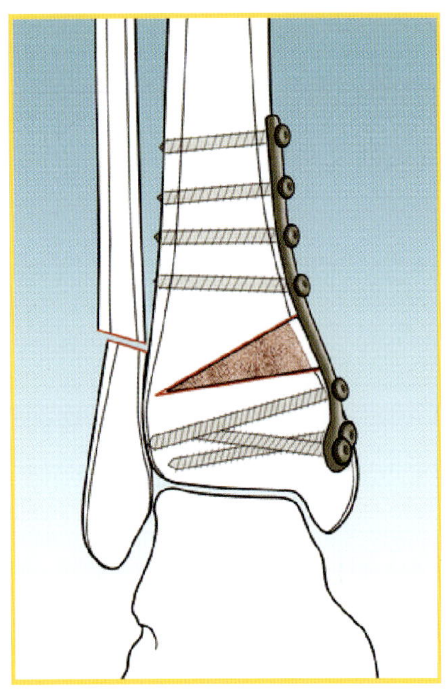

Figure 2. *Opening wedge supramalleolar osteotomy. Note the use of allograft to fill the defect (from Giannini et al., 2007).*

Posttraumatic malalignment predisposes to the development of chronic pain, functional impairment, and finally posttraumatic arthritis. Osteotomies can play an important role in re-establishing normal alignment and potentially delaying the need for arthrodesis or arthroplasty. Despite being a technically demanding surgical procedure, clinical outcomes support the role of supramalleolar osteotomy as an effective joint preservation procedure with few complications (Giannini *et al.*, 2010; Benthien and Myerson, 2004; Knupp, 2017). Once a correct alignment of the joint is achieved, redistribution of joint forces occurs and secondary surgery, if necessary, can be performed more easily, and with better results.

Takakura *et al.* (1995) designed an opening wedge low tibial osteotomy to correct the characteristic varus tilt and anterior opening of the distal tibial joint surface seen in primary ankle arthritis in their population (Figure 2). Follow-up of 18 patients at an average of 6 years and 11 months showed excellent results in 6 ankles, good in 9, and fair in 3 with no poor results. The authors recommend this technique for patients with intermediate primary arthritis with obliteration of the joint space and subchondral bone contact medially.

The success of total ankle arthroplasty depends largely on the alignment of the foot and ankle and osteotomies can be used in a staged manner as part of a reconstructive total ankle arthroplasty (Swords and Nemec, 2007; Gauvain *et al.*, 2017). Doets *et al.* (2008) reported excellent or good results in 12 of 14 arthritic ankles with varus malalignment in which medial malleolar lengthening osteotomy was done at the time of total ankle arthroplasty.

ANKLE FUSION

Even in the era of ankle arthroplasty, ankle fusion still has a role in the management of painful arthritic ankles with ankle malalignment and marked loss of motion. The purpose of ankle arthrodesis is to achieve a plantigrade, pain free and stable foot.

In the 1960s, ankle fusion was indicated to treat sequelae from poliomyelitis, osteoarticular tuberculosis, osteomyelitis, trauma, and spastic foot (Richter *et al.*, 1999; Thordarson *et al.*, 1997). Many of these indications are now very uncommon. Currently, the main indication for ankle fusion is a painful rigid ankle with functional impairment unresponsive to conservative treatment, secondary to previous fracture, infection, osteonecrosis, or primary arthritis. Other indications include rheumatoid arthritis, chronic ankle instability with severe chondral lesions, tumours, neuropathic arthropathy (including Charcot disease), and failed arthroplasty.

The most frequent indication for ankle fusion is posttraumatic arthritis that commonly affects young or middle-age patients who suffered a labour, sports, or traffic accident. Absolute indications for ankle fusion include severe osteopenia, talar collapse after avascular necrosis or neuropathy, and cartilage destruction secondary to recent infection in active patients younger than 45 years with a body mass index greater than 35 (Losch *et al.*, 2002; Jones *et al.*, 2018; Weatherall *et al.*, 2013).

Surgical Technique

Ankle fusion was first reported by Albert in 1879 to treat an equinus foot deformity in an 11-year-old girl with paralysis. A great advance in the surgical technique was the introduction of interfragmentary compression described by Charnley (Charnley and Lowe, 1959). Charnley's fixation system was uniplanar and did not allow rotational stability; therefore, Calandruccio designed a triangular frame to allow compression and motion control in three planes (Pickering, 2010).

The choice of the surgical technique depends on the underlying condition. Historically, large incisions and osteotomies were performed. Currently, both mini-open and arthroscopic techniques have achieved good results if the ankle deformity is less than 15° of varus or valgus. With minimal resections, the triplanar instability associated with large bony resections is minimised (Bozic *et al.*, 2008; Briggs and Stainsby, 1997; Ferkel and Hewitt, 2005). Open technique is used in cases with significant deformities and malalignment.

Ankle fixation has evolved so that now it is usually performed using compression of the prepared surfaces with interfragmentary screws (Anderson *et al.*, 1997; Holt *et al.*, 1991) (Figure 3). Placement of the screws in a crossed configuration increases the resistance to torsion when compared to parallel screws (Friedman *et al.*, 1994). Ogilvie-Harris *et al.* (1993) proved in a cadaver study that three screws provided more stability to torsion loads than two screws.

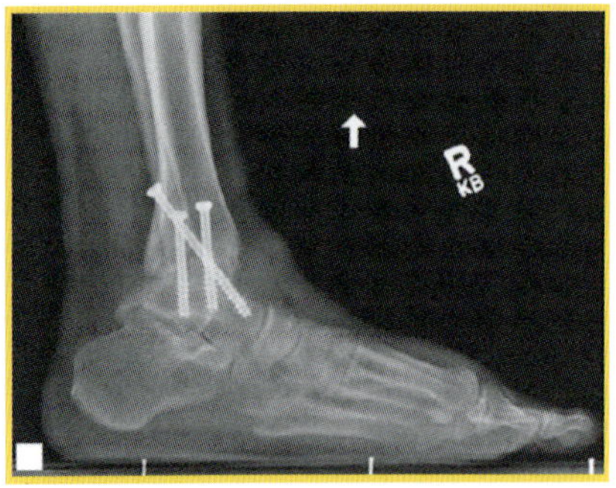

Figure 3. *Fixation after mini-incision ankle arthrodesis; note the use of a "home run" screw from the posterolateral tibia into the talar neck/head distally (from Murphy, 2013).*

The initial stiffness of ankle fusion with screws depends on the position of the joint, the mechanical properties of the fixation system, and the bone density. Brown and Seligson (2004) proved that fixation with cannulated screws in osteoporotic ankles is less rigid than with solid screws and requires greater diameter screws. Alonso-Vazquez *et al.* (2004) in a finite elements analysis proved that, when the medial and lateral screws are implanted with a lower than 45° angle over the axis of the tibia, they provide a greater initial stability.

In complex cases, where internal fixation is limited or even contraindicated, good results can be achieved using external fixators (Kiene *et al.*, 2009; Rochman *et al.*, 2008; Thordarson *et al.*, 1994). As a general rule, external fixators are preferred in patients with previous infection and severe osteopenia (Kollig *et al.*, 2003; Moeckel *et al.*, 1991; Ogut *et al.*, 2009). The techniques can be divided according to the surgical approach — anterior, transmalleolar, or posterior — and according to the fixation method — internal or external (Helm, 1990).

Open Ankle Fusion

More than 40 different surgical techniques have been described for open ankle fusion (Pickering, 2010; Abidi *et al.*, 2000; Mendicino *et al.*, 2017). Large incisions, wide bony resections, and different fixation methods were responsible for complication rates ranging from 13% to 60% in open ankle fusions, with a non-union rate up to 40% (Coester *et al.*, 2001; Cooper, 2001; Collman *et al.*, 2006; Morrey and Wiedeman, 1980; Muir *et al.*, 2002). These complications have been decreased or avoided using more rigid fixation devices, decreasing the amount of resected bone, increasing the contact between surfaces, and preserving soft-tissue attachments (Plaass *et al.*, 2009).

Compression and internal fixation with cannulated screws can be difficult in comminuted pilon fractures with associated bone defects (Bozic *et al.*, 2008). When using cannulated screws, care should be taken to avoid damage to the subtalar joint. A neutralising plate is a good alternative when using a posterior approach (Gentchos *et al.*, 2009; Sowa and Krackow, 1989). According to Nasson and Shuff (2001), posteriorly placed plates are less resistant to dorsal flexion and valgus forces than cannulated screws.

Arthroscopic Ankle Fusion

Arthroscopic ankle fusion was first described by Schneider (1983) who reported a faster consolidation time, earlier mobilisation, and lower morbidity (Figure 4). Myerson and Quill (1991) and O'Brien *et al.* (1999) compared arthroscopic with open techniques and favoured the former. With the arthroscopic technique, consolidation time was 4–8 weeks shorter, the hospital stay was also shorter, and there was a lower incidence of complications with a similar fusion rate. The shorter fusion time with the arthroscopic technique is due to the preservation of the periarticular blood supply (Collman *et al.*, 2006).

The arthroscopic technique is indicated in patients with minimal malalignment and good bone quality (Jones *et al.*, 2018;

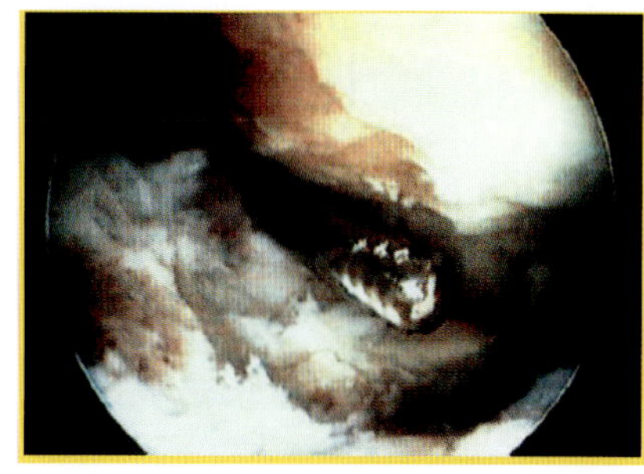

Figure 4. *Arthroscopic ankle arthrodesis. Motorised burr is used to remove a thin layer (approximately 2 mm) of sub-chondral bone (from Ishikawa, 2013).*

Hutchinson, 2016). Arthroscopy is also preferred over open surgery in elderly patients or patients with risk factors such as autoimmune diseases, diabetes, poor vascular supply, and dermatologic conditions. Maurer *et al.* (1991) reported successful ankle fusion through mini-arthrotomy in 15 patients. According to the authors, this technique preserved ankle anatomy and the periosteum and allowed rapid fusion.

Optimal Fixation Position in Ankle Fusion

Historically, there has been no consensus regarding the angle of plantar flexion at which the ankle should be fused. Barr and Record (1953) recommended fusion in 5° of equinus, Watson-Jones (Wilson and Watson-Jones, 1976) in 15° of equinus while Ratliff (1959) advocated fusion at right angles. Currently, the most widely accepted position in which to fuse the ankle is neutral plantar and dorsal flexion, 5° of valgus, and 5–10° of external rotation, mild posterior displacement of the talus, and 10–15° of pronation (Buck *et al.*, 1987).

Pronation is recommended because a fused ankle loses its capacity of hindfoot pronation, and there is usually a forefoot supination contracture which translates the load during weightbearing to the external margin of the hindfoot and forefoot. This position allows a better walking pattern and decreases loads in the knee (Collman *et al.*, 2006; Buck *et al.*, 1987; Mazur *et al.*, 1979); however, the position of the foot should always be compared with the contralateral foot before fusing the ankle. The most frequent malpositions are internal rotation, varus, and equinus.

Malposition in the Sagital Plane

If the ankle is fused in marked internal rotation, the patient suffers increased forces on the subtalar and midtarsal joints, which may cause pain and also affect the knee and hip secondary to the external rotation necessary to compensate the foot malposition.

If, on the other hand, there is marked external rotation, the patient increases weightbearing loads on the medial aspect of the first metatarsophalangeal joint, which may cause hallux valgus and increased load on the medial compartment of the knee.

Malposition in the Anteroposterior (AP) Plane

The angle of varus–valgus alignment should be related to the degree of mobility in the subtalar joint. If the joint is rigid and cannot compensate for malposition, it is necessary to fix the ankle in an angle of enough valgus to achieve a plantigrade position. If the ankle is fixed in varus, the patient will walk on the lateral border of his foot and will eventually develop rigidity and degenerative changes in the midtarsal joints.

Fixing the ankle in more than 5° of varus or valgus may increase the loads on the hindfoot and knee. When the valgus position of the ankle is excessive, there is increased load on the tibialis posterior tendon and ligamentous structures on the medial aspect of the foot with flat foot. These forces can be transmitted proximally to the medial compartment of the knee and distally to the medial column and the first metatarsophalangeal joint, causing stress fractures and early arthritis.

Varus malalignment of the fused ankle is poorly tolerated because it increases the loads on the subtalar joints, the peroneal tendons, the lateral ligamentous structures, and the lateral column of the foot, which may cause early subtalar joint arthritis, stress fracture of the fifth metatarsal, and peroneal tendon injuries.

Malposition in the Coronal Plane

When the ankle is fixed in more than 5° of plantar flexion, a genu recurvatum occurs during the stance phase. The patient externally rotates the lower limb, increasing the load on the medial compartment of the knee, the anterior aspect of the tibial plafond, and the midfoot causing stress fractures and metatarsalgia. The initial treatment of a fixed equinus deformity includes the use of a *solid ankle cushion heel* (SACH), to improve the gait and alleviate the symptoms. When conservative treatment fails, surgery is indicated (Chao *et al.*, 1994).

When the ankle is fused in marked dorsal flexion, the foot contacts the ground in a small area of the heel, which may cause chronic pain. During gait, knee flexion is necessary to achieve a plantigrade foot. If conservative treatment with an inverted sole shoe fails, surgery may be needed.

Revision surgery for sagittal plane deformities requires corrective opening or closing wedge osteotomies at the site of fusion. The latter are most commonly used because they decrease the tension on the soft tissues and neurovascular structures and have a higher fusion rate (Easley *et al.*, 2008; Midis and Conti, 2002; Raikin and Rampuri, 2008). The disadvantage is that closing osteotomies cause limb shortening.

Posterior translation of the talus at the time of fusion allows a better gait pattern and decreases knee disorders (Ogilvie-Harris *et al.*, 1993; Thomas *et al.*, 2006). Anterior displacement of the talus should be avoided to prevent increase in the lever arm of the ankle (Thomas *et al.*, 2006).

Complications of Ankle Fusion

Sheridan *et al.* (2006) reported hindfoot and midfoot degenerative changes in patients after ankle fusion. Mid-term and long-term studies have shown arthrofibrosis and subtalar arthritis to be the origin of the remaining alterations after ankle fusion (Lynch *et al.*, 1988; Jones *et al.*, 2018). Aaron (1990) reported a 31% incidence of subtalar arthritis while Thomas *et al.* (2006) found a 15% incidence. In the experience of Bertrand *et al.* (2001), following 37 cases of ankle fusion during 13 years, 45% were symptom-free and most were able to walk 1500m despite a 100% incidence of subtalar arthritis.

Jones *et al.* (2018) found at mean 86-month follow-up that 85% and 69% of patients had no change in talonavicular or subtalar grade of osteoarthritis, respectively (Jones *et al.*, 2018).

Provelengios *et al.* (2009) were unable to identify a relation between the position of the foot and the ipsilateral knee pain. They found that the incidence of tibial stress fracture was higher in patients with stiff subtalar and midtalar joints and in obese patients.

The non-union rate varies among authors and surgical techniques, ranging between 3% and 35% (Levine *et al.*, 1997; Mann and Rongstad, 1998; Jones *et al.*, 2018; Honnenahalli *et al.*, 2017). Risk factors include smoking, avascular bone, high-energy trauma, and non-compliant patients.

Painful Ankle Fusion

Most patients with a fused ankle achieve a pain-free gait soon after surgery; however, many studies have proved short-term and long-term functional impairment in activities such as climbing stairs, getting out of a chair, walking on uneven surfaces, and running (Morrey and Wiedeman, 1980; Lance *et al.*, 1979). The satisfaction level with ankle fusion has been poor in some studies and many patients need walking aids and permanent shoe modifications (Boobbyer, 1981; Fuchs *et al.*, 2003). A young patient who has his ankle fused has a great chance of developing hindfoot arthritis over the next 20 years and may eventually require a pantalar arthrodesis (Coester *et al.*, 2001).

The painful ankle arthrodesis is an unsolved clinical problem. Some authors have advocated converting painful ankle fusions into total ankle replacements in patients with good bone stock (Hintermann *et al.*, 2009). Greisberg *et al.* (2004) reported their experience with taking down ankle fusion and converting to total ankle replacement in 23 patients. They found that previous lateral malleolar resection was a relative contraindication to conversion of ankle fusion to total ankle replacement. They were able to follow 19 ankles for an average of 39 months. Three patients chose to have an amputation because of continued pain. In the remaining 16 ankles, the mean AOFAS ankle–hindfoot outcome score improved from 42 to 68. The authors concluded that for patients with a definable source of pain and who have not had previous malleolar resection, conversion of a failed ankle arthrodesis to total ankle arthroplasty may be a viable alternative to amputation. Similar results were reported by Barg and Hintermann (2008) in a series of 29 patients. The authors highlighted the importance of achieving intrinsic stability in the coronal plane, the use of wider talar components, and the difficulty in finding out the original rotation axis of the fused tibiotalar joint.

Several studies have compared functional outcomes of ankle fusion and total ankle replacement. Piriou *et al.* (2008) found that patients with a fused ankle could walk faster and had a longer footstep than patients with ankle replacement. They also found that the control group had higher knee flexion angles than those with arthrodesis or total ankle replacement. Kofoed (Kofoed and Stürup, 1994) reported that one-third of 14 patients with a fused ankle and none of 14 with ankle replacement had subtalar joint arthritis 7 years after surgery.

According to Soo-Ho *et al.* (2007), patients with ankle replacement have a lower risk of developing subtalar joint arthritis and a higher risk of infection or needing a revision surgery. In a meta-analysis of the papers published between 1990 and 2005, Haddad *et al.* (2007) evaluated 10 papers including 852 patients with ankle replacement and 39 papers including 1262 patients with ankle fusion. The incidence of radiographic subtalar arthritis was 1% in patients with ankle replacement and 5% after ankle fusion.

REFERENCES

Aaron, A. D. 1990. Ankle fusion: A retrospective review. *Orthopedics*, 13, 1249–1254.

Abidi, N. A., Gruen, G. S. & Conti, S. F. 2000. Ankle arthrodesis: Indications and techniques. *J Am Acad Orthop Surg*, 8, 200–209.

Alonso-Vazquez, A., Lauge-Pedersen, H., Lidgren, L. & Taylor, M. 2004. The effect of bone quality on the stability of ankle arthrodesis. A finite element study. *Foot Ankle Int*, 25, 840–850.

Anderson, J. G., Coetzee, J. C. & Hansen, S. T. 1997. Revision ankle fusion using internal compression arthrodesis with screw fixation. *Foot Ankle Int*, 18, 300–309.

Badahdah, H. M. & Zgonis, T. 2017. Ankle arthrodiastasis with circular external fixation for the treatment of posttraumatic ankle arthritis. *Clin Podiatr Med Surg*, 34, 425–431.

Barp, E. A., Erickson, J. G. & Hall, J. L. 2017. Arthroscopic treatment of ankle arthritis. *Clin Podiatr Med Surg*, 34, 433–444.

Barr, J. S. & Record, E. E. 1953. Arthrodesis of the ankle joint indications, operative technic and clinical experience. *N Engl J Med*, 248, 53–56.

Benthien, R. A. & Myerson, M. S. 2004. Supramalleolar osteotomy for ankle deformity and arthritis. *Foot Ankle Clin*, 9, 475–487, viii.

Bertrand, M., Charissoux, J. L., Mabit, C. & Arnaud, J. P. 2001. Tibio-talar arthrodesis: Long term influence on the foot. *Rev Chir Orthop Reparatrice Appar Mot*, 87, 677–684.

Boobbyer, G. N. 1981. The long-term results of ankle arthrodesis. *Acta Orthop Scand*, 52, 107–110.

Bozic, V., Thordarson, D. B. & Hertz, J. 2008. Ankle fusion for definitive management of non-reconstructable pilon fractures. *Foot Ankle Int*, 29, 914–918.

Briggs, P. J. & Stainsby, G. D. 1997. The Thomas method of ankle arthrodesis: 2 to 20 year follow-up. *The Foot*, 7, 14–18.

Brown, K. D. & Seligson, D. 2004. An optimal technique for ankle arthrodesis. *J Foot Ankle Surg*, 43, 64–66.

Buck, P., Morrey, B. F. & Chao, E. Y. 1987. The optimum position of arthrodesis of the ankle. A gait study of the knee and ankle. *J Bone Joint Surg Am*, 69, 1052–1062.

Chao, E. Y., Neluheni, E. V., Hsu, R. W. & Paley, D. 1994. Biomechanics of malalignment. *Orthop Clin North Am*, 25, 379–386.

Charnley, J. & Lowe, H. G. 1959. Compression arthrodesis of the ankle. *J Bone J Surg (Br)*, 41, 524–532.

Cheng, J. C. & Ferkel, R. D. 1998. The role of arthroscopy in ankle and subtalar degenerative joint disease. *Clin Orthop Relat Res*, 349, 65–72.

Coester, L. M., Saltzman, C. L., Leupold, J. & Pontarelli, W. 2001. Long-term results following ankle arthrodesis for post-traumatic arthritis. *J Bone Joint Surg Am*, 83-A, 219–228.

Collman, D. R., Kaas, M. H. & Schuberth, J. M. 2006. Arthroscopic ankle arthrodesis: Factors influencing union in 39 consecutive patients. *Foot Ankle Int*, 27, 1079–1085.

Cooper, P. S. 2001. Complications of ankle and tibiotalocalcaneal arthrodesis. *Clin Orthop Relat Res*, 391, 33–44.

Doets, H. C., Van Der Plaat, L. W. & Klein, J.-P. 2008. Medial malleolar osteotomy for the correction of varus deformity during total ankle arthroplasty. Results in 15 ankles. *Foot Ankle Int*, 29, 171–177.

Easley, M. E., Montijo, H. E., Wilson, J. B., Fitch, R. D. & Nunley, J. A., II, 2008. Revision tibiotalar arthrodesis. *J Bone Joint Surg Am*, 90, 1212–1223.

Felson, D. T. 1990. The epidemiology of knee osteoarthritis: Results from the Framingham Osteoarthritis Study. *Semin Arthritis Rheum*, 20, 42–50.

Ferkel, R. D. & Hewitt, M. 2005. Long-term results of arthroscopic ankle arthrodesis. *Foot Ankle Int*, 26, 275–280.

Friedman, R. L., Glisson, R. R. & Nunley, J. A., II 1994. A biomechanical comparative analysis of two techniques for tibiotalar arthrodesis. *Foot Ankle Int*, 15, 301–305.

Fuchs, S., Sandmann, C., Skwara, A. & Chylarecki, C. 2003. Quality of life 20 years after arthrodesis of the ankle. A study of adjacent joints. *J Bone Joint Surg Br*, 85, 994–998.

Gauvain, T. T., Hames, M. A. & Mcgarvey, W. C. 2017. Malalignment correction of the lower limb before, during, and after total ankle arthroplasty. *Foot Ankle Clin*, 22, 311–339.

Gentchos, C. E., Bohay, D. R. & Anderson, J. G. 2009. Technique tip: a simple method for ankle arthrodesis using solid screws. *Foot Ankle Int*, 30, 380–383.

Giannini, S., Buda, R., Faldini, C., Vannini, F., Romagnoli, M., Grandi, G. & Bevoni, R. 2007. The treatment of severe posttraumatic arthritis of the ankle joint. *J Bone Joint Surg Am*, 89(Suppl 3), 15–28.

Giannini, S., Faldini, C., Acri, F., Leonetti, D., Luciani, D. & Nanni, M. 2010. Surgical treatment of post-traumatic malalignment of the ankle. *Injury*, 41, 1208–1211.

Greisberg, J., Assal, M., Flueckiger, G. & Hansen, S. T., Jr. 2004. Takedown of ankle fusion and conversion to total ankle replacement. *Clin Orthop Relat Res*, 424, 80–88.

Haddad, S. L., Coetzee, J. C., Estok, R., Fahrbach, K., Banel, D. & Nalysnyk, L. 2007. Intermediate and long-term outcomes of total ankle arthroplasty and ankle arthrodesis. A systematic review of the literature. *J Bone Joint Surg Am*, 89, 1899–1905.

Hassouna, H., Kumar, S. & Bendall, S. 2007. Arthroscopic ankle debridement: 5-year survival analysis. *Acta Orthop Belg*, 73, 737–740.

Helm, R. 1990. The results of ankle arthrodesis. *J Bone Joint Surg Br*, 72, 141–143.

Hintermann, B., Barg, A., Knupp, M., Valderrabano, V. 2009. Conversion of painful ankle arthrodesis to total ankle arthroplasty. *J Bone Joint Surg Am*, 91(4), 850–858.

Holt, E. S., Hansen, S. T., Mayo, K. A. & Sangeorzan, B. J. 1991. Ankle arthrodesis using internal screw fixation. *Clin Orthop Relat Res*, 268, 21–28.

Honnenahalli, C. M., Hajibandeh, S. & Hajibandeh, S. 2017. Ankle arthrodesis — open versus arthroscopic: A systematic review and meta-analysis. *J Clin Orthop Trauma*, 8, S71–S77.

Hutchinson, B. 2016. Arthroscopic ankle arthrodesis. *Clin Podiatr Med Surg*, 33, 581–589.

Inda, D. J., Blyakher, A., O'Malley, M. J. & Rozbruch, S. R. 2003. Distraction arthroplasty for the ankle using the Ilizarov frame. *Tech Foot Ankle Surg*, 2, 249–253.

Ishikawa, S. N. 2013. Arthroscopy of the foot and ankle. In S. T. Canale & J. H. Beaty (eds.), *Campbell' Operative Orthopaedics*, 12th Edition, Elsevier, Philadelphia, p. 2385.

Jones, C. R., Wong, E., Applegate, G. R., Ferkel, R. D. 2018. Arthroscopic ankle arthrodesis: A 2-15 year follow-up study. *Arthroscopy*, 34(5), 1641–1649.

Kiene, J., Schulz, A. P., Hillbricht, S., Jurgens, C. & Paech, A. 2009. Clinical results of resection arthrodesis by triangular external fixation for posttraumatic arthrosis of the ankle joint in 89 cases. *Eur J Med Res*, 14, 25–29.

Kimizuka, M., Kurosawa, H. & Fukubayashi, T. 1980. Load-bearing pattern of the ankle joint. Contact area and pressure distribution. *Arch Orthop Trauma Surg*, 96, 45–49.

Knupp, M. 2017. The use of osteotomies in the treatment of asymmetric ankle joint arthritis. *Foot Ankle Int*, 38, 220–229.

Kofoed, H. & Stürup, J. 1994. Comparison of ankle arthroplasty and arthrodesis. *Foot*, 4, 6–9.

Kollig, E., Esenwein, S. A., Muhr, G. & Kutscha-Lissberg, F. 2003. Fusion of the septic ankle: Experience with 15 cases using hybrid external fixation. *J Trauma*, 55, 685–691.

Lafeber, F. P. J. G., Veldhuijzen, J. P., Vanroy, J. L. A. M., Huber-Bruning, O. & Bijlsma, J. W. J. 1992. Intermittent hydrostatic compressive force stimulates exclusively the proteoglycan synthesis of osteoarthritic human cartilage. *Rheumatology*, 31, 437–442.

Lance, E. M., Paval, A., Fries, I., Larsen, I. & Patterson, R. L., Jr. 1979. Arthrodesis of the ankle joint. A follow-up study. *Clin Orthop Relat Res*, 142, 146–158.

Levine, S. E., Myerson, M. S., Lucas, P. & Schon, L. C. 1997. Salvage of pseudoarthrosis after tibiotalar arthrodesis. *Foot Ankle Int*, 18, 580–585.

Losch, A., Meybohm, P., Schmalz, T., Fuchs, M., Vamvukakis, F., Dresing, K., Blumentritt, S. & Sturmer, K. M. 2002. Functional results of dynamic gait analysis after 1 year of hobby-athletes with a surgically treated ankle fracture. *Sportverletz Sportschaden*, 16, 101–107.

Lynch, A. F., Bourne, R. B. & Rorabeck, C. H. 1988. The long-term results of ankle arthrodesis. *J Bone Joint Surg Br*, 70, 113–116.

Mann, R. A. & Rongstad, K. M. 1998. Arthrodesis of the ankle: A critical analysis. *Foot Ankle Int*, 19, 3–9.

Marco Sanz, C. 2003. *Marcha Patológica. Revista del pie y tobillo*, 17, 1–7.

Marijnissen, A. C., Van Roermund, P. M., Van Melkebeek, J., Schenk, W., Verbout, A. J., Bijlsma, J. W. & Lafeber, F. P. 2002. Clinical benefit of joint distraction in the treatment of severe osteoarthritis of the ankle: Proof of concept in an open prospective study and in a randomized controlled study. *Arthritis Rheum*, 46, 2893–2902.

Marijnissen, A. C., Van Roermund, P. M., Van Melkebeek, J. & Lafeber, F. P. 2003. Clinical benefit of joint distraction in the treatment of ankle osteoarthritis. *Foot Ankle Clin*, 8, 335–346.

Maurer, R. C., Cimino, W. R., Cox, C. V. & Satow, G. K. 1991. Transarticular cross-screw fixation. A technique of ankle arthrodesis. *Clin Orthop Relat Res*, 268, 56–64.

Mazur, J. M., Schwartz, E. & Simon, S. R. 1979. Ankle arthrodesis. Long-term follow-up with gait analysis. *J Bone Joint Surg Am*, 61, 964–975.

Mendicino, S. S., Kreplick, A. L., Walters, J. L. 2017. Open ankle arthrodesis. *Clin Podiatr Med Surg*, 34, 489–502.

Midis, N. & Conti, S. F. 2002. Revision ankle arthrodesis. *Foot Ankle Int*, 23, 243–247.

Moeckel, B. H., Patterson, B. M., Inglis, A. E. & Sculco, T. P. 1991. Ankle arthrodesis. A comparison of internal and external fixation. *Clin Orthop Relat Res*, 78–83.

Morrey, B. F. & Wiedeman, G. P., Jr. 1980. Complications and long-term results of ankle arthrodeses following trauma. *J Bone Joint Surg Am*, 62, 777–784.

Muir, D. C., Amendola, A. & Saltzman, C. L. 2002. Long-term outcome of ankle arthrodesis. *Foot Ankle Clin*, 7, 703–708.

Murphy, G. A. 2013. Ankle arthrodesis. In S. T. Canale & J. H. Beaty (eds.), *Campbell' Operative Orthopaedics*, 12th Edition, Elsevier, Philadelphia, p. 513.

Myerson, M. S. & Quill, G. 1991. Ankle arthrodesis. A comparison of an arthroscopic and an open method of treatment. *Clin Orthop Relat Res*, 268, 84–95.

Nasson, S., Shuff, C., Palmer, D., Owen, J., Wayne, J., Carr, J., Adelaar, R. & May, D. 2001. Biomechanical comparison of ankle arthrodesis techniques: crossed screws vs. blade plate. *Foot Ankle Int*, 22(7), 575–580.

O'Brien, T. S., Hart, T. S., Shereff, M. J., Stone, J. & Johnson, J. 1999. Open versus arthroscopic ankle arthrodesis: A comparative study. *Foot Ankle Int*, 20, 368–374.

Ogilvie-Harris, D. J., Lieberman, I. & Fitsialos, D. 1993. Arthroscopically assisted arthrodesis for osteoarthrotic ankles. *J Bone Joint Surg Am*, 75, 1167–1174.

Ogilvie-Harris, D. J. & Sekyi-Otu, A. 1995. Arthroscopic debridement for the osteoarthritic ankle. *Arthroscopy*, 11, 433–436.

Ogut, T., Glisson, R. R., Chuckpaiwong, B., Le, I. L. & Easley, M. E. 2009. External ring fixation versus screw fixation for ankle arthrodesis: A biomechanical comparison. *Foot Ankle Int*, 30, 353–360.

Osti, L., Del Buono, A. & Maffulli, N. 2016. Arthroscopic debridement of the ankle for mild to moderate osteoarthritis: A midterm follow-up study in former professional soccer players. *J Orthop Surg Res*, 11, 37.

Paley, D. & Lamm, B. M. 2005. Ankle joint distraction. *Foot Ankle Clin*, 10, 685–698, ix.

Paley, D., Lamm, B. M., Purohit, R. M. & Specht, S. C. 2008. Distraction arthroplasty of the ankle — How far can you stretch the indications? *Foot Ankle Clin*, 13, 471–484, ix.

Pickering, R. M. 2010. Arthrodesis of the ankle, knee and hip. In S. T. Canale & J. H. Beaty (eds.), *Campbell's Orthopaedic Surgery*, 11th edition, Elsevier, Barcelona. Chapter 3. 163–207.

Piriou, P., Culpan, P., Mullins, M., Cardon, J. N., Pozzi, D. & Judet, T. 2008. Ankle replacement versus arthrodesis: A comparative gait analysis study. *Foot Ankle Int*, 29, 3–9.

Plaass, C., Knupp, M., Barg, A. & Hintermann, B. 2009. Anterior double plating for rigid fixation of isolated tibiotalar arthrodesis. *Foot Ankle Int*, 30, 631–639.

Provelengios, S., Papavasiliou, K. A., Kyrkos, M. J., Kirkos, J. M. & Kapetanos, G. A. 2009. The role of pantalar arthrodesis in the treatment of paralytic foot deformities. A long-term follow-up study. *J Bone Joint Surg Am*, 91, 575–583.

Raikin, S. M. & Rampuri, V. 2008. An approach to the failed ankle arthrodesis. *Foot Ankle Clin*, 13, 401–416, viii.

Ratliff, A. H. 1959. Compression arthrodesis of the ankle. *J Bone Joint Surg Br*, 41-b, 524–534.

Richter, D., Hahn, M. P., Laun, R. A., Ekkernkamp, A., Muhr, G. & Ostermann, P. A. 1999. Arthrodesis of the infected ankle and subtalar joint: Technique, indications, and results of 45 consecutive cases. *J Trauma*, 47, 1072–1078.

Rochman, R., Jackson Hutson, J. & Alade, O. 2008. Tibiocalcaneal arthrodesis using the Ilizarov technique in the presence of bone loss and infection of the talus. *Foot Ankle Int*, 29, 1001–1008.

Schneider, D. 1983. Arthroscopic ankle fusion. *Arthros Video J*, 3, 11.

Sheridan, B. D., Robinson, D. E., Hubble, M. J. & Winson, I. G. 2006. Ankle arthrodesis and its relationship to ipsilateral arthritis of the hind- and mid-foot. *J Bone Joint Surg Br*, 88, 206–207.

SooHoo, N. F., Zingmond, D. S. & Ko, C. Y. 2007. Comparison of reoperation rates following ankle arthrodesis and total ankle arthroplasty. *J Bone Joint Surg Am*, 89, 2143–2149.

Sowa, D. T. & Krackow, K. A. 1989. Ankle fusion: A new technique of internal fixation using a compression blade plate. *Foot Ankle*, 9, 232–240.

Swords, M. P. & Nemec, S. 2007. Osteotomy for salvage of the arthritic ankle. *Foot Ankle Clin*, 12, 1–13.

Takakura, Y., Tanaka, Y., Kumai, T. & Tamai, S. 1995. Low tibial osteotomy for osteoarthritis of the ankle. Results of a new operation in 18 patients. *J Bone Joint Surg Br*, 77, 50–54.

Tellisi, N., Fragomen, A. T., Kleinman, D., O'malley, M. J. & Rozbruch, S. R. 2009. Joint preservation of the osteoarthritic ankle using distraction arthroplasty. *Foot Ankle Int*, 30, 318–325.

Thomas, R., Daniels, T. R. & Parker, K. 2006. Gait analysis and functional outcomes following ankle arthrodesis for isolated ankle arthritis. *J Bone Joint Surg Am*, 88, 526–535.

Thordarson, D. B., Markolf, K. L. & Cracchiolo, A., III. 1994. External fixation in arthrodesis of the ankle. A biomechanical study comparing a unilateral frame with a modified transfixion frame. *J Bone Joint Surg Am*, 76, 1541–1544.

Thordarson, D. B., Patzakis, M. J., Holtom, P. & Sherman, R. 1997. Salvage of the septic ankle with concomitant tibial osteomyelitis. *Foot Ankle Int*, 18, 151–156.

Tochigi, Y., Rudert, M. J., Saltzman, C. L., Amendola, A. & Brown, T. D. 2006. Contribution of articular surface geometry to ankle stabilization. *J Bone Joint Surg Am*, 88, 2704–2713.

Van Roermund, P. M., Marijnissen, A. C. & Lafeber, F. P. 2002. Joint distraction as an alternative for the treatment of osteoarthritis. *Foot Ankle Clin*, 7, 515–527.

Weatherall, J. M., Mroczek, K., Mclaurin, T., Ding, B. & Tejwani, N. 2013. Post-traumatic ankle arthritis. *Bull Hosp Jt Dis* (2013), 71, 104–112.

Wilson, J. N. & Watson-Jones, R. 1976. Injuries of the Ankle. In JN Wilson & R Watson-Jones (eds), *Fractures and Joint Injuries*, 5th edition, Churchill Livingstone, Edinburgh, Vol 2, 1146.

Zhao, H., Qu, W., Li, Y., Liang, X., Ning, N., Zhang, Y. & Hu, D. 2017. Functional analysis of distraction arthroplasty in the treatment of ankle osteoarthritis. *J Orthop Surg Res*, 12, 18.

HISTORICAL EVOLUTION OF TOTAL ANKLE REPLACEMENT

CHAPTER 7

J. Kirkup and A. J. Goldberg

Summary

One of the last major joints to be replaced by a modern prosthesis has proved to be a formidable technical challenge. This brief historical survey recalls the fundamental surgical and technical advances underlining modern prosthetic procedures, and the importance of hip surgery in encouraging and perhaps misleading early total ankle replacement (TAR) surgeons to insert spherical components and cement. Yet, disappointment of initial prostheses has stimulated functional research to define ankle function more accurately, leading to improved designs. The majority of the really epoch-making operations of surgery have passed through a certain number of phases in their life-history (Todd, 1923).

History confirms that further research and improvements will follow.

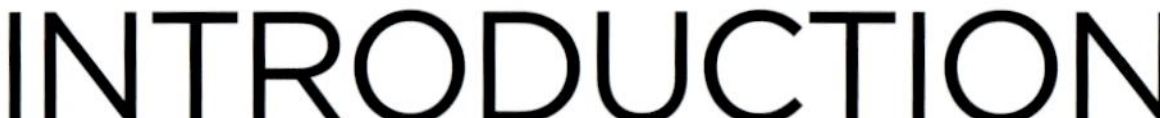

INTRODUCTION

Successful joint replacements have a considerable pedigree indebted to the concepts and courage of pioneering surgeons, to vital medical and surgical discoveries, and especially to new materials and bioengineering research. Consideration of this background may remind today's surgeons of the historical base underpinning their operative success and, additionally, signal future changes for nothing stands still.

Indeed, innovations can be described as two types. Disruptive innovations are completely new ways of doing things or game changers, in contrast to incremental innovations, which are iterative improvements in the way things are done. As with most of orthopaedics, ankle replacements are very much of the iterative incremental form across many years, countries, and continents.

Ankle resembles *ankel* and *enkel* of Germanic and Scandinavian languages and may relate to the Latin *angulus* meaning angle or corner. Arthroplasty, by derivation joint moulding or formation, is noted in 1881 (Ollier and Ollier, 1885) and was designated either joint excision or reconstruction by means of fascia lata interposition until the 1920s (Todd, 1923); today, arthroplasty includes prosthetic substitution, also termed total joint replacement. Unlike the hip joint, the ankle has three distinct articular facets involving the tibia, fibula, and talus, all heavily dependent on stabilising ligaments.

FUNDAMENTAL DISCOVERIES

Medical, Bacteriological, and Technical

Surgery progressed decisively in the 19th century stimulated by the advantages of general anaesthesia in 1846, chemical antisepsis in 1867, thermal asepsis in 1888 following bacteriological discoveries and, finally, X-rays in 1895. Later World War experiences, blood transfusion, chemotherapy, antibiotics, and sophisticated pharmaceutical products extended surgery to the wider spectrum of an ageing population (Table 1).

Surgical

Partial excision of the ankle by removal of the talus for compound dislocation was described in 1607 by Wilhelm Fabry (1560–1634) (Le Vay, 1990) and of the lateral or medial malleolus, or both, for

Table 1. Significant discoveries advancing prosthetic surgery.

Discoveries		Date	Discoverer
Tourniquet	Screw Pneumatic	1705 1904	Petit (1741) Cushing (1904)
Anaesthesia	Ether Chloroform	1846 1847	WTG Morton (Duncum, 1947) J Simpson (Duncum, 1947)
Chemical antisepsis		1867	Lister (1867)
Bacterial discoveries	Multiple Staphylococcus Tubercle bacillus	1877–1886 1881 1882	L Pasteur (Foster, 1970a) A Ogston (Foster, 1970a) R Koch (Foster, 1970a)
Thermal asepsis		1888–1892	Redard (1888) Bergman (1890)
X-rays		1895	Röntgen (1895)
Blood groups		1900	Landsteiner (Foster, 1970b)
Penicillin		1928	Fleming (1929)
Sulphonamides		1932	Domagk (1935)
Laminar air-flow theatres		1962	Charnley (1964a,b)

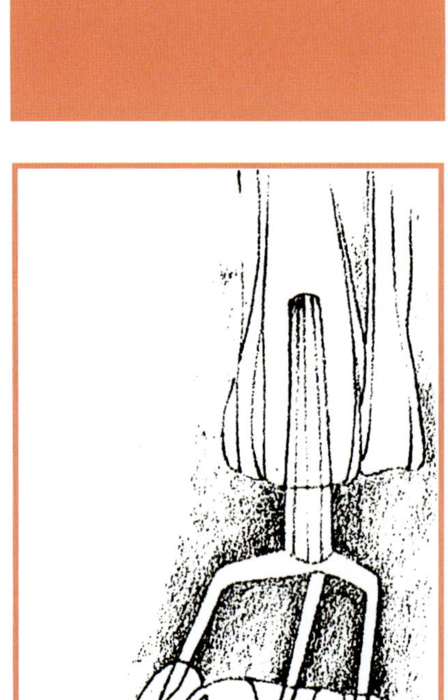

Figure 1. *Gluck's proposed prosthesis for excised ankle and tarsal joints; said to have ankle movement (Bick, 1948).*

compound fractures by 18th and 19th century surgeons (Cooper, 1844). Mons. Moreau (*c.*1740–1799) undertook partial excisions for infected ankle fractures in 1782 and, more importantly, the first total ankle joint excision in 1792, for "arthritis" (Moreau, 1803), with a favourable outcome, yet without approval from French colleagues who preferred below knee amputation. Leon Ollier (1830–1900) stated Robert Liston (1794–1847) performed the first total ankle resection for tuberculosis in 1818, removing tibia, fibula, talus, navicular, and two cuneiforms, and that Johann Heyfelder (1798–1869) noted only 22 total ankle resections published worldwide, six for compound injuries in 1862 (Ollier and Ollier, 1885). Leonard Peltier (*c.*1920–2003) stated the first arthrodeses of the foot were undertaken by L. von Lesser in 1879 and Eduard Albert (1841–1900) reported an ankle arthrodesis for paralysis in 1882 (Peltier, 1841–1900).

With the benefit of asepsis, Themistocles Gluck (1853–1942) inserted several joint prostheses from 1890, including an ivory plug for excision of a metatarsus and tarsus except the proximal talus and calcaneum (Anon, 1890) and he also illustrated, and perhaps inserted, a total ankle prosthesis of nickel-plated steel with a "glue" of plaster, pumice, and resin (Figure 1). As the joints selected were tuberculous or malignant, failure was inevitable reinforcing his peer's sharp criticism of his unconventional approaches and he suspended further attempts. Of course years later, he was considered a pioneer.

In 1908, Erich Lexer (1867–1937) replaced damaged and diseased joints with intact joints derived from amputated or postmortem limbs (Lexer, 1908); many were half joints and of his cases of 300 in 1925, only 10 involved the ankle, although he provided no details. Poor results lead to abandonment of this technique.

In 1962, Dr Larson in Iowa inserted a vitallium dome resurfacing talar cap onto a posttraumatic talus in a 38-year-old male following trauma. This was a one-off customised solution. Clinical examination at 40-year follow-up showed mild hindfoot malalignment with slightly decreased ROM (25° plantar flexion), AOFAS score of 85, no pain, and no activity limitation (Muir *et al.*, 2002).

Technical

When Gluck experimented with ivory, plated steel, aluminium, wood, glass, and celluloid, materials science as applied to surgery was in its infancy and progress towards durable prostheses was frustrated for many decades.

Interpositional material (Table 2)

Gluck's failure persuaded others to conserve damaged joints and improve function by interposing the patient's muscle, fascia or fat, or pig's bladder, or metallic films of gold foil or magnesium (Verneuil, 1860; Bick, 1948). Only fascia secured wide approval and John Murphy's (1857–1916) reconfiguration of the hip joint by reaming and lining with fascia lata became popular from 1912 to the early 1930s though partial ankylosis usually resulted (Murphy, 1912). Marius Smith-Petersen's (1886–1953) trials of interposed hip moulds or cups in viscaloid, glass, and bakelite proved disappointing but, in 1938 chrome–cobalt alloy (Vitallium) cups remained inert and generally effective (Smith-Petersen, 1939).

Table 2. Evolution of joint interposition materials.

Material	Date and surgeon	Joint
Muscle	1860, Verneuil (1860)	Temporo-mandibular
Gold foil	1895, Jones (Bick, 1948)	Hip
Magnesium	1900, Chlumsky (Bick, 1948)	Animal joints
Fascia lata	c. 1905, Murphy (1912)	Hip
Pig's bladder	1918, Baer (1918)	Hip, knee, ankle
Glass	1923, Smith-Petersen (1939)	Hip
Bakelite	1937, Smith-Petersen (1939)	Hip
Vitallium	1938, Smith-Petersen (1939)	Hip

Prosthetic material (Table 3)

Nickel-plated steel and ivory components were soon abandoned whereas low alloy stainless steel and acrylic resin achieved short-lived popularity before failure. However, chrome–cobalt alloys and high alloy stainless steel proved tissue compatible and resistant to corrosion, both persisting with polyethylene, titanium, and ceramic as prosthetic materials of choice.

Table 3. Evolution of prosthetic replacement materials.

Material	Date and surgeon	Joint
Nickel-plated steel	1891, Gluck (1890)	Possible Ankle+
Ivory	1923, Groves (1927)	Hip (hemi)
Stainless steel — low alloy	1938, Wiles (1958)	Hip (total)
Vitallium, chrome–cobalt	1940, Moore (Moore, 1952; Moore and Bohlman, 1943)	Hip (hemi)
Acrylic resin	1946, Judet (Judet and Judet, 1949)	Hip (hemi)
Vinertia, chrome–cobalt	1956, McKee (1974)	Hip (total)
Titanium	1957, Leventhal (1957)	Hip (hemi)
Stainless steel — high alloy	1960, Charnley (1961)	Hip (total)
Polyethylene	1962, Charnley (Waugh, 2012)	Hip (total)
Ceramic	1970, Boutin (1972)	Hip (total)

Prosthetic fixation

Gluck's "glue" was replaced by Philip Wiles (1899–1967) with stabilising metal screws, by Kenneth McKee (1906–1991) with uncemented femoral and acetabular screw fixation and, in 1960, by John Charnley (1911–1982) with revolutionary intramedullary methyl methacrylate cement. More recently, others have rejected cement in favour of sintered surfaces and hydroxyapatite coating to integrate directly with bone, and some surgeons even went further to add screw fixation (for example, the initial designs of the Hintegra prosthesis).

EVOLVING PATHOLOGY AND INDICATIONS

Indications for ankle joint surgery have changed with time. In the 18th century, partial excision was performed commonly for compound fractures and dislocations, total excision rarely for chronic sepsis and ankylosis while excision was exceptional for tuberculosis and club foot. During the Crimean War gunshot fractures of the talus encouraged talectomy, with indifferent results until antiseptic techniques improved. A survey in America, by Melvin Henderson in 1918, obtained information from 51 surgeons on 395 fascia interposition arthroplasties mainly for ankylosis which included 22 ankles (5%) with discouraging results (Henderson, 1918). In 1924, Ernest Hey Groves (1872–1944) advised indications in order of suitability for interposition arthroplasty as trauma, pyaemia, gonorrhoea, tubercle, osteoarthritis, and rheumatoid arthritis (Groves, 1923). However, Vittorio Putti (1880–1940) and Russel and Andrew MacAusland (20th century) avoided tubercle and rheumatoid arthritis, stating ankylosis due to burnt out sepsis was the primary indication, doubtless influenced by many disabled gunshot victims after World War One, though few ankle arthroplasties were attempted. In 1929, the MacAuslands wrote *"under no circumstances is arthroplasty to be considered in the ankle-joint"* and surprisingly, for today's surgeons, they emphasised avoidance of primary osteoarthritis and rheumatoid arthritis as indications for arthroplasty (MacAusland and MacAusland, 1929). While ankle arthroplasty stalled, Wiles undertook total hip replacement for severe juvenile rheumatoid arthritis (Still's disease) in 1938, modified in 1951, with low-alloy stainless steel prostheses without cement and indifferent results (Wiles, 1958). McKee accepted osteoarthritic hips for total replacement in 1951, utilising a stainless steel components but after one case changed to a vitallium Thompson femoral prosthesis and was much encouraged after 1956, despite lacking cement (McKee, 1974). Following several trials for methyl methacrylate cemented osteoarthritic hips, Charnley abandoned teflon (PTFE) for polyethylene (HMWP) cups and small high-alloy steel femoral heads (Charnley, 1961), whose results were to have a dramatic effect on joint replacement history, and prompting surgeons to consider replacement of other joints.

Thus in 1970, Gerald Lord and J.-H.Marotte (20th century) first undertook modern replacement for a postfracture arthritic ankle (Lord and Marotte, 1973) although, subsequently, rheumatoid arthritis became a prominent indicator for TAR's, some series being entirely for this diagnosis commonly complicated with bilateral ankle disability combined with tarsal ankylosis. Only in more modern times have primary or posttraumatic osteoarthritis proved the commonest indicator, in part stimulated by long-term problems following ankle fusion.

FIRST-GENERATION TOTAL ANKLE REPLACMENT

Unconstrained Prostheses

Up until this point we have emphasised the pioneering aspects of total hip replacement, for its ultimate success proved the inspirational model for other joint replacements including the ankle. Unsurprisingly, Lord and Marotte's ankle prosthesis of 1970, closely resembled a miniature hip prosthesis, by utilising a steel spherical tibial component articulating with a plastic talar component though, unlike hips, these materials were reversed (Lord and Marotte, 1973) (Figure 2).

After the talus had been completely removed, they implanted a cemented acetabular cup in the calcaneus. This procedure was performed in 25 consecutive patients and only 7 patients reported satisfaction postoperatively (Lord and Marotte, 1980). Around 12 of the 25 arthroplasties failed early, and therefore the authors did not recommend the further use of this prosthesis design (Table 4).

Table 4. Examples of two-part cemented prostheses — Unconstrained.

Model	Years in use*	Published cases	Range of: RA %	OA %	Satisfaction rate %
Lord (Lord and Marotte, 1973)	1970–1973	15	—	—	—
Smith (Dini and Bassett, 1980; Kirkup, 1985)	1972–1979	21 + 24	14–82	86–18	46–61
Newton (1982)	1973–1978	50	20	80	57
Bath & W. (Kirkup, 1990; Carlsson *et al.*, 2001)	1980–1996	25 + 72	90–100	10–0	70–39

Note: *End date approx.

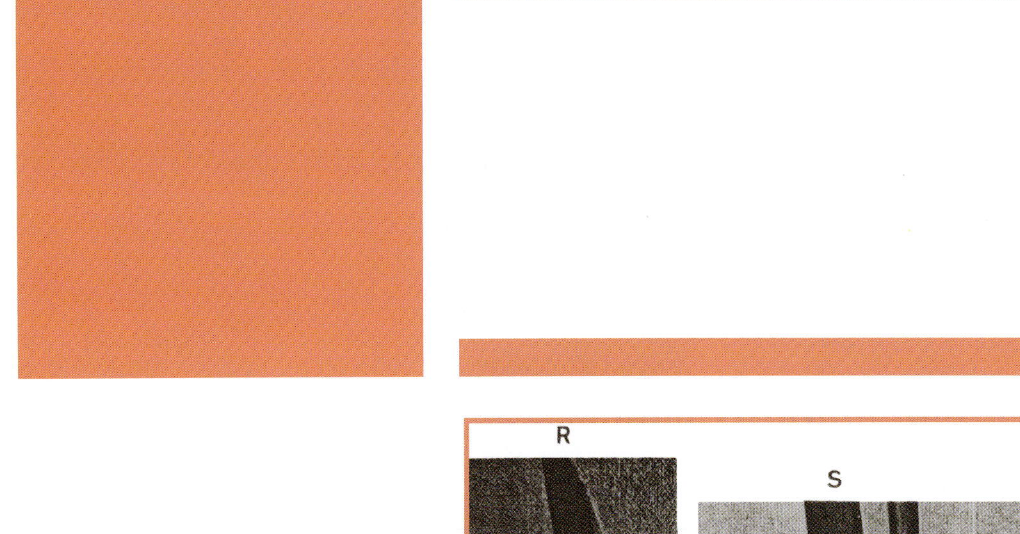

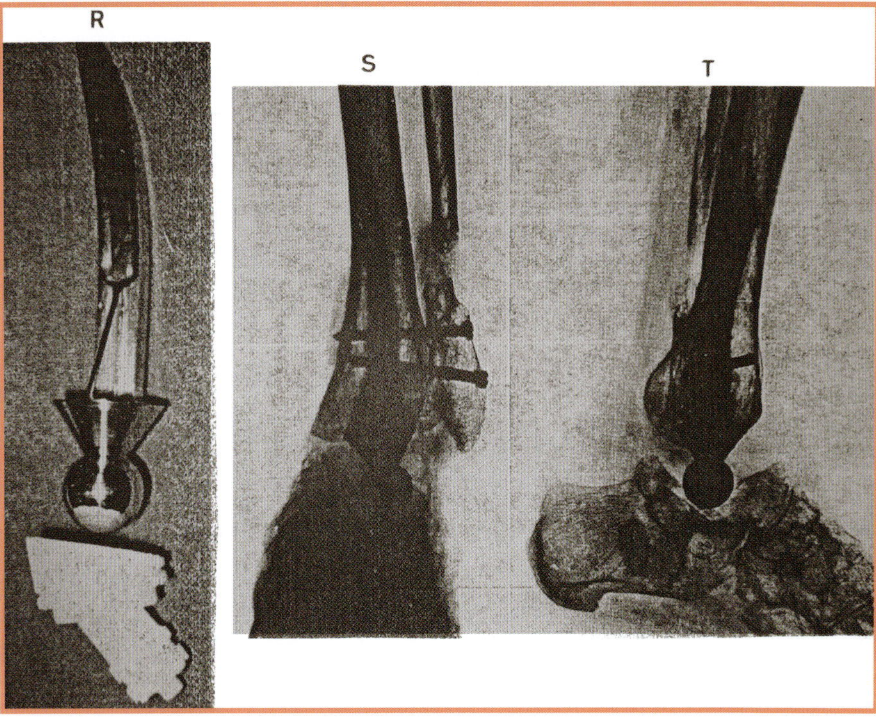

Figure 2. *(R) Lord & Marotte's total ankle of steel and polyethylene; (S) Antero-posterior X-ray showing fixation of the syndesmosis after osteotomising the fibula; (T) lateral X-ray showing the subtalar joint had been fused and the talar component went into the calcaneum (Waugh, 2012).*

The spherical concept of the hip was also evident in the Smith (Figure 3), Newton, and Bath and Wessex (Figure 4) prostheses, in expectation of providing multiaxial movement. Stimulus for choice of a sphero-centric Bath and Wessex prosthesis, in part at least, was due to observations firstly, that children with congenital tarsal fusions and spherical-shaped ankle joints developed additional compensatory tarsal movement at the ankle (Figure 5) and secondly, that some rheumatoid and Still's disease patients with spontaneous tarsal fusions, due to longstanding disease, also developed radiological evidence of spherical ankle joints.

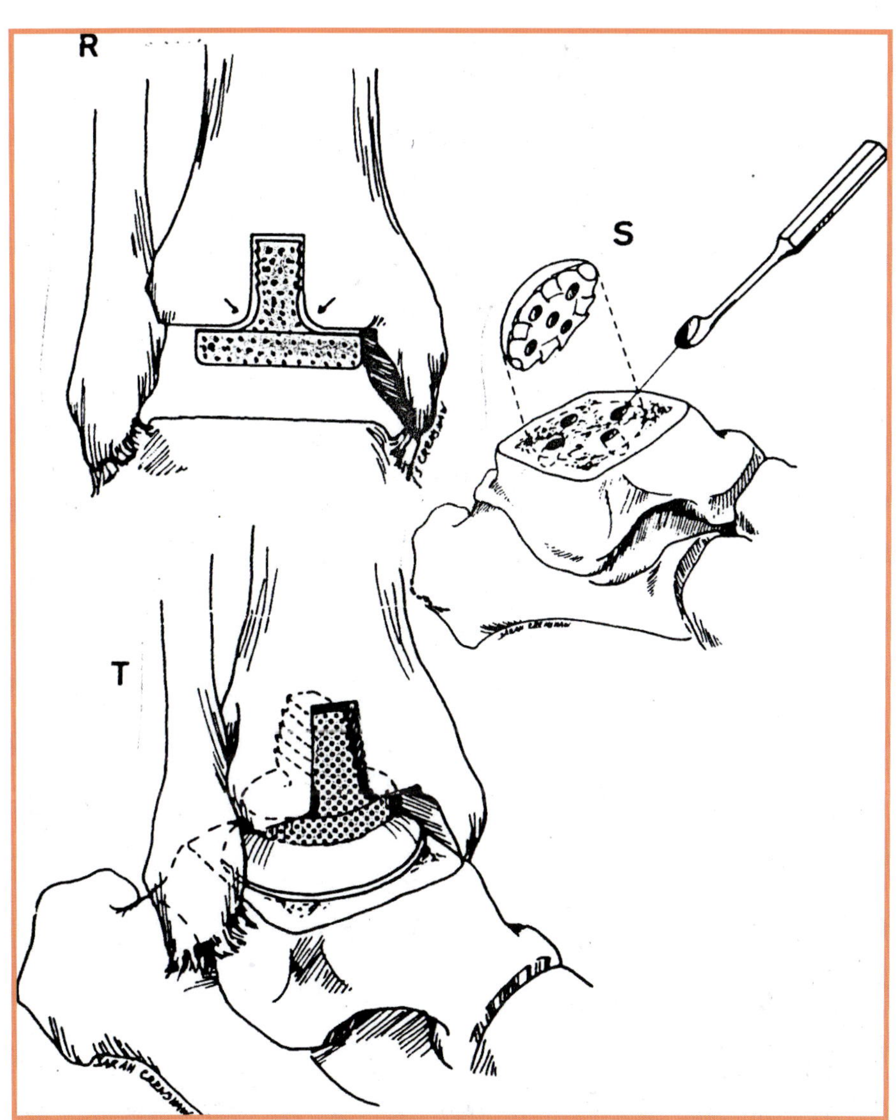

Figure 3. *Smith total ankle. (R) bone resected and tibial steel component in situ; (S) talar polyethylene component and prepared bed; (T) final position after cementation (courtesy Zimmer Orthopaedic Ltd., 1974).*

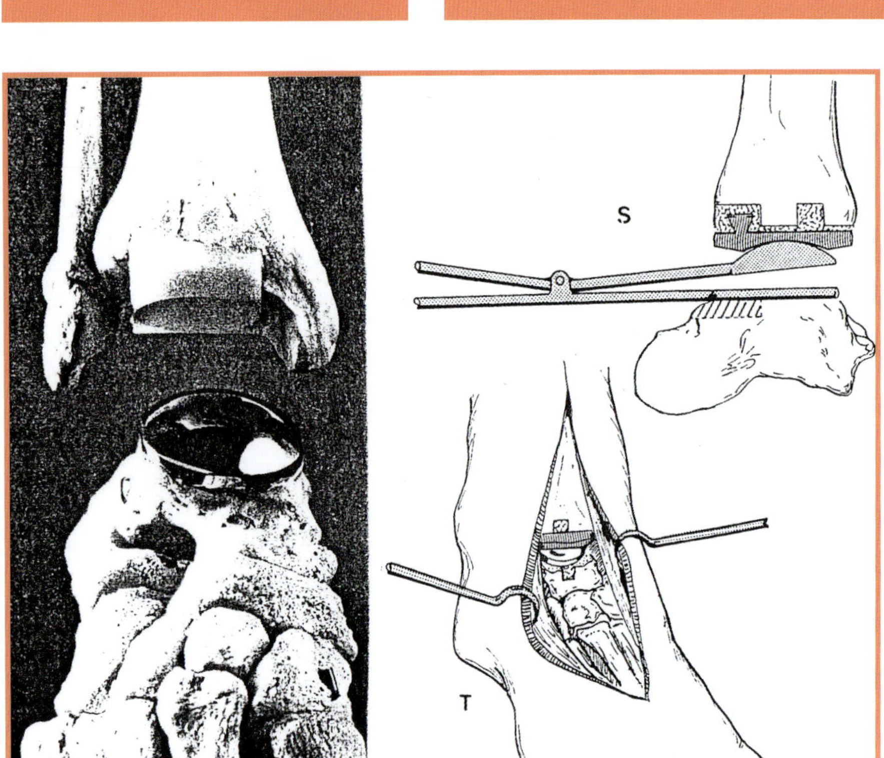

Figure 4. *R, Bath and Wessex total ankle in skeleton; S, lateral view demonstrating pressurised implantation of polyethylene tibial component; T, completed insertions before suturing (courtesy Howmedica (UK) Ltd., 1982).*

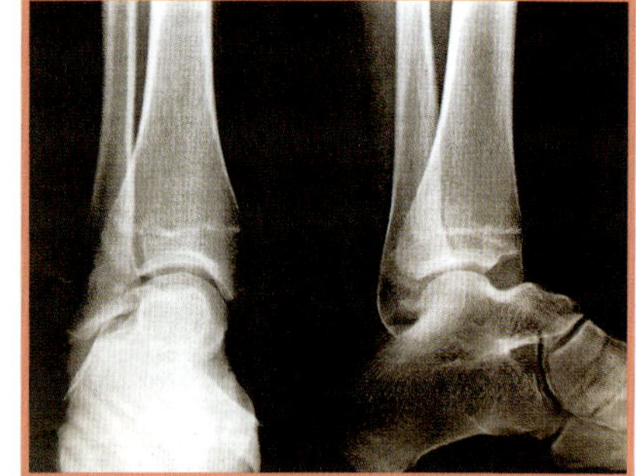

Figure 5. *X-rays of congenital tarsal fusion with sphero-centric ankle formation. (private collection of J. Kirkup).*

The Irvine Ankle TAR (Howmedica prosthesis) followed similar thinking (Waugh and Evanski, 1976), but in practice, the earliest generation of ankle prostheses did not have good results. That said, they often relieved rheumatoid patients even when radiologically they could have been loose, for their low demands were satisfied by improved mobility, enabling them to drive a car, and more importantly, rise from a chair or a lavatory seat.

Semiconstrained Prostheses

These models attempted to provide a more anatomical joint with some axial movement in addition to dorsiplantar flexion (Figures 6 and 7). Later studies demonstrated loosening and abnormal wear (Table 5).

Table 5. Examples of two-part cemented prostheses — Semiconstrained.

| Model | Years in use* | Published cases | Range of: | | Satisfaction rate (%) |
			RA (%)	OA (%)	
St Georg 1 (Smith, 1994; Buchholz *et al.*, 1973)	1973–1978	15	53	47	13
TPR (Kaukonen and Raunio, 1983; Tillman *et al.*, 1998)	1976–1996	28 + 67	100	0	93–94
STAR 1 (Kofoed and Sorensen, 1998)	1981–1985	28	52	48	—

Note: *End date approx.

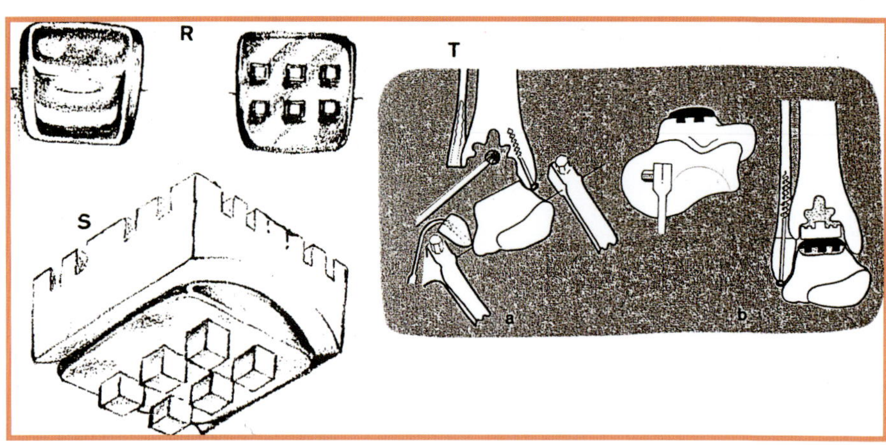

Figure 6. *St Georg total ankle, R, Superior and inferior surfaces of chrome–cobalt tibial component; S, under-surface of polyethylene talar component; T, operative approach via osteotomy of fibula, stabilisation of medial malleolus and implantation of components.*

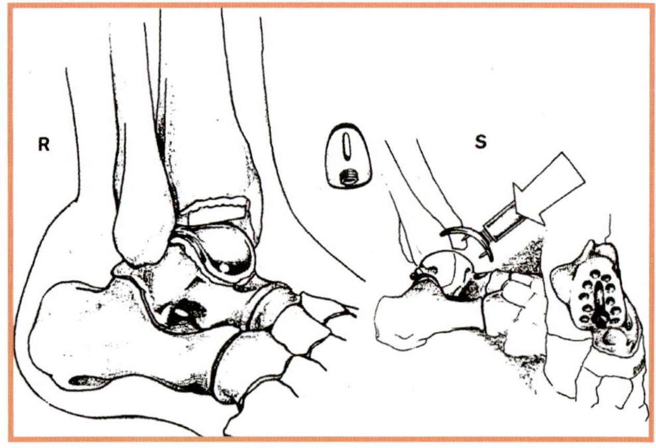

Figure 7. *TPR total ankle, R, implantation of polyethylene tibial component and either steel or chrome–cobalt talar component; S, talus template and insertion of component into well-preserved talus (courtesy Richards Manufacturing Co Inc, 1975).*

Constrained Prostheses

These aimed to reproduce the talocrural joint and its predominant dorsiplantar flexion movement (Figure 8). Constraint stressed these prostheses abnormally especially when intertarsal joints were spontaneously fused due to rheumatoid disease (Table 6).

Since the 1980s, recognition of the long-term uncertainty of the early cemented two part joints stimulated new concepts including three-part uncemented prostheses and later a rethink of an uncemented two-part joint.

Table 6. Examples of two-part cemented prostheses — Constrained.

Model years in use*	Published cases	RA (%)	Range of:		Rate (%)
			OA (%)	Satisf. n	
ICLH (Bolton-Maggs *et al.*, 1985; Helm and Stevens, 1986; Kempson *et al.*, 1975; Freeman *et al.*, 1978)	1972–1989	41 + 19	54–100	46–0	31–69
Conaxial (Wynn and Wilde, 1992)	1974–1977	36	50	50	8
Mayo 1 (Kitaoka and Patzer, 1996)	1974–1988	160	60	40	19
TNK (Takakura, 1990)	1975–1987	30	33	67	27

Note: *End date approx.

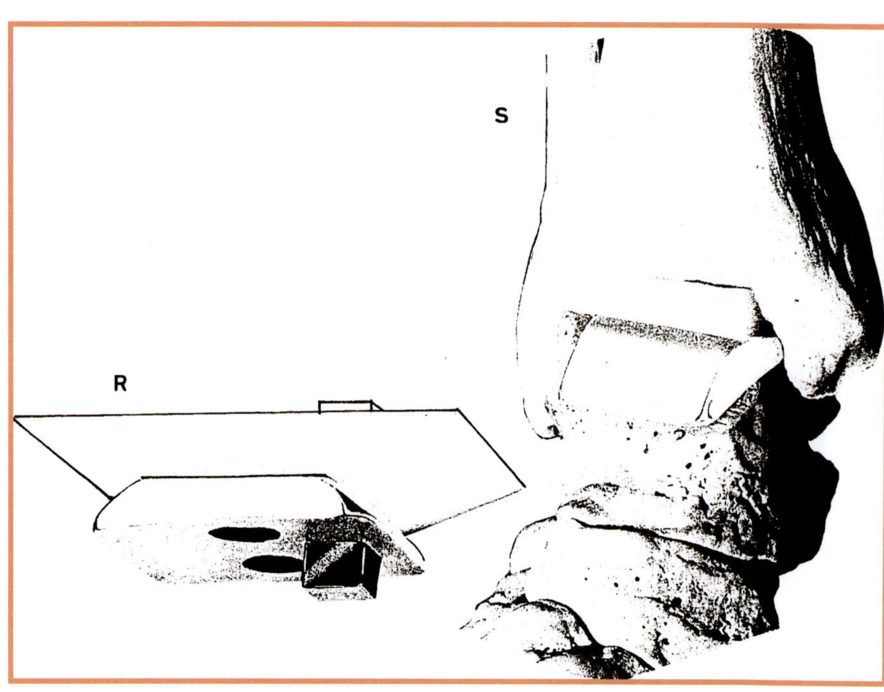

Figure 8. *R, ICLH total ankle in polyethylene and vitallium; S, their completed insertions with cement (courtesy Howmedica Management & Technical Services Ltd).*

MODERN ANKLE REPLACEMENTS

The New Jersey Experience — The BP Ankle

One of the crucial pioneers in ankle replacement technology came from the USA. In 1974, Fred Buechal, a second year resident in New Jersey, working under Dr Anthony DePalma, was very interested in joint replacement and so made a trip up to visit the Mayo Clinic and also to Cincinnati researching his ideas. He also went to see Dr Pappas a postdoc at the School of Engineering, which was the beginning of a relationship that would spark numerous orthopaedic inventions including those in the shoulder, knee, and ankle. They initially carried out anatomical surveys on animals such as pigs and sheep and in 1975 started the first human trial. Their first ankle implant was the cylindrical fixed bearing cemented New Jersey device. However, even in its first year, there were already early signs of loosening. In a quest to solve this, Fred continued his world tour with a survey of all the world's experts on ankle replacement and presented his findings in 1977 at the AOFAS residents section. Buechal and Pappas (BP) went through several iterations and refinements using spherical (1975) instead of cylindrical components, trunions (1976), shallower sulcuses (1978), and sliding cylindrical surfaces (1986) of the BP ankle replacement.

Meanwhile, across the Atlantic two British counterparts were working on ideas that would create a race to the finish line that would compete with many of the great international invention disputes like that of the invention of television.

Orthopaedic surgeon, John Goodfellow and engineer John O'Connor from Oxford in the United Kingdom, were travelling in a car on return from a conference where they first conceived the idea for a mobile bearing implant. Following a huge amount

of work they finally submitted a patent on September 14th 1994 (prosthetic knee joint device US 5871545A). This patent was not granted until 1999. In contrast, Michael Pappas (interestingly, Fred Buechel did not have his name on the patent) filed his patent on March 13th 1995 (US 5683468A), 6 months after Goodfellow and O'Connor. However, the Patent Office granted Buechal and Pappas their patent in 1997, two years earlier than the British team. The laws of patents are complex and far too detailed for the scope of this textbook, but needless to say, it provides another example of the US versus British invention controversy. The UK filed the patent first but the Americans were first to grant. This timing, however, had a significant impact on wealth creation for Buechal and Pappas later on.

In terms of clinical practice, BP moved to a three-part meniscal-bearing implant in 1978. Fred Buechal also recalls conceiving the idea for the windowing of the tibia, a concept that would become popularised by later implant designs. In addition, they produced the first implant that had a central fin on the talus; however, after experiencing subsidence they revised this into a double finned implant. The sulcus started shallow but was deepened to improve stability. Of interest, Fred Buechal replaced Joe Ascencio's ankle (Joe was the inventor of the AES ankle) in New Jersey and this lasted about 8 years but has since been revised; however, Ascencio says that at the time he used to jump up and down on a stage to show off Fred's good work.

The Scandinavian Experience — The STAR

Hakon Kofoed, a young surgeon in Denmark had his Eureka moment in 1978, aged 35. In a similar vein to Fred Buechal, he first researched the anatomy by measuring 100 skeletons in Stockholm in 1978. He found lots of variability in the sizes and angles of the articular surface of the talus. In the zoological museum in Copenhagen, he studied ankles of animals. Only the brown bear, the elephant, and the gibbon ape had a rotating fibula. Further studies revealed that also the Indonesian swamp swine had a free rotation fibula. Hans Malmgren, an engineer, had experience in making products for Volvo so Hakon asked Hans for some help. They took 316 L stainless steel and carved a talar prosthesis. The tibial component was made of polyethylene. Hans' contribution was reversing the normal tibial crest into a groove in the tibial component now corresponding to a crest on top of the talus component.

At the time, Denmark would not allow importing of pigs. Indonesian swamp swines were sent to the Veterinary High School in Stockholm. After that they were reclassified as experimental animals, and could be transported to the Royal Veterinary High School in Copenhagen. Experiments took place in the Institute for Experimental Surgery in Copenhagen. Hakon recalls the first study where they learnt at pace. All five pigs died, and this taught them that halothane was lipophilic and stored in the pigs fat and they all died in the stables after surgery, a mistake that lost them 2 years in development. Professor Arnoldi, the Chief in Copenhagen managed to find Hakon some patients. The first implant took place in 1981 and was a severe rheumatoid who had not walked for 5 years. He had a major valgus deformity but could be realigned, and they judged the case to be a success. They did four more cases in the first year. They put in 28 of the STAR1 prostheses (1981–1985) and published the results several years later in 1995 (Kofoed, 1995).

Unhappy with the technique however, he conceived the idea for a three-component device in 1985, and first implanted this in a patient in 1986. Despite this being 8 years after the three-part BP ankle was first implanted in 1978, Hakon recalls being unaware of the BP design at this point. By 1988, the founding developers entered into a deal with Waldemer Link and subsequent development was taken over by industry. The STAR three uncemented three component device came

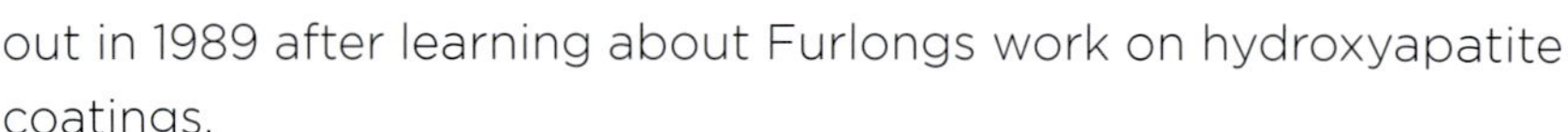

out in 1989 after learning about Furlongs work on hydroxyapatite coatings.

Ownership of the STAR prosthesis has changed hands several times over the years. Initially owned by Waldemar LINK GmbH & Co. KG, Hamburg, Germany, it was then acquired by Small Bone Innovations Inc in 2009 so that FDA approval for the first mobile bearing implant in the US could be achieved. They then sold the intellectual property to Stryker Corporation, Michigan, USA, in 2014.

When reviewing the clinical evidence, it is important to be aware that there are more than 5 different versions of the STAR ankle. Four of these have been implanted since 1981 outside of the USA. Since 1998, a fifth design was introduced into the US market which had subtle differences again.

In 1998, the base coating of the STAR implant was changed to a rough Titanium plasma so that it could be used in the USA. This is the design used in the US clinical trials for FDA approval (Mann *et al.*) and is the current design used in the USA & Canada. This is different from the current design used outside of the USA and Canada, as of 1999, which has Calcium Phosphate on top of the Titanium plasma spray (referred to as double coat).

The Agility Ankle System

Frank Alvine was an orthopaedic surgeon working in private practice in Sioux Falls, South Dakota, USA, the place he grew up in. Like many other surgeons, he was frustrated by early ankle designs and felt the answer related to poor implant integration. His thinking was that if a larger surface area could be achieved, a better result may follow. He designed the Agility TAR System and although work started on this in the late 1970s and a prototype was developed by 1983, the patent was not filed until 1992. The first patient implantation was in 1984, seemingly 8 years before the patent was filed for this prosthesis.

The Agility ankle is a semiconstrained two-component ankle prosthesis, which relied on a fusion of the distal tibiofibular joint to increase surface area for implant support and bony ingrowth (Pyevich *et al.*, 1998). The patent was granted in 1994, but before this had happened, Alvine had already entered into a long-term relationship with DePuy, a Johnson and Johnson company. The implant was cleared by the FDA as the DePuy Alvine Total Ankle Prosthesis under K920802, in December 17, 1992 and rapidly became the market leading product in the USA. Since its original introduction, the Agility went through several design modifications and in 2007, DePuy launched the Agility LP Total Ankle System, as the fourth-generation design. The design changes included a redesigned broader based talar component; the ability to mismatch component sizes; and a front loading polyethylene. The published results of medium-term outcomes of the Agility were in the main positive (Pyevich *et al.*, 1998; Knecht *et al.*, 2004; Kopp *et al.*, 2006; Cerrato and Myerson, 2008), although others published less promising results with a 5-year survival rate with reoperation defined as their end point being 54% (Spirt *et al.*, 2004). Nonetheless, the sheer technical challenges of implanting and revising the Agility, led to its demise, initially in Europe and later through the FDA approval of the STAR prosthesis and the development of newer implants, its use fell off in the USA.

The Ankle Evolutive System (AES)

Joe Ascencio, a surgeon from Nimes' story was similar to others, namely a surgeon frustrated by his use of other implants on the market. In 1994, he met Fred Buechal at AOFAS but he recalls Buechal being too busy working on the knee to take interest in Joe's ideas. In hindsight, we know that is only half the story but this story is being written as though it is recalled through the inventors'

eyes. Joe came back to Nimes where he had an established private practice.

He met an engineer and after initial struggles to find a manufacturer he managed to obtain an investor and also get Trans-Systems in France to manufacture. Patents were filed and trials took place initially in cadavers. The product hit the market in 1999, soon after the Salto.

The Salto and STAR were the main products on the market at the time. The AES grew a large share of the market but in 2009 concerns were raised in relation to the presence of periprosthetic cysts (Besse *et al.*, 2009) and in July 2012, the MHRA (Medicines and Healthcare products Regulatory Authority) in Europe issued a medical device alert due to higher than expected frequency of osteolytic lesions in patients implanted with the AES implants. Although the AES is no longer on the market, between 2002 and 2009, there were approximately 450 of these devices implanted within the UK. A much larger number across Europe, the exact amount is unknown however.

The Box Ankle — The Bologna–Oxford Experience

In the early 1990's, Fabio Catani, a surgeon from Bologna, Italy, heard engineer John O'Connor from Oxford, speak at a conference and asked him afterwards if they could collaborate on an ankle project. John O'Connor jested "I would, but I'm not actually sure where in the body the ankle lies…".

In 1994, Catani and his colleague, Professor Sandro Giannini went to Oxford to see John O'Connor where a swap was made for one of the Oxford fellows to go to Bologna in return for a young

Italian researcher, Alberto Leardini to travel to Oxford. Leardini stayed in Oxford from 1995 to 2000 carrying out his PhD in ankle biomechanics. In 1999, they collectively filed a patent which was not published until 2006 (Prosthesis device for the ankle articulation US 20060020345 A1) — This gave them intellectual property on a curved tibial surface. With the granted patent, they approached Cremascoli to develop the implant whose concept was that it was the first implant that was capable of retaining ligamentous tension.

The first components were produced using rapid prototyping made of a form of plaster but when implanted into a cadaver in 1999. The result was a stiff ankle whose movement did not replicate their mathematical model. Fabio Catani recalls adding a drop of olive oil to the construct and it moved beautifully demonstrating that friction was too high and with some tweaks they felt they were on to something. The company, Cremascoli, however, soon sold to Wright who had earlier bought the distribution rights for the BP ankle and so the BOX ankle was dropped. Eventually, it was taken on by Mike Tooke's engineering and distribution company, Finsbury in 2002. At that stage, a meeting took place to decide on the name for the Oxford and Bologna collaboration. The "Bol-Ox" ankle was coined by the Italians, much to John O'Connor's amusement. He politely suggested that the team should consider the "Ox-Bol" although the team settled on the BOX ankle which is a glorious story of how language barriers can interfere with branding. The BOX ankle was first implanted in July 2003. Finsbury later sold out to DePuy and the BOX implant moved hands to Matt Ortho, which was Finbury's Founder, Mike Tuke's new company once he had sold on Finsbury. The BOX was one of the most popular implants used in the UK but latterly has lost some of its market share to newer implants (NJR Annual Reports 2016–2019).

The SALTO and SALTO-Talaris

In 1995, DePuy, a Johnson & Johnson company, stopped selling the BP in France due to cost pressures. Bonin had been doing the STAR ankle and in 1995 a Dutch company, Tornier approached Bonin & Columbier to develop an ankle replacement of their own. The two involved Thierry Judet at the Hospital Raymon in Paris, because he had extensive experience in hips and knees along with his father's track record of joint development. Judet's experience at that point involved removal and revision of many ankle replacements. Judet recalls having already taken out Lord, ICLH, Ramses, Agility, AES, STAR & Integra implants (personal communication). The three design surgeons met with the engineers and the result was the Salto ankle, first implanted in 1997. Their key objective was reproducibility and they focused heavily on instrumentation, something that they felt BP and STAR had been lacking.

The name SALTO was decided by the company. In July 2006, Warburg Pincus acquired Tornier from Alain Tornier, the company's former President and owner, and the US market became a key focus. Shortly afterwards a decision was made to modify the three component European Salto implant by fixing the mobile bearing onto the tibial component to create a two part fixed bearing design subsequently to be called the Salto Talaris ankle. The Salto-Talaris received a 510k premarket approval in February 2009. To achieve this approval, the French development team carried out some studies. One was a kinematic study using dynamic X-rays on patients walking and the other was a non-randomised retrospective review comparing their fixed with mobile bearing implants (Leszko *et al.*, 2008; Gaudot *et al.*, 2014). They concluded that there was little advantage of the mobile bearing and the company's focus on the US market grew. In 2015, Wright Medical Technology merged with Tornier which meant a change in direction for the Salto-Talaris. Because Wright Medical had their own ankle system, the rights to the Salto-Talaris in the USA were sold to Integra LifeSciences.

The Hintegra Prosthesis

Beat Hintermann, a Swiss Orthopaedic surgeon, qualified from Bern's University Medical School and underwent specialist orthopaedic training in Switzerland before completing a research fellowship in biomechanics in Calgary, Canada, as well as other travelling fellowships. He returned to Switzerland to set up practice in Kantonsspital in Liestal where he started doing TAR in 1995 using the STAR ankle. After the first 60 cases, he realised that many of his complications were unrelated to his learning curve. He felt there were issues especially with the instrumentation and so contacted the manufacturer, LINK several times but felt they were not interested in listening to him and so he stopped doing ankles for 1 year in 1998 to find a better solution (personal communication). After joining a group of experts set up by a different company, NewDEAL® SA (Lyon, France), he developed renewed interest in TAR and a product called the HINTEGRA Ankle. In May 2000 he started using the HINTEGRA TAR, but since his colleagues did very few of them, Hintermann became the lead for the Hintegra TAR. Also involved were Dr Dereymaeker (Pellenberg, Belgium); Dr Viladot (Barcelona, Spain); and Dr Diebold (Maxeville, France). Their criteria were anatomical surfaces with optimal bony support. It was the first implant on the market with a conical-shaped talus. It had a greater contact area between implant and insert than the STAR ankle and did not allow inversion or eversion in order to afford frontal plane stability.

The HINTEGRA® Total Ankle Prosthesis is a non-constrained, three-component system. The initial design had screw fixation but since 2002 the talar implant screws were stopped. However, from 2002 to about 2007 the tibial plate had an anterior lip through which screws were inserted into the tibia. After 2007, the anterior lip remained but they discouraged the use of screws and the implant was modified to have sharp pegs for tibial fixation.

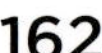

The HINTEGRA® went through several iterations. The first generation in 2001 was single coated (05/2000–03/2001). The second generation was a double-coated titanium implant (04/2001–09/2002), and the third generation was a pegged talus double-coated titanium (10/200) implant. In 2004, Integra LifeSciences (Plainsboro, NJ) acquired Newdeal Technologies and thus became the distributor for the Hintegra prosthesis. Despite, positive medium-term results (Barg *et al.*, 2013; Nery *et al.*, 2015), in 2016, Integra stopped distributing the Hintegra implant and ownership moved to DTMedtech LLC.

DTMedtech LLC, working with the inventor, later received FDA premarket approval for a two-component version, entitled the H2. DT Medtech LLC then used 18 years of non-US data of their three-component design to obtain FDA premarket approval of the H3 prosthesis, which was granted in June 2019. The Indications for Use (IFU) differ for the H2 and H3 depending on whether it is sold in the USA or outside of the USA.

The Lateral Approach Ankle

The lateral approach to the ankle has been explored on several occasions.

In the 1980s, Dr. Rudigier working with Eska Medical Gmbh & Co in Germany developed the ESKA TAR implanted through the lateral approach with fibular osteotomy, or in special cases, a medial malleolar approach was used for component implantation (Rudigier *et al.*, 2001). The ESKA ankle was never popularised.

Similarly in 2006, Kinetikos Medical inc remarkably obtained 510k FDA clearance for the Eclipse Total Ankle Implant on the basis that it was substantially equivalent to the Agility ankle even though it was a completely different implant and was implanted from the lateral (or medial) approach in contrast to the anteriorly implanted predicate. Kinetikos was acquired by Integra Lifesciences prior to the FDA clearance and small numbers of the Eclipse were implanted, but for a host of reasons the implant was shelved and there were no published outcome data.

To demonstrate the way innovation is like rain and tends to occur at the same time in different places, in 1999, a US surgeon from Baltimore, Lou Schon, began to explore the lateral approach once more. In 2001, Schon, alongside his engineer Brent Parks, and Chris Chiodo, his fellow at the time, designed a jig to allow resection of the curved surface of the talus and tibia from the lateral side, using a curved oscillating saw and curved chisels (personal communication). The jig was used for both donors and recipients. Later on, Schon decided to develop this concept into an ankle replacement, and started to involve his next round of fellows, Johnny Lau and Steven Herbst. They jointly wrote a patent in or around 2003, and decided to start discussions with industry.

Meanwhile, roughly in the same timeframe, US surgeons, Jonathan Deland, Charles Saltzman and Al Bernstein were heavily involved in ankle research. They approached American industry giant, Zimmer, who funded a feasibility study to develop a design that replicated the kinematics of the ankle. Saltzman was working at the University of Iowa at that time, and in 2001, the University entered into contract to develop the implant and a method for implantation. Saltzman worked with Tom Baer and Yuki Tochigi in their labs over the next couple of years. Their findings were presented to Zimmer in 2003, who identified that Schon *et al.*'s patent potentially blocked their freedom to operate (personal communication).

When Schon et al. approached Zimmer, it immediately became clear that the two groups had similar ideas and so a collaboration was born that formed the development team to develop the lateral

approach ankle, and after another 2 years had the final design locked. Towards the end of the development, another patent filed by Sandro Giannini from Bologna needed to be brought into the fold, and so Giannini, joined the team. It took another 7 years before the first implant was performed, known as the Zimmer® Trabecular Metal™ Total Ankle implant. More than 5000 have been performed since and the first early results were submitted for publication in 2017 (Barg *et al.*, 2018).

The INBONE

In 2005, Dr Mark Reiley, an orthopaedic surgeon from California, brought the novel INBONE ankle replacement to the market. He filed a provision patent in March 2005, although due to nuances in patent law, the final patent was only published in July 2017 (US2017189198 (A1)). Mark had gained experience in business from his previous involvement in Kyphon, where he had been involved as one of the original inventors behind kyphoplasty (US6716216 (B1)) in the late 1990s which was a huge commercial success and later sold to Medtronic for billions of dollars. He used his experience to set up INBONE® Technologies which had several other patented products and his ankle replacement was being trialled by several surgeons known to Mark including Duke Health in North Carolina. INBONE® Technologies was acquired by Wright Medical in 2008. The INBONE®, was the first ankle system to use intramedullary guidance and pegs inserted through the joint to create a stem rather than through an anterior cortical window. The team at Wright had also acquired a European implant known as the CCI® (inventor Kees Doets) but as an American company with an eye on the US market, they ended up developing a new implant from scratch that involved many of the leading key opinion leaders in the US. The new development team led by Wright Medical's engineering team, went on to develop what was later to become the market leading product the Infinity Total Ankle System®, and that coupled with the INBONE® and a later revision solution, known as Invision®, were to become a more complete primary and revision solution. This system rapidly gained global market dominance and is proving to become a formidable force in ankle replacement history.

The Future

From 2010 onwards, many new innovations and implants came to the fore including the use of Patient-Specific Instrumentation (PSI) as well as improved revision instrumentation to get us to where we are today. Exciting developments such as robotic ankles, custom prostheses and subtalar joint replacements are ongoing.

What is clear is that the evolution from the earliest designs to modern thinking has involved a patchwork quilt of ideas and innovations from several different countries and individuals, and because much of this was prior to the Internet generation, often the inventors lacked any awareness of similar ideas happening simultaneously elsewhere. Indeed two of the godfather's of ankle replacement, Hakon Kofoed and Fred Buechal, independent of each other went on to develop a mobile bearing ankle implant and it is said that only years later in 1994 did they first meet, in Basel where they were invited to go head to head to discuss tibial peg's versus tibial stems.

Ultimately, truly innovative ideas from the real pioneers of ankle replacement like Hakon Kofoed, Fred Buechal, Frank Alvine, and Mark Reiley, led to an explosion of "me-too" ideas that are are known as incremental improvements, mainly around instrumentation.

Most striking is, that like most innovations in orthopaedics, iterations and invention invariably result from surgeon frustration with existing

technology or with industry behaviour. Indeed, many surgeons that went onto develop their own implants were frustrated by the performance of the implants they were using. Surgeons like Ascencio, Hintermann, Rippstein, Wood, and many others are all examples of this, each approaching industry with better ways of doing things, but on rejection decided to do it alone. This is unlikely to ever change nor is the fact that the best ideas only come to fruition when the surgeon meets the engineer. That coupled with drive, determination and dedication to improve patient care, will mean that innovations in ankle replacement are likely to continue for many years.

REFERENCES

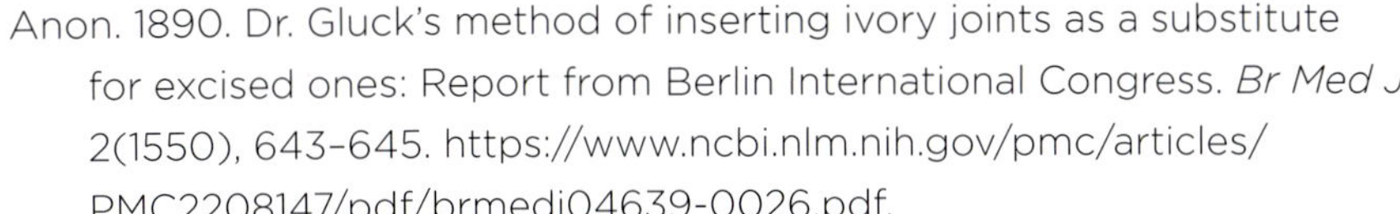

Anon. 1890. Dr. Gluck's method of inserting ivory joints as a substitute for excised ones: Report from Berlin International Congress. *Br Med J*, 2(1550), 643–645. https://www.ncbi.nlm.nih.gov/pmc/articles/PMC2208147/pdf/brmedj04639-0026.pdf.

Baer, W. S. 1918. Arthroplasty with the aid of animal membrane. *J Bone Joint Surg*, 2(3), 171–199.

Barg, A., Bettin, C. C., Burstein, A. H., Saltzman, C. L. & Gililland, J. 2018. Early clinical and radiographic outcomes of trabecular metal total ankle replacement using a transfibular approach. *J Bone Joint Surg Am*. 100(6), 505–515. doi: 10.2106/JBJS.17.00018.

Barg, A., Zwicky, L., Knupp, M., Henninger, H. B. & Hintermann, B. 2013. Hintegra total ankle replacement: Survivorship analysis in 684 patients. *J Bone Joint Surg Am,* 95(13), 1175–1183.

Bergman, E. 1890. Methode aseptique suivie a la clinique de Berlin. *Rev Chir*, 10, 844–845.

Besse, J. L., Brito, N. & Lienhart, C. 2009. Clinical evaluation and radiographic assessment of bone lysis of the AES total ankle replacement. *Foot Ankle Int*, 30(10), 964–975.

Bick, E. M. 1948. *Source Book of Orthopaedics*, Williams & Wilkins, Baltimore.

Bolton-Maggs, B. G., Sudlow R. A. & Freeman M. A. 1985. Total ankle arthroplasty. A long-term review of the London Hospital experience. *J Bone Joint Surg Br*, 67(5), 785–790.

Boutin, P. 1972. Total arthroplasty of the hip by fritted aluminum prosthesis. Experimental study and 1st clinical applications. *Rev Chir Orthop Reparatrice Appar Mot*, 58(3), 229–246.

Buchholz, H. W., Engelbrecht, E. & Siegel, A. 1973. Complete ankle joint endoprosthesis type "St. Georg". *Der Chirurg Zeitschrift fur alle Gebiete der operativen Medizen*, 44(5), 241–244.

Carlsson Å. S., Henricson, A., Linder, L., Nilsson, J. Å. & Redlund-Johnell, I. 2001. A 10-year survival analysis of 69 Bath and Wessex ankle replacements. *Foot Ankle Surg*, 7(1), 39–44.

Cerrato, R. & Myerson, M. S. 2008. Total ankle replacement: The Agility LP prosthesis. *Foot Ankle Clin*, 13(3), 485–494, ix.

Charnley, J. 1961. Arthroplasty of the hip: A new operation. *The Lancet*, 277(7187), 1129–1132.

Charnley, J. 1964a. A sterile-air operating theatre enclosure. *Br J Surg*, 51, 195–202.

Charnley, J. 1964b. A clean-air operating enclosure. *Br J Surg*, 51(3), 202–205.

Cooper, A. 1844. *A Treatise on Dislocations and Fractures of the Joints,* Lea & Blanchard, Philadelphia, until 1851.

Cushing, H. 1904. Pneumatic tourniquets with special referrence to their use in craniotomies. *Med News*, 84, 557.

Dini, A. A. & Bassett, F. H. 1980. Evaluation of the early result of Smith total ankle replacement. *Clin Orthop Relat Res,* 146, 228–230.

Domagk, G. 1935. Ein beitrag zur chemotherapie der bakteriellen infektionen. *DMW — Dtsch Med Wochenschr*, 61(07), 250–253.

Duncum, B. M. 1947. *The Development of Inhalation Anaesthesia,* Oxford Univeristy Press, London.

Fleming, A. 1929. On the antibacterial action of cultures of a penicillium, with special reference to their use in the isolation of *B. influenzae. Br J Exp Pathol*, 10(3), 226.

Foster, W. D. 1970a. *A History of Medical Bacteriology and Immunology,* Butterworth-Heinemann, Oxford, UK.

Foster, W. D. 1970b. *A Short History of Clinical Pathology*, Livingstone, Edinburgh.

Freeman, M. A. R., Kempson, G. E., Tuke, M. A. & Samuelson, K. M. 1978. Total replacement of the ankle with the ICLH prosthesis. *Int Orthop,* 2(4), 327–331.

Gaudot, F., Colombier, J. A., Bonnin, M. & Judet, T. 2014. A controlled, comparative study of a fixed-bearing versus mobile-bearing ankle arthroplasty. *Foot Ankle Int,* 35(2), 131–140.

Gluck, T. 1890. Referat uber die durch das monderne chirurgische experiment gewonnenen positiven resultate, betreffend die naht und den ersatz von defecten hcherer gewebe, sowie uber die verwerthung vesorbirbarer und lebendiger tampons in der chirurgie. *Arch Klinische Chirurgie*, 41, 187–239.

Groves, E. W. H. 1923. Arthroplasty. *Br J Surg*, 11(2), 234–250.

Groves, E. W. H. 1927. Some contributions to the reconstructive surgery of the hip. *Br J Surg*, 14(55), 486–517.

Hay, S. M. & Smith, T. W. D. 1994. Total ankle arthroplasty: A long-term review. *The Foot,* 4(1), 1–5.

Helm, R. & Stevens, J. 1986. Long-term results of total ankle replacement. *The J Arthroplasty*, 1(4), 271–277.

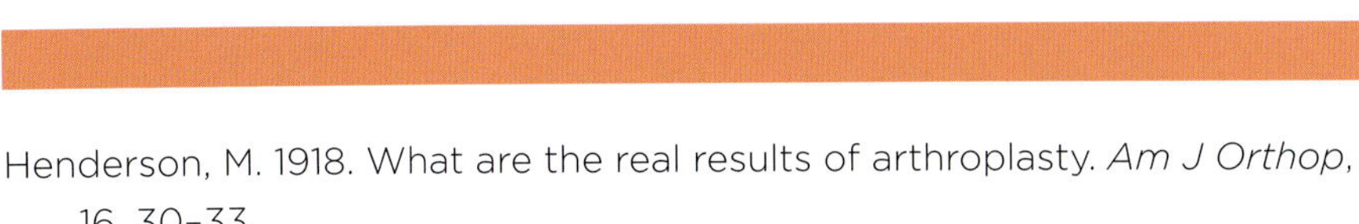

Henderson, M. 1918. What are the real results of arthroplasty. *Am J Orthop*, 16, 30–33.

Judet, J. & Judet, R. 1949. Essais de reconstruction prothétique de la hanche après résection de la tête fémorale. *J Chir*, 65, 17–24.

Kaukonen, J. P. & Raunio, P. 1983. Total ankle replacement in rheumatoid arthritis: A preliminary review of 28 arthroplasties in 24 patients. *Ann Chir Gynaecol*, 72(4), 196–199.

Kempson, G. E., Freeman, M. A. & Tuke, M. A. 1975. Engineering considerations in the design of an ankle joint. *Biomed Eng*, 10(5), 166–171, 80.

Kirkup, J. 1985. Richard Smith ankle arthroplasty. *J R Soc Med*, 78(4), 301–304.

Kirkup, J. 1990. Rheumatoid arthritis and ankle surgery. *Ann Rheum Dis*, 49 Suppl 2, 837–844.

Kitaoka, H. B. & Patzer, G. L. 1996. Clinical results of the Mayo total ankle arthroplasty. *J Bone Joint Surg Am*, 78(11), 1658–1664.

Knecht, S. I., Estin, M., Callaghan, J. J., Zimmerman, M. B., Alliman, K. J. & Alvine, F. G., *et al.* 2004. The Agility total ankle arthroplasty. Seven to sixteen-year follow-up. *J Bone Joint Surg Am*, 86-a(6), 1161–1171.

Kofoed, H. & Sorensen, T. S. 1998. Ankle arthroplasty for rheumatoid arthritis and osteoarthritis: Prospective long-term study of cemented replacements. *J Bone Joint Surg Br*, 80(2), 328–332.

Kofoed, H. 1995. Cylindrical cemented ankle arthroplasty: A prospective series with long-term follow-up. *Foot Ankle Int*, 16(8), 474–479.

Kopp, F. J., Patel, M. M., Deland, J. T. & O'Malley, M. J. 2006. Total ankle arthroplasty with the Agility prosthesis: Clinical and radiographic evaluation. *Foot Ankle Int*, 27(2), 97–103.

Le Vay, D. 1990. *The History of Orthopaedics: An Account of The Study And Practice of Orthopaedics From The Earliest Times To The Modern Era*, Parthenon Publishing, Nashville TN.

Leszko, F., Komistek, R. D., Mahfouz, M. R., Ratron, Y. A., Judet, T. & Bonnin, M., *et al.* 2008. In vivo kinematics of the salto total ankle prosthesis. *Foot Ankle Int,* 29(11), 1117–1125.

Leventhal, G. S. 1957. Titanium for femoral head prosthesis. *Am J Surg*, 94(5), 735–740.

Lexer, E. 1908. Substitution of whole or half joints from freshly amputated extremities by free plastic operation. *Surg Gynecol Obstet*, 6, 601–607.

Lister, J. 1867. On the antiseptic principle in the practice of surgery. *The Lancet*, 90(2299), 353–356.

Lord, G. & Marotte, J. H. 1973. Prothese total de cheville: Technique et premier resultats. *Rev Chir Orthop Reparatrice Appar Mot,* 59, 139–151.

Lord, G. & Marotte, J. H. 1980. Total ankle replacement (author's transl). *Rev Chir Orthop Reparatrice Appar Mot,* 66(8), 527–530.

MacAusland, W. A. & MacAusland, A. R. 1929. T*he Mobilisation of Joints by Arthroplasty*, Lea & Febiger, Philadelphia.

McKee, G. 1974. The Norwich method of total hip replacement: Development and main indications. *Ann R Coll Surg Engl*, 54(2), 53–62.

Moore, A. T. & Bohlman, H. R. 1943. Metal hip joint: A case report. *J Bone Joint Surg*, 25(3), 688–692.

Moore, A. T. 1952. Metal hip joint: A new self-locking vitallium prosthesis. *South Med J,* 45(11), 1015.

Moreau, P. 1803. *Observations pratiques relatives à la résection des articulations affectées de carie: pr" sentée et soutenue à l'Ecole de Médecine de parsi, le 30 floréal en XI*, Paris. https://archive.org/details/b22408757/page/10.

Muir, D. C., Amendola, A. & Saltzman, C. L. 2002. Forty-year outcome of ankle "cup" arthroplasty for post-traumatic arthritis. *The Iowa Orthop J*, 22, 99–102.

Murphy, J. B. 1912. The surgical clinics of John B. Murphy, M.D. at Mercy Hospital, Chicago. Clinics of John B Murphy, MD at Mercy Hospital, Chicago. Vol. 1(4), pp. 243–255.

Nery, C., Fernandes, T. D., Ressio, C., Fuchs, M. L., Godoy Santos, A. L. & Ortiz, R. T. 2015. Total ankle arthroplasty: Brazilian experience with the hintegra prosthesis. *Rev Bras Ortop*, 45(1), 92–100.

Newton, S. E. 1982. Total ankle arthroplasty. Clinical study of fifty cases. *J Bone Joint Surg A*, 64A(1), 104–111.

Ollier, L. X. É. L. & Ollier, L. 1885. *Traité des résections et des opérations conservatrices qu'on peut pratiquer sur le système osseux*: G. Masson.

Peltier, L. F. 1890. *Orthopedics: A History and Iconography*, Norman Publishing.

Petit, J.-L. 1741. D'un nouvel instrument de chirurgie. *Hist Acad R Sci*, 199–202.

Pyevich, M. T., Saltzman, C. L., Callaghan, J. J. & Alvine, F. G. 1998. Total ankle arthroplasty: A unique design. Two to twelve-year follow-up. *J Bone Joint Surg Am*, 80(10), 1410–1420.

Redard, P. 1888. De la désinfection des instruments chirurgicaux et les objets de pansement. *Rev Chir*, 8, 360–494.

Röntgen, W. 1895. *Über eine neue Art von Strahlen: Vorläufige Mitteilung. Sitzungsber Phys Med Gesell*.

Rudigier, J., Grundei, H. & Menzinger, F. 2001. Prosthetic replacement of the ankle in posttraumatic arthrosis: 10-year experience with the cementless ESKA ankle prosthesis. *Eur J Trauma*, 27, 66–74.

Smith-Petersen, M. N. 1939. Arthroplasty of the hip: A new method. *J Bone Joint Surg*, 21(2), 269–288.

Spirt, A. A., Assal, M. & Hansen, S. T. Jr. 2004. Complications and failure after total ankle arthroplasty. *J Bone Joint Surg Am*, 86-a(6), 1172–1178.

Takakura, Y., Tanaka, Y., Sugimoto, K., Tamai, S. & Masuhara, K. 1990. Ankle arthroplasty. A comparative study of cemented metal and uncemented ceramic prostheses. *Clin Orthop Relat Res*, (252), 209–216.

Tillmann, K., Schirp, M., Schaar, B. & Fink, B. 1998. Cemented and uncemented ankle endoprosthesis: Clinical and pedobarographic results. In H. Kofoed, (ed.), *Current Status of Ankle Arthroplasty*, Springer, Berlin, pp. 22–25.

Todd, A. H. 1923. Arthroplasty. *Br J Surg*, 11, 319–326.

Verneuil, A. S. 1860. De la creation d'une fausse articulation par section ou resection partielle de l'os l'ankylose vraie ou fausse de la machoire inferieure. *Arch Gen Med*, 15, 174–195.

Waugh, T. R. & Evanski, P. M. 1976. Irvine ankle arthroplasty: Prosthetic design and surgical technique. *Clin Orthop Relat Res*, 114, 180–184.

Waugh, W. 2012. *John Charnley: The Man and The Hip,* Springer Science & Business Media, Berlin, Germany.

Wiles, P. 1958. The surgery of the osteo-arthritic hip. *Br J Surg*, 45(193), 488–497.

Wynn, A. H. & Wilde, A. H. 1992. Long-term follow-up of the Conaxial (Beck-Steffee) total ankle arthroplasty. *Foot Ankle,* 13(6), 303–306.

TOTAL ANKLE REPLACEMENT DESIGNS

P. H. Cooke, A. J. Goldberg, A.-A. Najefi, A. Navi,
A. Ramasamy and R. Zaidi

AKILE ANKLE REPLACEMENT

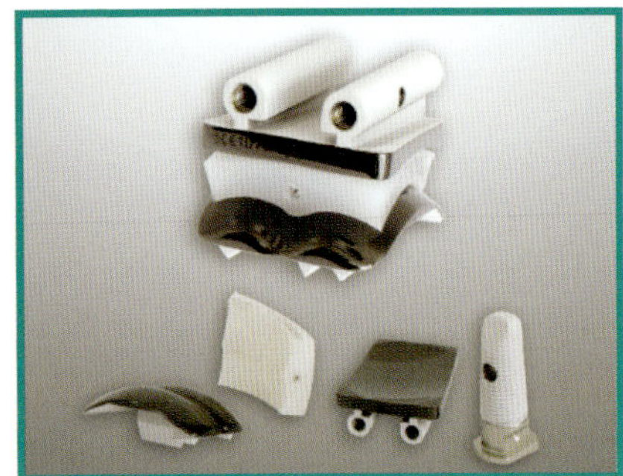

Manufacturer	I.CERAM, LIMOGES, FRANCE
Inspiration behind name	N/A
Surgeon inventor/ designer(s)	Prof Chauveaux, Dr Laffenetre, Dr Lucas, Dr Toullec, France
FDA approved, date	N/A
CE mark, date	1995
First operation date	1995
Number implanted to date	Unknown
Generation	Third
Type	Three component mobile bearing implant

Evidence	
Hernandez *et al.* (2013) *Designer series*	Designers reviewed outcomes and CT scans for 68 new generation implants. Average follow-up of 81 months, minimum 36 months. 5-year survivorship 79.4% for in situ implants, and 62% for revision-free implants. AOFAS score improved from an average of 33.7 to 77.1. CT assessment found type A cysts <200 mm^2 close to the components of the tibia (50%) and talus (52%).

	Material	Fixation	Sided
Tibial component	Stainless steel: M30NW.	Cemented or uncemented. Uncemented bone–implant interface is an alumina coating. Surfaces in contact with the polyethylene are coated with a diamond-like carbon material to reduce the coefficient of friction (Carbioceram®). Optional tibial locking keel.	No
Talar component	Stainless steel: M30NW.	Cemented or uncemented. Uncemented bone–implant interface is an alumina coating. Surfaces in contact with the polyethylene are coated with a diamond-like carbon material to reduce the coefficient of friction (Carbioceram®). Trochlea-spherical talar dome.	No
Insert	High density polyethylene dual curvature.		

History of Implant

First generation released in 1995. Second generation released in 2005 with highly cross-linked polyethylene and ceramic-coated bearing surfaces.

Design Rationale

Double curvature of the polyethylene allows movement along two planes. Large contact surface area between components. All components are compatible with every other size of another component. Modular components allow use of cement or tibial keel as required.

Technique

Anterior approach with tibial bone window if keel used.

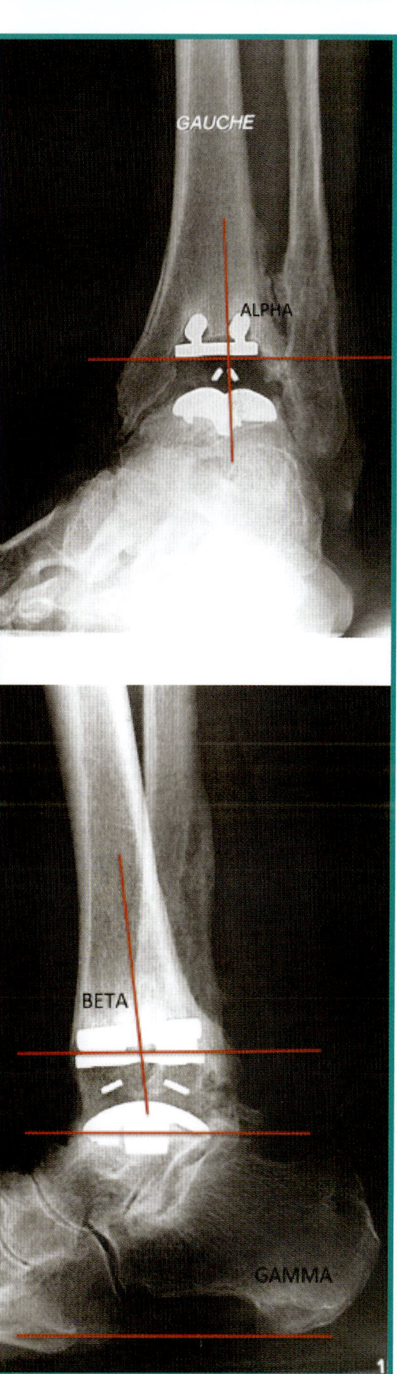

ALPHA ANKLE REPLACEMENT (TRIPLE A)

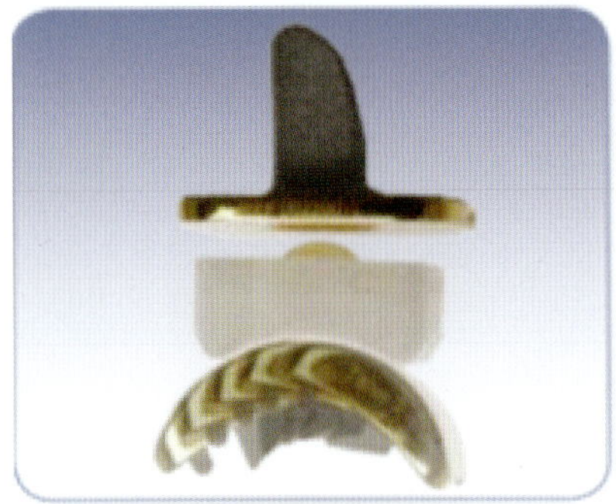

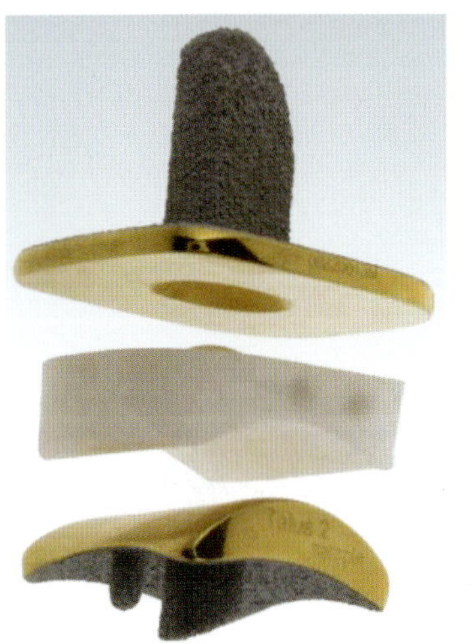

Photo — oblique and side view.

Manufacturer	**Implantcast GmbH / Alphanorm**
Inspiration behind name	Alpha Ankle Arthroplasty (Triple A)
Surgeon designer(s)	Univ.Doz.Dr. Ernst Orthner Univ.Prof.Dr. Michael Fellinger Prim.Dr. Robert Siorpaes
FDA approved, date	N/A
CE mark, date	1996
First operation date	1996
Number implanted to date	First implanted 2008. More than 1000 implanted
Generation	Third
Type	Three-component semi-constrained mobile bearing design

Evidence	
No evidence available	No published outcome data available at the time of publication.

	Material	Fixation	Sided
Tibial component	Cobalt chrome alloy with a titanium nitride plasma spray porous coating, covered with the Bonit® Biphasic Calcium Phosphate coating.	Uncemented.	No
Talar component	Cobalt chrome alloy with a titanium nitride plasma spray porous coating, covered with the Bonit® Biphasic Calcium Phosphate coating.	Uncemented.	No
Insert	A longitudinal oval depression in the tibial component and a corresponding bump on the polyethylene meniscus provides for semi-constrained rotation and anterior translation between tibial component and the bearing.		

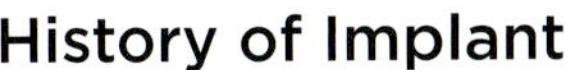

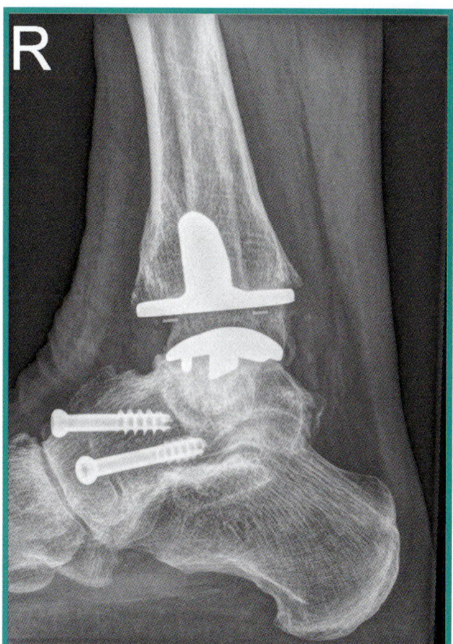

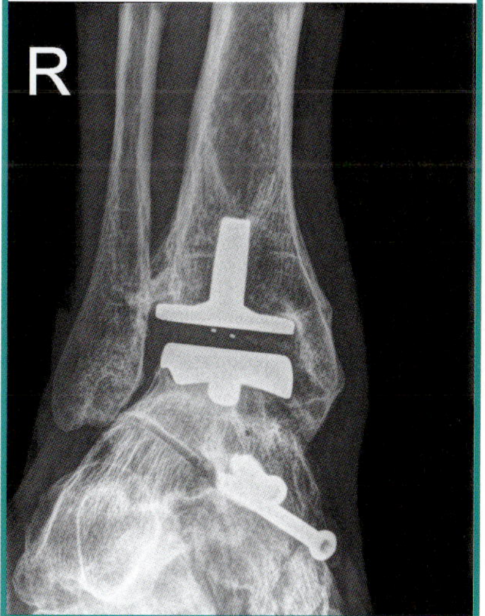

History of Implant

The design was developed by a German surgeon designer team with a patented guiding geometry such that most of the movements do not take place between tibial component and bearing but between the polyethylene bearing and the talar component. Their aim was to possibly reduce wear and hence the chance of cyst formation.

Design Rationale

The Triple A ankle system is a semi constrained Buechel–Pappas type design with a 90° tibial stem without inclination. Before developing the Alphanorm TAR for use, the designers had experience with the TPR prosthesis, New Jersey prosthesis, and STAR prosthesis between 1976 and 1998.

Additional Info

Implantcast GmbH of Buxtehude, Germany manufacture the implants but distribution is via Alphanorm Medizintechnik GmbH, Lassnitzhöhe, Austria.

PSI (patient specific instrumentation since 2018) with special cutting blocks. The tibia has 5 sizes. The talus has 4 sizes. The meniscus is sized 6mm-12mm in 2mm increments.

Technique

Anterior approach.

APEX 3D™ TOTAL ANKLE REPLACEMENT SYSTEM

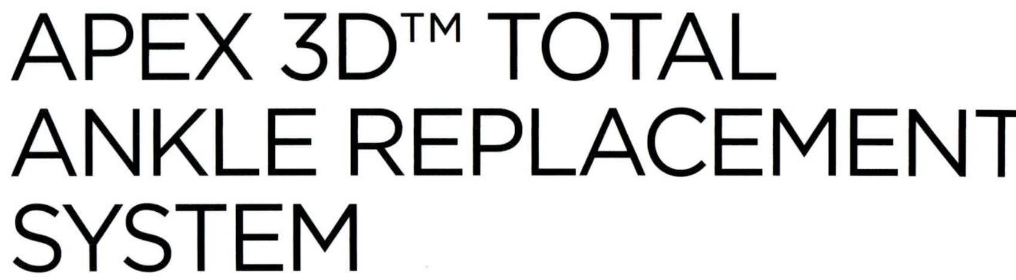

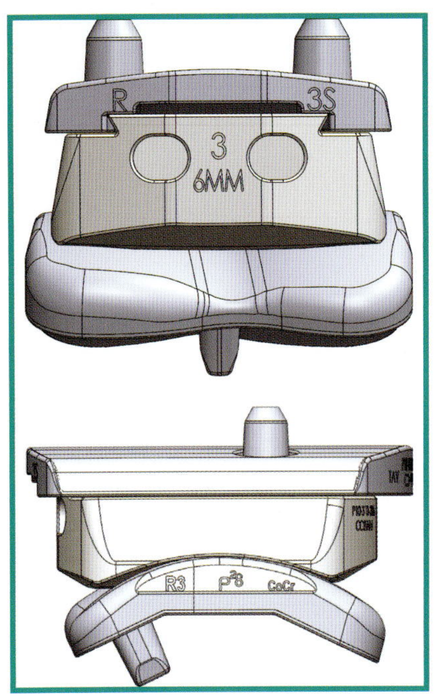

Manufacturer	Paragon 28, Inc. Englewood, CO
Design surgeons	Mark Myerson, MD, Baltimore, Maryland Michael Houghton, MD, Fort Collins, Colorado Mark Dalton, MD, Austin, Texas Jeff Christensen, DPM, Everett, Washington
FDA clearance	Pending
CE mark	Pending
First operation	Pending Launch Q3 2020
Generation	Fourth
Type	Fixed-bearing

Evidence

Premarket implant

Component	Material	Fixation	Sided
Tibial tray	3D printed titanium (FDA).	Cemented.	Right and left sided.
Talar dome	Cobalt-chromium.	Cemented.	
Poly insert	Vitamin E cross-linked UHMWPE (FDA).	Fixed to tibial component.	

History of the Implant

The APEX 3D™ Total Ankle Replacement System was designed by experienced surgeons who aim was to address the recognized current modes of failure, whilst improving the ease of technique and reproducibility for surgeons.

Design Rationale

Through third party partnerships, CT based talar morphology research, Paragon 28® found that Inman (1976), Seigler (2013), Barnett and Napier (1952), were all correct in part with their assessments of ankle kinematics. Paragon 28® found that the healthy ankle joint experiences varying, tri-axial rotation during simulated

gait (data on file with Paragon28). In Early stance the foot is in slight plantarflexion and the medial condyle surface is larger than the lateral but shifts to slight dorsiflexion in late stance so that the lateral condyle surface is larger than the medial (Myerson, 2019). This proprietary "S" like curve is unique to the APEX 3D™ Total Ankle Replacement System.

Additional Info

The APEX 3D™ Total Ankle Replacement System offers several alignment guides ranging from traditional standard guides but also fast track guides and Patient Specific Instrumentation (PSI). They include novel strategies to assess varus/valgus alignment such as laser adjustments to avoid violation of tibial tubercle bone and dovetailed attachments for combined tibia cutting block and joint line height reference.

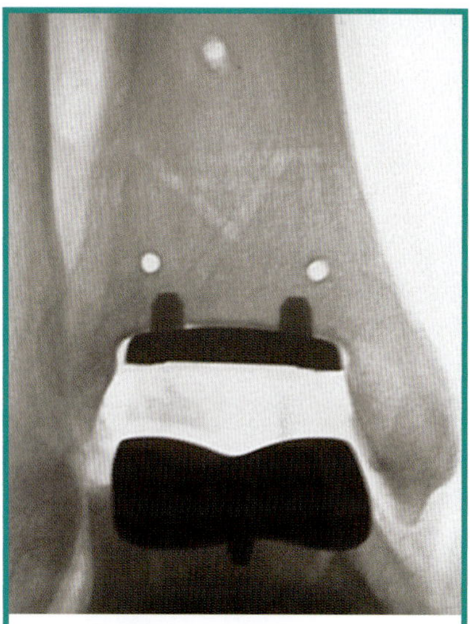

The left and right talar domes are available in both chamfer and flat cuts with a sulcus design. Right and left tibial trays are offered in a gentle arc whose aim is to provide additional rotational stability and mitigate edge loading. The smooth axial pegs are placed slightly posterior to midline where the peak bone strength is located (Hvid *et al.*, 1985). The tibial tray includes standard and long lengths for optimal tibial bone coverage. In non-CE regulated markets, the tibial tray is 3D printed which has increased porosity and surface area compared to that of Titanium Plasma Spray (MacBarb *et al.*, 2017). The 3D manufacturing process allows for controlled trabecular like roughened surfaces that aim to promote earlier cell proliferation which trends toward higher calcium production than of TPS coating (MacBarb *et al.*, 2017). The semi constrained, highly crosslinked poly comes in multiple thickness with additional anterior, central, and posterior biased options.

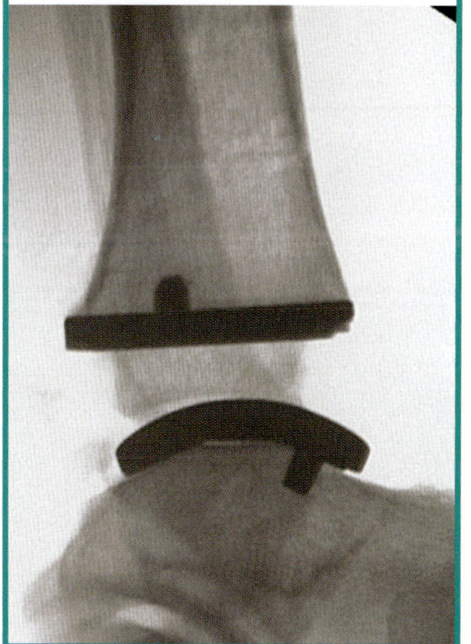

BOX® TOTAL ANKLE REPLACEMENT

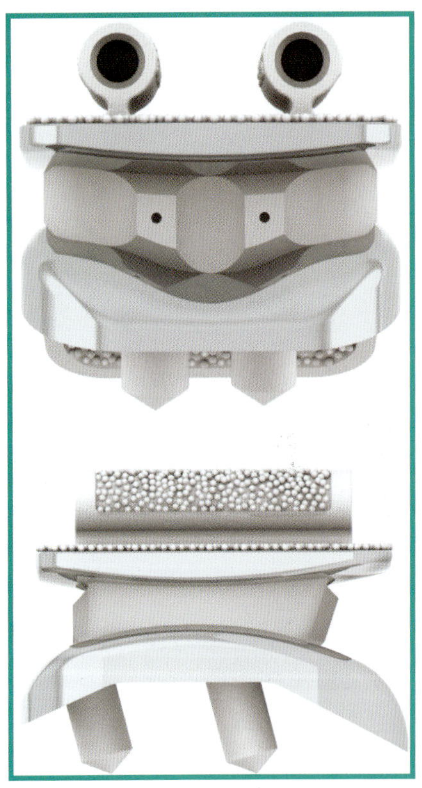

Photo — AP and lateral view.

Manufacturer	MatOrtho® Limited
Inspiration behind name	Collaboration of the inventor group, from Bologna and Oxford — BOX®
Surgeon inventor/ designer(s)	Prof Sandro Giannini, Prof Fabio Catani, Dr Alberto Leardini (Rizzoli Orthopaedic Institute, Bologna, Italy), Prof John J O'Connor (Oxford University)
FDA approved, date	N/A
CE mark, date	March 2003
First operation date	June 2003
Number implanted to date	More than 2000
Generation	Third
Type	Mobile bearing

Evidence	
Giannini *et al.* (2017) *Designer series*	Series of 75 BOX ankle replacements at mean 6.5 years follow-up. The mean AOFAS score achieved at last follow-up was 78. Radiographs showed no loosening and little signs of radiolucency. Two revisions necessitated component removal, neither for implant loosening. The overall survival rate was 97.3%.
Bianchi *et al.* (2012)	62 consecutive implants were placed with an average of 3.5 years follow-up. Survivorship was 91.9%, with radiolucencies of more than 2 mm seen around tibial and talar components in 16 and 4 ankles, respectively.
Giannini *et al.* (2011b) *Designer series*	Multicentre study (9 centres, including inventor surgeon). Included 158 prostheses with mean 17 months (6–48 months) follow-up. Kaplan–Meier survivorship of over 97% at 3 years, over 96% remaining functional when examined 4 years postoperatively.
Giannini *et al.* (2010a) *Designer series*	51 patients with minimum follow-up of 2 years showed improvement in AOFAS scores and survival 97%.

	Material	Fixation	Sided
Tibial component	Cobalt chromium.	Low-profile resurfacing design with rails. Uncemented "as-cast" beaded fixation with HAP coating.	No
Talar component	Cobalt chromium.	Low-profile resurfacing design with pegs. Uncemented "as-cast" beaded fixation with HAP coating.	No
Insert	UHMWPE fully conforming meniscal bearing with spherical concave upper surface and saddle-shaped lower surface.		

History of Implant

The BOX® ankle was developed by the inventor group and Finsbury Orthopaedics Ltd. It was first used in July 2003 in Bologna, Italy. In 2011, following a sale of Finsbury, the BOX® implant was transferred to MatOrtho®, which operates on the same premises and with the same personnel as Finsbury.

Design Rationale

Research by the designers argued that physiological mobility at the ankle involves rolling as well as sliding. The BOX® Total Ankle Replacement was devised to reproduce physiological mobility so that the ligaments continue to function normally. They claimed that the implant enabled movement of isometric fibres within the calcaneofibular and tibiocalcaneal ligaments to restore physiological motion, and that the joint surfaces can have full congruence at the articulating surfaces over the entire motion arc, leading to less wear.

Technique

Anterior approach, fully instrumented technique. Joint tensioning device is used so that ligament balance and tension is taken into account prior to performing the tibial cuts.

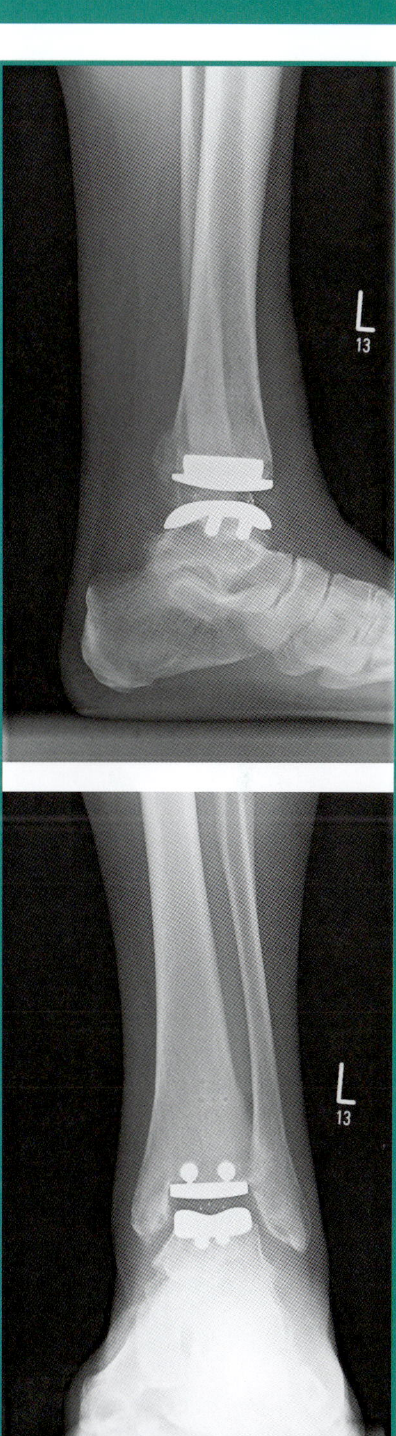

Photo — AP and lateral view.

CADENCE ANKLE REPLACEMENT

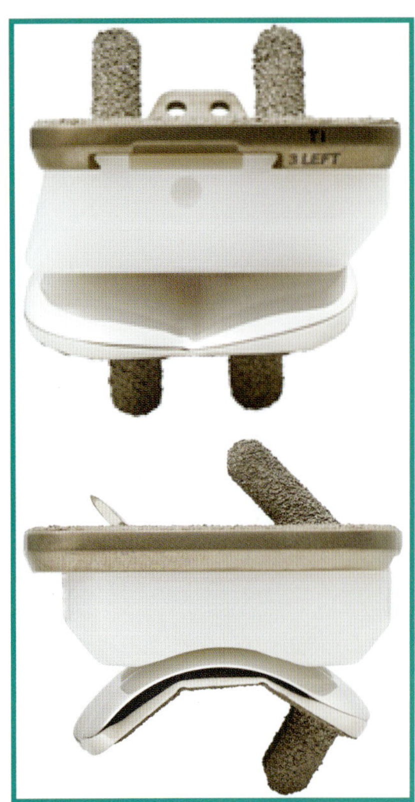

Manufacturer	**Integra Lifesciences**
Inspiration behind name	Cadence = Regular rhythm, reproducibility, streamlined surgical technique
Surgeon inventor/ designer(s)	Timothy R. Daniels MD Selene G. Parekh MD David I. Pedowitz MD Chris Hyer DPM
FDA approved, date	August 31, 2015
CE mark, date	March 21, 2016
First operation date	In the US: March 8, 2016 In EMEA: July 13, 2016
Number implanted to date	More than 100 worldwide
Generation	Third
Type	Two component fixed bearing

Evidence	
Daniels *et al.* (2019)	Two year follow up of Cadence™ prosthesis, manufactured by Integra LifeSciences. Designer series. 31 consecutive patients included. Improved pain and AOS disability scores. No revisions. No radiological concerns but 40 ancillary procedures performed on 24 TAR's.

	Material	Fixation	Sided
Tibial component	Titanium alloy.	Initial fixation with pegs and a posterior fin. 9 sizes of tibial component. US Cemented and outside US cemented or uncemented use.	Yes
Talar component	Cobalt chrome alloy.	Initial fixation with pegs. Cemented use US but cemented or uncemented outside of US.	Yes
Insert	Highly cross-linked ultra high molecular weight polyethylene. Five sizes, 7 heights, left foot and right foot specific each with neutral, anterior biased or posterior biased options.		

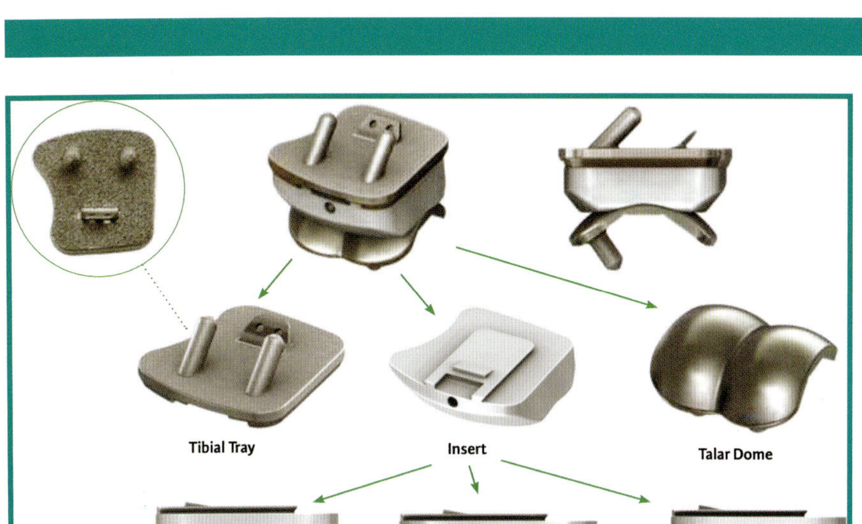

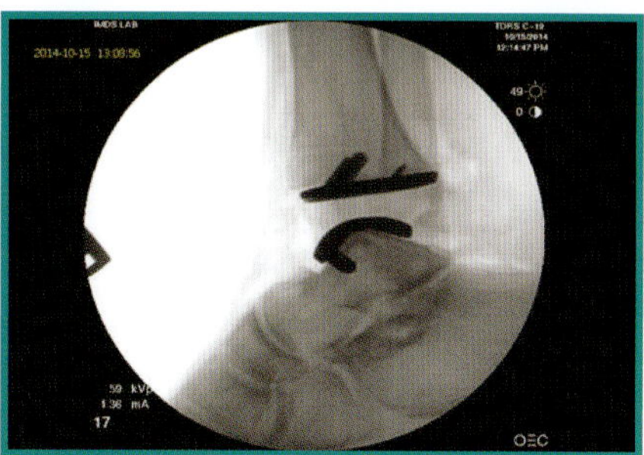

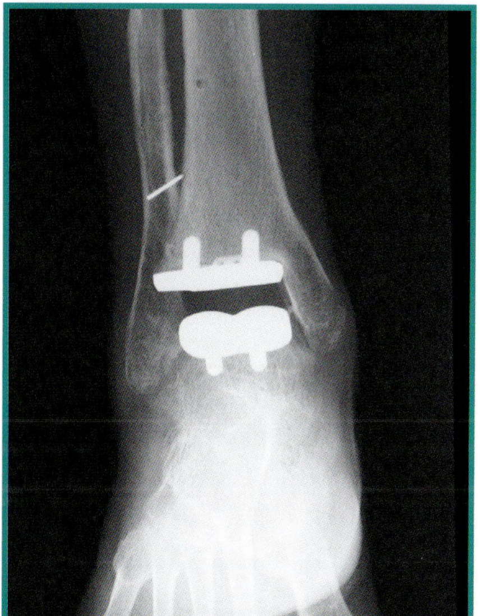

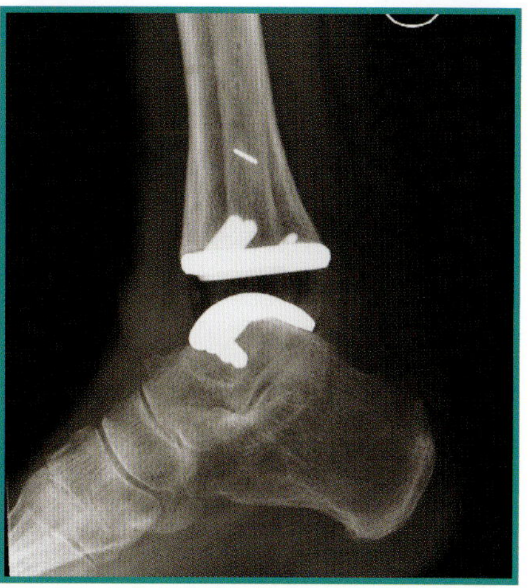

History of Implant

An industry driven project using a design team comprised of surgeons and a surgical podiatrist.

Design Rationale

On top of the usual features of minimal bone resection and natural kinematics the Cadence had some specific rationale:

(1) **Anatomic** — to be sided aiming for tricortical coverage with a cut out for the incisura on the tibial component.
(2) **Safe** — aim to avoid damage to tarsal canal artery by pins.
(3) **Reduce dissymmetry** with modular anterior and posterior biased implants.
(4) **Instrumentation** — to simplify and make reliable.

Technique

Anterior approach.

HINTEGRA ANKLE REPLACEMENT

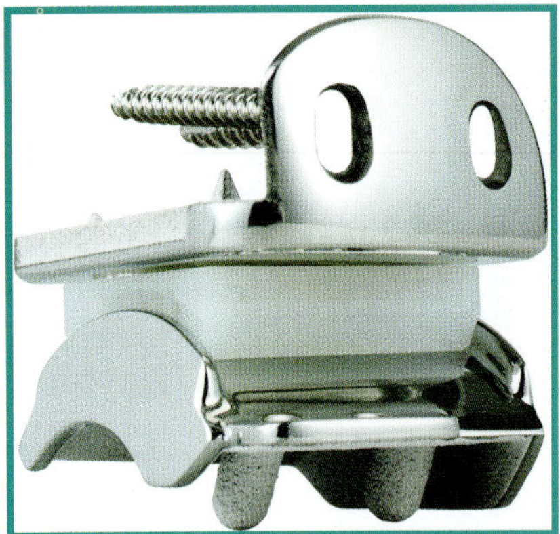

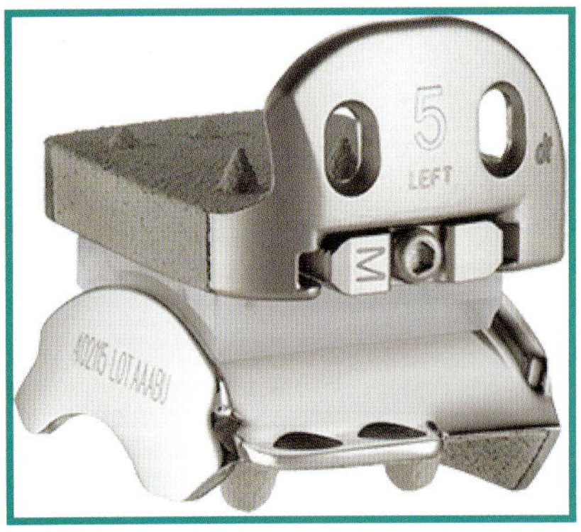

Photo — above original Hintegra (now called H3), below new fixed H2 implant.

Manufacturer	DTMedtech LLC
Inspiration behind name	Combination of inventor name and manufacturer
Surgeon inventor/ designer(s)	Prof Hintermann (Basel, Switzerland)
FDA approved, date	H2 2017; H3 2019
CE mark, date	2000
First operation date	2000
Number implanted to date	Unknown
Generation	Third
Type	H3 three component design; H2 two component design

Evidence	
Yang *et al.* (2019)	Single surgeon series of 205 consecutive patients (210 ankles) with mean follow-up of 6.4 years (2.0 to 13.4). Improvement in clinical scores with implant survivorship of 91.7%. Complication rate 15.7% with 12 failures (5.7%). 9% osteolysis.
Lefrancois *et al.* (2017)	Mean improvement in total AOS score was 29.7, pain AOS score was 29.0, and disability AOS score was 30.4. Survival rates and improvements in pain and function were comparable to Agility and STAR implants, and superior to Mobility. Survival 92% at mean 3.5 years.
Jung *et al.* (2015)	Retrospective comparative study looking at Hintegra versus the mobility in 52 patients with average 28.3 months follow-up. VAS and AOFAS improvements were similar. More impingement reported with Hintegra (38% vs 9.1%), but more malleolar fractures with the mobility (15% vs 0%).
Deleu *et al.* (2015)	Average 45 months follow-up of 50 Hintegra ankle replacements. Survival 90%, with asymptomatic osteolysis in 48%.
Yoon *et al.* (2014)	99 ankle replacements followed up for a mean of 40.8 months. 37% had radiologic evidence of osteolysis which were asymptomatic, with 10% developing progressive bone loss. No major association between bone loss and clinical symptoms.
Barg *et al.* (2013) *Designer series*	Analysis of 722 Hintegra implants with a mean follow-up of 6.3 years. Survival was 94% and 84% after five and ten years respectively.
Hintermann *et al.* (2013) *Designer series*	Review of 117 revision arthroplasties converted to a Hintegra replacement. Average follow-up 6.2 years, with 83% survival for the revised implant.

Bai _et al._ (2010)	67 patients divided into two groups of posttraumatic OA (37 ankles) and primary OA (30 ankles). At mean follow-up of 38 months, clinical and radiographic outcomes were comparable, but the posttraumatic group had a higher rate of complications (37% vs 27% respectively).
Hintermann _et al._ (2004, 2006) _**Designer series**_	Review of 122 Hintegra implants with mean 19 months follow-up. Survival 93.5%, with AOFAS improvement from 40 to 85 points. Later study looked at mid-term results for 271 cases with average 36 month follow-up. Of these, 39 required revision surgery including arthrolysis, TA lengthening, and ligament reconstruction.

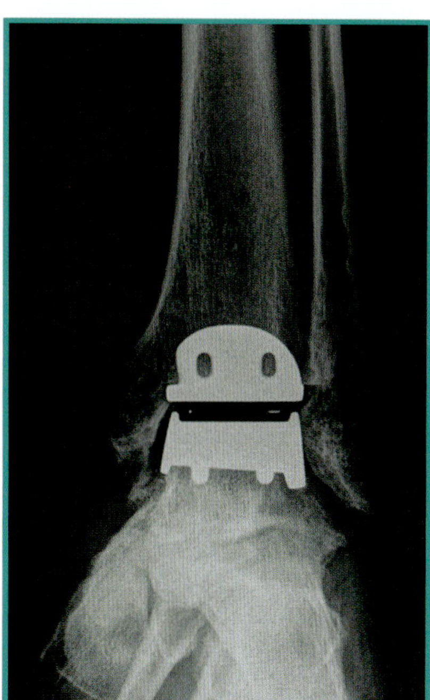

	Material	Fixation	Sided
Tibial component	Cobalt chrome coated with titanium plasma and hydroxyapatite (HaP) for uncemented or biological fixation. Pyramidal peaks for anchoring in subchondral bone. Additional fixation may be achieved with screws.	Uncemented fixation.	Yes
Talar component	Cobalt chrome with dual titanium HA coating. Smaller radius medially than laterally. Anterior pegs to improve sagittal stability and positioning. Medial and lateral rims to guide anteroposterior movement of the meniscus. Anterior shield to increase primary support and potentially reduce adherent scar tissue. Polished overhangs on the medial and lateral side serve as anatomical articular surfaces.	Uncemented fixation.	Yes
Insert	Ultra-high molecular weight polyethylene.	Fixed (H2) or Mobile (H3).	

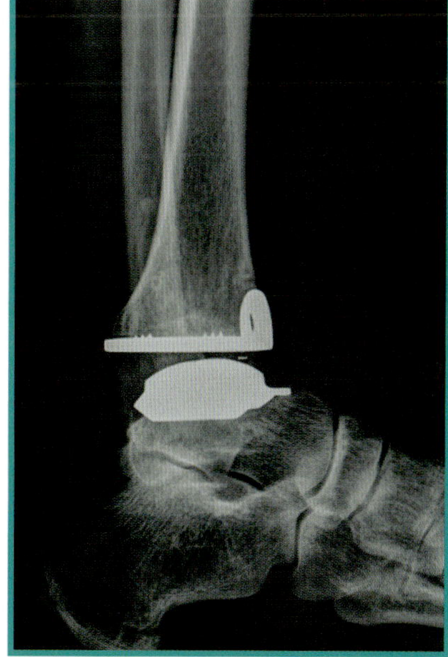

History of Implant

The Hintermann Series Total Ankle Replacements began life as the Hintegra distributed by Integra Lifesciences with the first implant in 2000. In 2016 ownership moved to DTMedtech LLC who received FDA premarket approval for a two component version, entitled the H2. DT Medtech LLC then used 18 years of non US data of their three component design to obtain FDA premarket approval of the H3 prosthesis which was granted in June 2019.

The Indications for Use (IFU) differs for the H2 and H3 depending on whether it is sold in the USA or outside of the USA.

See Chapter 7 for further history.

Technique

Anterior approach. Instrumented technique.

This page was left blank intentionally

INBONE ANKLE REPLACEMENT

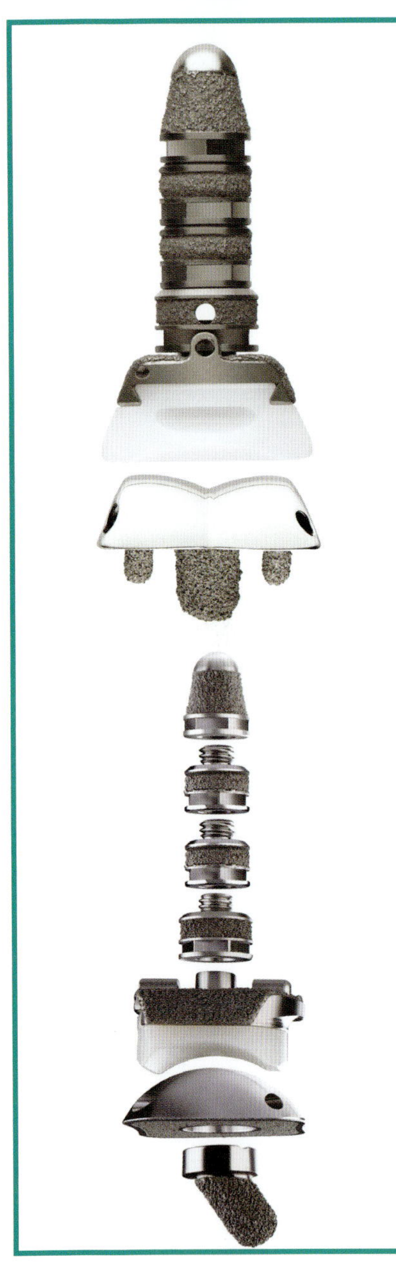

Manufacturer	**Wright Medical**
Inspiration behind name	Tibial components can be built up as a stem for internal fixation within the tibia
Surgeon inventor/designer(s)	INBONE 1 Mark A Reiley, MD INBONE 2 — See Infinity Development Team
FDA approved, date	2005
CE mark, date	2011
First operation date	2005
Number implanted to date	More than 10,000
Generation	Third
Type	Fixed-bearing modular system

History of Implant

The INBONE® Total Ankle System was developed by Mark Reiley. The implant is the only one on the market to offer intramedullary instrumentation and modular designs. The implants are guided by a screwdriver or impaction rod that is channelled through the heel and across the subtalar joint (although in many cases misses the articular surface and traverses the sinus tarsi). The actual implant however is placed in modularly through the incision at the front of the ankle.

Design Rationale

Fixed bearing two-component system. Modular stem for both metallic components. Intramedullary guidance system allows potential for more reproducible bone cuts.

The INBONE 2 system was developed by the same development team as behind the Infinity ankle system and incorporates design modifications of sulcus articulation, additional subtalar fixation, long AP tibial trays, and talar trial reductions.

The INBONE2 can be implanted using a specialized foot holder which is assembled prior to the surgery by the scrub team or using the Prophecy patient specific instrumentation (PSI) system.

Evidence	
Harston *et al.* (2017)	A consecutive series of 149 patients with INBONE 1. Significant improvements in pain and function. Survivorship of 90.6% at mean 5.9 years follow-up. No difference in outcome if severe varus or valgus deformity preoperatively. Catastrophic talar component collapse occurred in 2.7% of cases.
Daigre *et al.* (2017)	Radiographic assessment of inbone 2 in 44 patients. In 79.5% of patients, the postoperative implant position of the tibia corresponded to the preoperative plan of the tibia within 3° of the intended target, and within 5° in 100% of patients.
Coetzee *et al.* (2017)	Significantly improved outcomes at 2 years in VAS, SF-36, and AOFAS scores at 2 years. Similar results to Salto and STAR.
Williams *et al.* (2015)	Review of agility TAR revised to inbone. 31.5% complication rate. Therapeutic level 4.
Brigido *et al.* (2015)	The mean implant migration was 0.7 mm at 1 year and 1.0 mm at 2 years.
Lewis *et al.* (2015)	Comparison of first- and second-generation inbone implants. Implant failure rate 2.6% at 2 years in second-generation group (compared with 6% in first-generation group). Rate of reoperation 15.9% at 2 years in second-generation group (compared with 18.5% in first-generation group).
Hsu *et al.* (2015)	Follow-up average 35 months for 59 implants. 96% 2-year survival (91% inbone 1, 100% inbone 2), and 20% required reoperation but no component revision.
Adams *et al.* (2014)	Mean 3.7 years follow-up of 194 inbone ankle replacements. Improvement in functional, pain, and quality of life scores. Overall implant survival 89%.
Brigido *et al.* (2014)	3-year outcomes of 23 patients. Pain, function, and disability significantly improved. Nine patients had complications (39.1%). Three patients had a further procedure (13%).
DeVries *et al.* (2013)	Agility to inbone (revision) — two early failures and high complication rates.

	Material	Fixation	Sided
Tibial component	Titanium with a porous titanium plasma spray coating.	Cementless. Long modular stem in tibia which can be varied in length.	No
Talar component	Cobalt chrome with a porous titanium plasma spray coating. Highly polished bearing surface.	Cementless. Modular talar stem which can be lengthened across a subtalar fusion.	No
Insert	Fixed bearing polyethylene insert.		

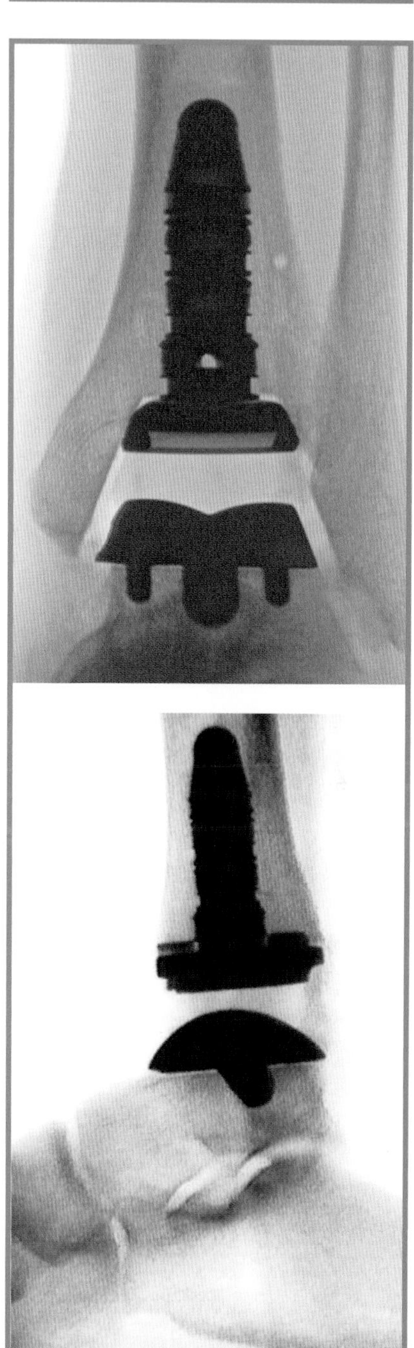

X-ray — AP and lateral view.

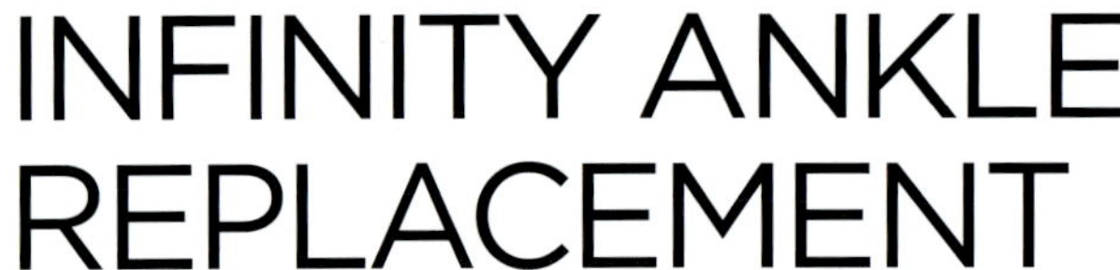

INFINITY ANKLE REPLACEMENT

Manufacturer	Wright Medical Technology, Memphis, TN
Inspiration behind name	The quality or state of being infinite in its performance
Surgeon inventor/ designer(s)	Robert B. Anderson, MD, *Charlotte*; Gregory C. Berlet, MD, *Columbus*; W. Hodges Davis, MD, *Charlotte*; Steven L. Haddad, MD, *Chicago*; Thomas H. Lee, MD, *Columbus*; Murray J. Penner, MD FRCSC, *Vancouver*. Prophecy comes under Wright Medical Research and Development
FDA approved, date	2014
CE mark, date	2014
First operation date	2014
Number implanted to date	More than 5000
Generation	Third
Type	Fixed-bearing modular system

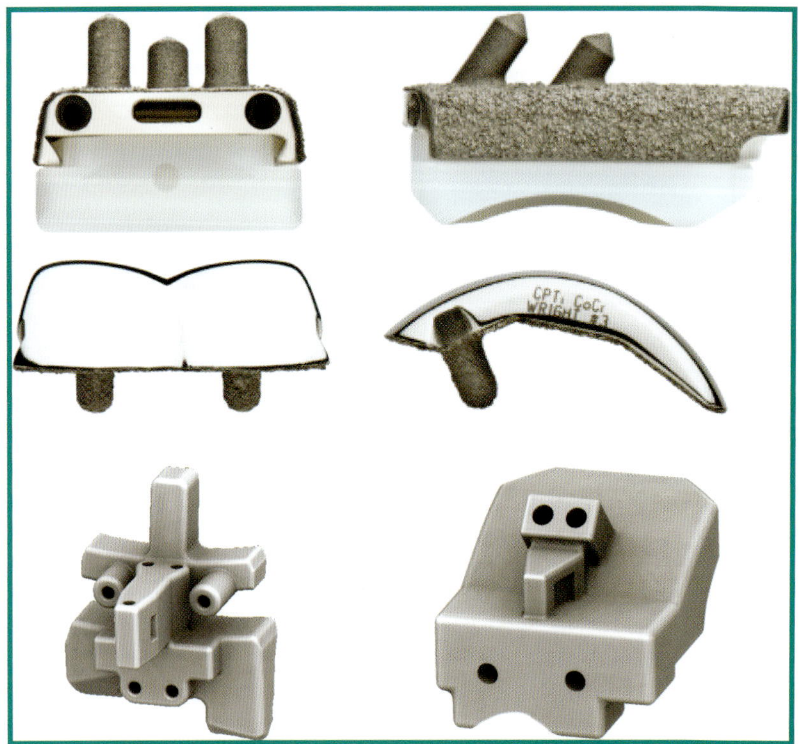

Tibial and talar components from front and side. Below are patient specific guides for the PSI technique.

History of Implant

Guiding principles include bone–implant interface visibility and INBONE® compatibility for a continuum of care from primary to revision.

Design Rationale

Low profile tibial implant design; Resurfacing talar component designed for improved fluoroscopic visualization; Talar component interchangeability including compatibility with INBONE 2 system; and implantable using instrumented or patient specific instrumentation technique.

Additional Info

The PROPHECY® Preoperative Navigation Guides is a system of patient specific instrumentation where the patients receive a preoperative CT according to a specific protocol which includes their ankle and knee. Using special software, a patient-specific preoperative plan is developed. PROPHECY® Preoperative Navigation Guides which are custom nylon jigs are then provided to the surgeon at the time of surgical implantation to reproduce the preoperative plans.

In 2020 Wright Medical Introduced a new coating called ADAPTIS® but no outcome data is available.

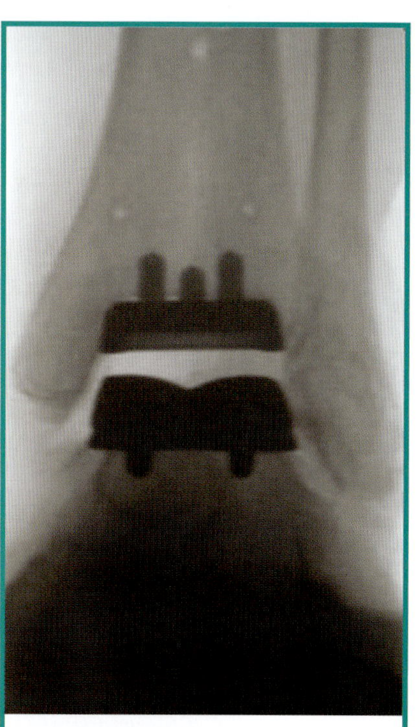

Technique

Anterior incision — prophecy guided or via external jig.

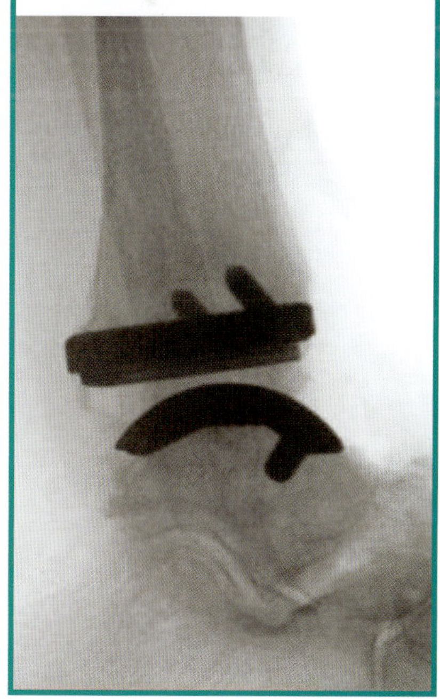

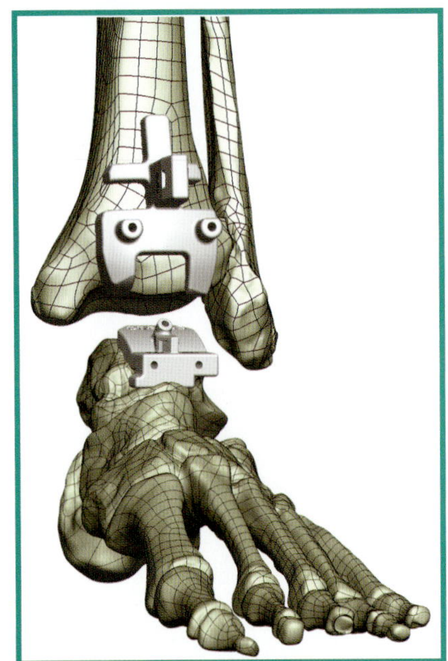

Patient specific instrumentation.

Evidence	
Infinity TAR follow-up (ITAR)	Currently recruiting in USA.
UK Infinity post-market clinical follow-up study	A multicentre, non-inventor, prospective observational study of 504 implants. All patients had improvement in clinical scores at 6 months, maintained up to 2 year follow up but only 104 patients had reached this milestone at initial reports in 2020.
Cody *et al.* (2019)	A review of 159 primary Infinity TAR with a mean follow up of 20 months. Sixteen ankles (10%) underwent revision at a mean 13 months postoperatively. The most common reasons for revision were symptomatic tibial component loosening (3.8%) and deep infection (3.8%).
King *et al.* (2019)	Early follow up of 19 patients (20 implants) with minimum of 2 year follow up. Improved clinical scores. 15% complication rate. No revisions.
Saito *et al.* (2018)	A retrospective analysis of 64 primary Infinity TAR's with an average follow-up of 24.5 months. Survivorship of the implant was 95.3%. Fourteen ankles (21.8%) presented a total of 17 complications with a 17.1% re-operation rate and a 4.7% revision rate. Periprosthetic radiolucent lines were observed around the tibial component in 31%.
Hsu *et al.* (2015)	Accurate postoperative alignment after using patient specific instrumentation.
Berlet *et al.* (2014)	Deviation of final implant placement from the preoperative plan was less than 2° in all angular degrees of freedom, providing greater accuracy than other implant systems.

	Material	Fixation	Sided
Tibial component	Titanium with a porous titanium plasma spray coating.	Cementless. Three-angled tibial pegs.	No
Talar component	Cobalt chrome with a porous titanium plasma spray coating. Bearing surface is highly polished.	Cementless pegged insertion.	No
Insert	Polyethylene insert.	Fixed.	

This page was left blank intentionally

INVISION ANKLE REPLACEMENT

Manufacturer	**Wright Medical Technology, Memphis, TN**
Inspiration behind name	A merger of the names INBONE and revision
Surgeon inventor/ designer(s)	Robert B. Anderson, MD, OrthoCarolina, Charlotte, NC; Gregory C. Berlet, MD, Orthopedic Foot and Ankle Center Columbus, OH; W. Hodges Davis, MD, OrthoCarolina, Charlotte, NC; Steven L. Haddad, MD, Illinois Bone and Joint Institute, Chicago, IL; Thomas H. Lee, MD, Orthopedic Foot and Ankle Center Columbus, OH; William McGarvey, MD FRCSC, Houston Orthopedic & Spine Hospital Houston, TX; Murray J. Penner, MD FRCSC, Providence Health Care, Vancouver, BC
FDA approved, date	2018
CE mark, date	June 2016
First operation date	July 2016
Number implanted to date	More than 100
Generation	Fourth
Type	Fixed-bearing implant

Evidence

No published evidence as yet

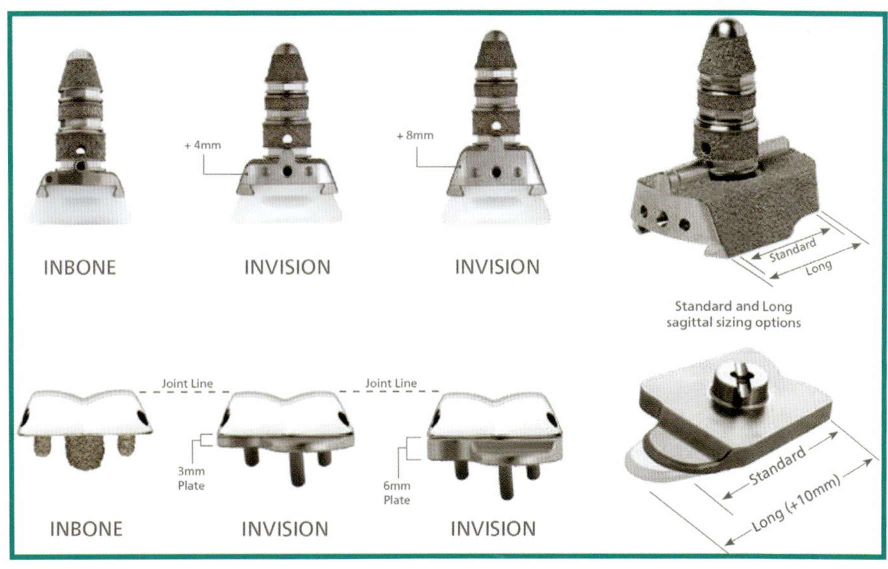

Photo — AP and oblique views.

History of Implant

Extension of portfolio derived from INBONE 2 for revisions requiring unique metal replacement for large bone losses. Indicated for patients with a failed previous ankle replacement.

Design Rationale

The INVISION™ Total Ankle Revision System is the first bespoke modern revision ankle system. The system retains all the design principles of the INBONE® total ankle system but enables the management of bone deficiencies. The INVISION™ Total Ankle Revision System offers universal tibial trays; with four sizes (2–5), three lengths (standard, long, and extra-long), and two thicknesses. The tibial trays are manufactured from titanium (Ti) alloy and utilise a similar trapezoidal profile as the INBONE® tibial trays. On the superior surface, a Morse taper identical to INBONE® is utilised for compatibility with the INBONE® tibial stems.

Technique

Can be guided by the PROPHECY® Preoperative Navigation Guides. The polyethylene options range from 6 to 20mm. The talar plates have two thicknesses to help restore joint height and can be fixed with additional screw fixation outside of the USA.

	Material	Fixation	Sided
Tibial component	Titanium.	Cementless.	No
Talar component	Cobalt chrome.	Cementless pegged insertion.	Talar plate is sided, with two thicknesses to manage position of the joint line.
Insert	Polyethylene insert.		

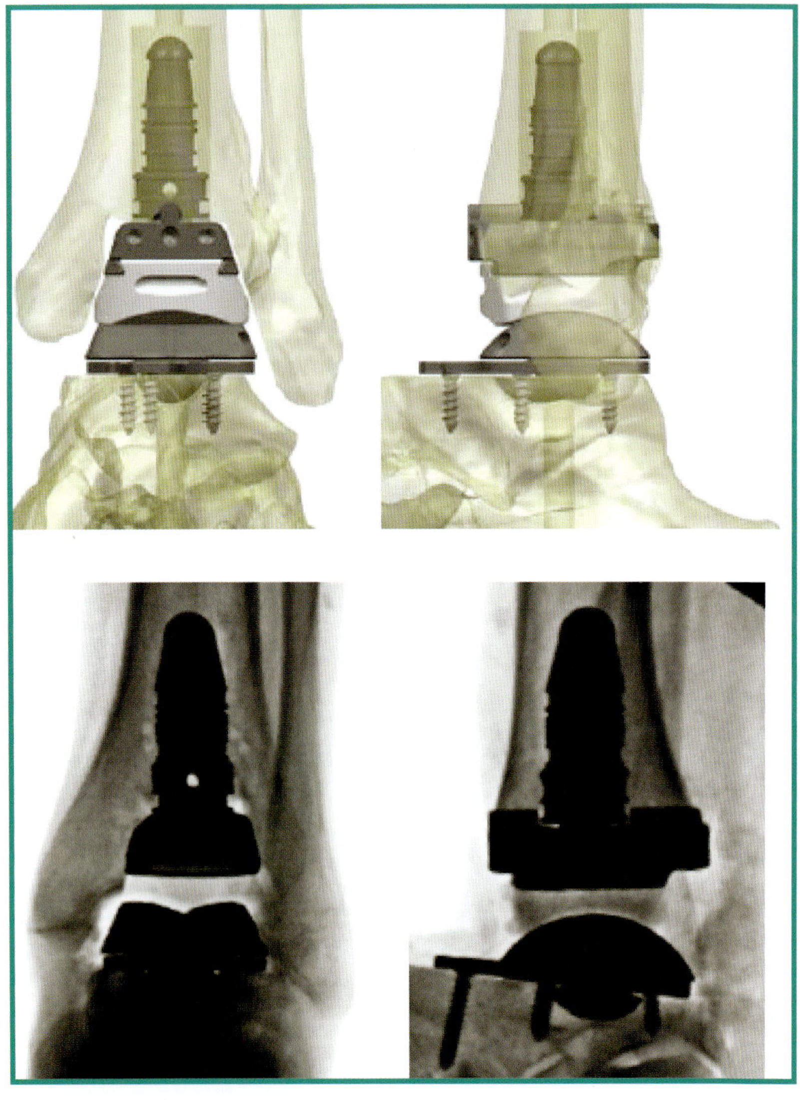

X-ray — AP and lateral view.

This page was left blank intentionally

SALTO & SALTO TALARIS ANKLE REPLACEMENT

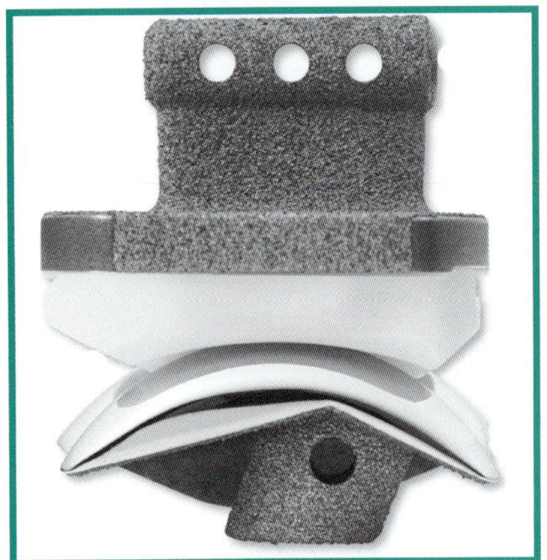

Manufacturer	**Tornier SA, Montbonnot, France** **After merger with Wright Medical in 2015, the rights to the Salto outside of the US moved to Wright Medical. In the USA the rights moved to Integra.**
Inspiration behind name	
Surgeon inventor/ designer(s)	Michel Bonnin (Lyon, France), Jean-Alain Colombier (Lyon, France), Thierry Judet (Paris, France) developed the Salto implant. The US subsidary of Tornier brought in Brian Donley MD from the Cleveland Clinic to help design the Salto Talaris
FDA approved, date	2006 Salto Talaris
CE mark, date	1997 (Salto) and 2007 (Salto-Talaris)
First operation date	1997 (salto) and 2006 (Salto-Talaris)
Number implanted to date	Unknown but more than 5000
Generation	Third
Type	Mobile bearing (Salto) and Fixed bearing (Salto-Talaris)

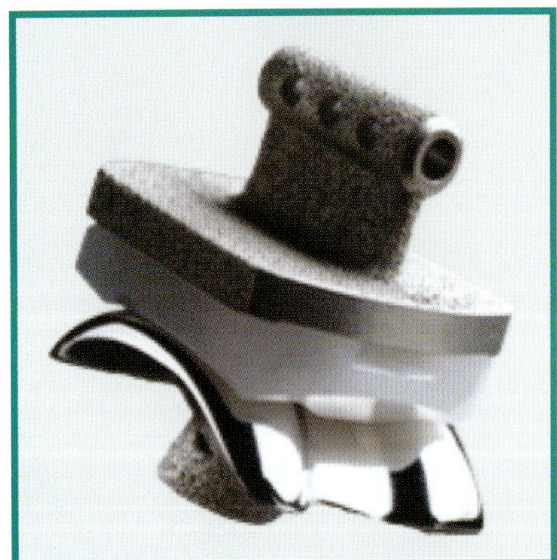

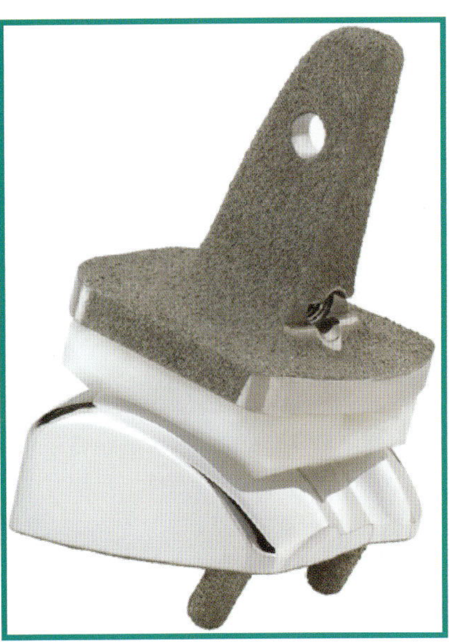

Evidence	
Bonnin *et al.* (2011)	87 Salto implants with mean follow up of 8.9 years (Designer series). The survival rate 85% at a mean of 8.9 years.
Schenk *et al.* (2011)	Follow up of 413 Salto implants. 5-year estimated survivorship was 86.6%. The AOFAS score increased from 50.9 preoperatively to 82.2 at follow up ay 2 years. Visual analogue scale for pain decreased from 7.4 preoperatively to 2.0 postoperatively at 2 years. Flexion/extension ROM increased from 25.2 degrees to 33.1 degrees.
Schuberth *et al.* (2011)	Range of motion of 97 Salto Talaris implants. The overall mean increase in the range of motion from 6 weeks to 12 months was 8.25°.
Schweitzer *et al.* (2013)	Follow up of 67 Salto Talaris implants. Implant survival at a mean follow-up time of 2.8 years was 96%. Significant improvement in AOFAS score.
Gaudot *et al.* (2014)	SALTO (mobile bearing) versus SALTO Talaris (Fixed bearing) Clinical performance of both was equivalent.
Nodzo *et al.* (2014)	Follow up of 75 Salto implants. Survivorship was 98% at a mean of 43 months. Average ankle dorsiflexion and plantar flexion improved from 4.3 to 8.7 degrees and 24 to 29 degrees respectively. Significant improvements in FAOS, SF-12 and VAS scores.

Chao _et al._ (2015)	Review of 23 Salto-Talaris implants with mean follow up of 3 years. Statistically significant improvements in VAS, AOFAS ankle/hindfoot scores, and SF36 scores. Survivorship of the implant was 82.6% with any reoperation as the endpoint and 95.6% for revision or removal of components.
Hofmann _et al._ (2016)	A review of 81 Salto-Talaris implants. Implant survival 97.5% at mean 5.2 year follow up. 22% additional surgery rate. Maintained improved outcome scores at 5 years.
Oliver _et al._ (2016)	A review of 245 Salto-Talaris implants with a mean follow up 38.9 months. There were significant improvements in clinical scores. Two patients underwent revision TAA at a minimum of 36 months; 8 patients failed the primary TAA and were converted to ankle fusions at a mean of 20.1 months.
Coetzee _et al._ (2017)	Significantly improved outcomes at 2 years in VAS, SF-36 and AOFAS scores at 2 years after a Salto-Talaris. Similar results to STAR and Inbone TAR.
Stewart _et al._ (2017)	Review of 72 patients with a Salto Talaris at mean 81 month follow up. Survivorship 95.8% with those with at least 5 year follow up. 19% needed additional surgery. Significant improvements in pain and function scores.
Wan _et al._ (2018)	A review of 59 Salto implants some with very short follow up — Survival of 94.9% at mean of 35.9 months. There were significant improvements in pain, range of movement and function.

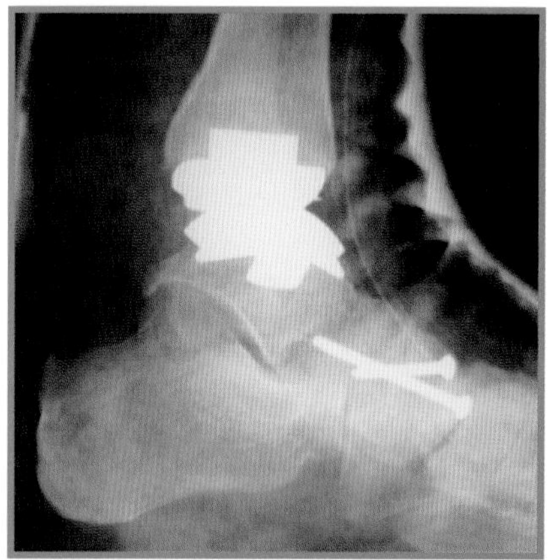

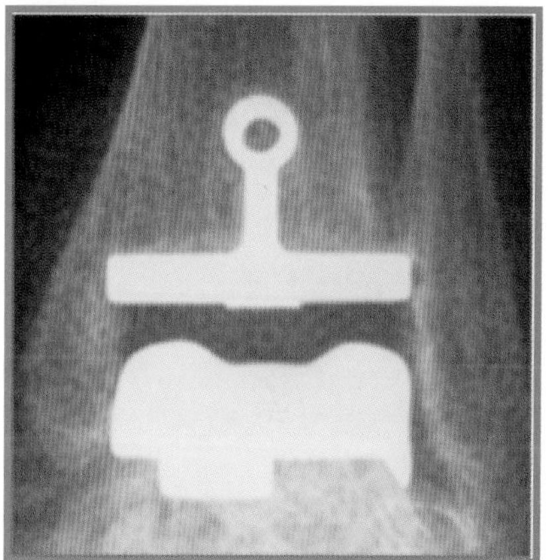

	Material	Fixation	Sided
Tibial component	Cobalt-chrome with dual titanium HA coating. Flat surface that faces the mobile bearing, allowing free translation and rotation.	Uncemented. Tibial central fin with hollow end.	No
Talar component	Cobalt-chrome with dual titanium HA coating.	Uncemented. Talo-fibular facet replacement. Smaller medial radius allows inversion, eversion. Anterior width is wider than the posterior width and the lateral flange has a larger curvature radius than the medial.	Yes
Insert	UHMWPE.		

History of Implant

Developed by French designers in the late 1990's. Approximately 10 years later a venture capital group acquired Tornier and its focus became the USA where mobile bearing implants could not be used, hence the fixed bearing version where the polyethylene liner was fixed onto the tibial component was born. This device known as the Salto-Talaris became FDA approved in 2006 on the basis of a 510k application on the basis it was substantially equivalent to the Agility (DePuy) Implant. A revision implant entitled the Salto-XT was developed later but then the name changed to the Integra XT revision implant.

Design Rationale

Used in the USA since December 2006. It is a variant of the SALTO ankle replacement, a three-component mobile-bearing design used in Europe since 1997. The Initial Salto design was mobile-bearing, but lack of motion led to the fixed bearing Salto Talaris. A key feature of this fixed-bearing implant is that the mobile- bearing concept has been incorporated into the trial reduction stage. During the trial reduction, the mobile tibial trial component is allowed to rotate into proper position during ankle range of motion.

Technique

Anterior approach. Instrumented technique.

This page was left blank intentionally

STAR ANKLE REPLACEMENT

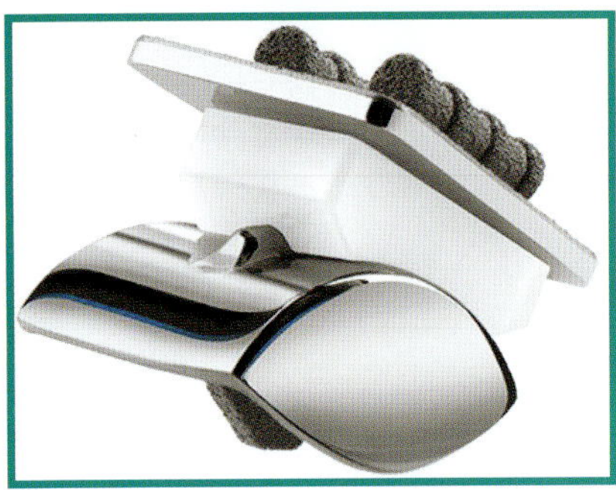

Manufacturer	**Stryker Corporation, Michigan, USA** acquired the rights in 2014. Prior to that Small Bone Innovations Inc. acquired the rights in 2009 from Waldemar LINK GmbH & Co. KG, Hamburg, Germany
Inspiration behind name	Scandinavian Total Ankle Replacement (STAR)
Surgeon inventor/designer(s)	Dr Hakon Kofoed
FDA approved, date	2009
CE mark, date	Unknown
First operation date	1981
Number implanted to date	Greater than 30,000 patients worldwide
Generation	Third
Type	Mobile bearing

Evidence	
Palanca *et al.* (2018)	Metal implant survival was 73% at 15 years. In 70.7%, there was no change in prosthetic alignment from the immediate postoperative radiograph. More than half (52.4%) of patients with retained implants required an additional surgical procedure; three required two additional procedures.
Frigg *et al.* (2017)	Minimal 10-year follow-up in 46 patients. 10-year survival was 94%, but exchange of any component including the inlay (due to breakage or wear) was needed in 22%. 19-year survival was 91%, but exchange of any component was needed in 45%. Mean Kofoed score was 89 after 16 years.
Koivu *et al.* (2017b)	93.9% survival at 5 years. 63.6% survival at 15 years. 44% revision rate.
Coetzee *et al.* (2017)	Significantly improved outcomes at 2 years in VAS, SF-36, and AOFAS scores at 2 years. Similar results to Salto Talaris and Inbone TAR.
Lefrancois *et al.* (2017)	Mean improvement in total AOS score was 28.5, pain AOS score was 29.1, and disability AOS score was 27.8. Survival rates and improvements in pain and function were comparable to Agility and Hintegra implants, and superior to mobility. Survival 92% at mean 6.2 years.
Kerkhoff *et al.* (2016)	Cumulative survival 78% after 10 years. 10.4% had polyethylene fractures. Removal of implant and arthrodesis in 14.9%. Secondary procedure rate 15.9%. Osteolytic cysts seen in 59.8% at 10 years.
Daniels *et al.* (2015)	111 ankles with average follow-up 9 years showed 12% metal component revision and 18% polyethylene-bearing failure.

Haytmanek *et al.* **(2015)**	Reported on 79 of the 4th generation STAR implants with a mean follow-up was 8.0 years. There was a 31.6% rate of secondary surgery. 10.1% revision rate (higher in complicated cases). Heterotopic ossification rate was 100%.
Jastifer and Coughlin (2015)	Follow-up of 18 patients showed 94.4% survival at a mean of 12.6 years. 39% required additional procedures, survival defined as tibial or talar metallic replacement. AOFAS improvement 32.8 to 78.1 at latest F/U.
Schimmel *et al.* **(2014)**	Compared first 50 STAR ankle replacement with their most recent 50 in a consecutive series of 134 cases. Surgery time decreased, fewer perioperative fractures, and the tibial component orientation. No difference in clinical outcome between the two cohorts.
Brunner *et al.* **(2013)**	Follow-up of 11–15 years of 72 consecutive patients who had smooth single coat HA (3rd generation). They showed an implant survivorship of 70.7% and 45.6% at 10 and 14 years, respectively. The main causes for erosion were aseptic loosening, talar subsidence, and progressive cyst formation, with polyethylene fractures in 11 patients.
Mann *et al.* **(2011)**	Pivotal FDA study. Follow-up of 84 STAR (4th generation titanium sprayed) ankle replacements. Survival was 96% at 5 years and 90% at 10 years. Improvement in mean AOFAS score from 43 to 82 points. 10 patients (13%) developed concerning osteolytic lesions.
Karantana *et al.* **(2010)**	Follow-up of 52 ankles STAR prostheses. Survival was 90% at 5 years and 84% at 8 years.
Wood *et al.* **(2009)**	Randomised, prospective study of Buechel–Pappas versus the STAR. 200 ankle replacements were followed up for 36 months. The 6-year survivorship of the BP design was 79% and of the STAR 95%. The authors concluded that preoperative deformity was the most likely predictor of failure.
Wood *et al.* **(2008)**	The same cohort of 200 replacements were reviewed.
Wood and Deakin (2003)	200 STAR total ankle replacements (in the main 4th generation double coat). 5-year cumulative survival was 92.7%. A later publication of the same cohort resulted in a 10-year survivorship of 80.3%.
Kofoed (2004)	Study cohort compared 33 patients who had a cemented implant against 25 patients who subsequently had uncemented 3 piece (Smooth HA coated) implants. The average follow-up was 9.4 years, with 12-year survivorship in the cemented group 70%, and in the uncemented group 95.4%.
Kofoed (1995) *Designer series*	First-generation 2 piece implants used in 28 patients with 12-year survivorship of 70%.

	Material	Fixation	Sided
Tibial component	Cobalt chromium with titanium plasma spray coating alone (in USA) and an additional calcium phosphate coating (referred to as a double coat) outside of USA. Trapezoidal shape with rounded corners. The plate is 2.5 mm thick, flat, and polished.	On the proximal surface of the tibial component, two parallel cylindrical barrels are positioned equidistant from the centre of the plate running anterior to posterior for bone fixation.	No
Talar component	Cobalt chromium with titanium plasma spray coating alone (in USA) and an additional calcium phosphate coating (referred to as a double coat) outside of USA. Dome-shaped talus with walls. A small, raised half-cylindrical ridge runs from anterior to posterior in the medial–lateral centre of the dome to constrain the medial/lateral motion of the Mobile bearing.	Single talar fin.	Yes
Insert	The proximal surface of the UHMWPE mobile bearing is flat. The talar surface is concave and has a central radial groove running from anterior to posterior. The walls of the bearing component are straight. A 0.5 mm stainless steel X-ray marker wire is placed 2 mm from the proximal surface.		

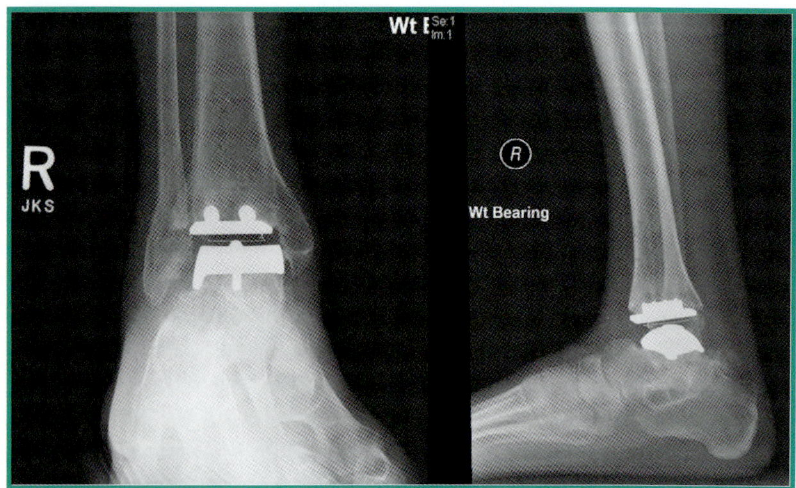

History of Implant

There are more than 5 different versions of the STAR ankle. Four of these have been implanted since 1981 outside of the USA. Since 1998 a fifth design was introduced into the US market which had subtle differences again. Although the first STAR ankle was a 2 component cemented design and was implanted between 1981–1986, Kofoed then developed the 3 component mobile bearing implant to replace this from 1986–2012. In 1989 the 3rd generation 3 piece design but with HA coating was introduced. Kofoed published improved results from the 3rd generation implant with 12 year survival of 95.4%. In 1998, the base coating of the STAR implant was changed to a rough Titanium plasma so that it could be used in the USA. This is the design used on the US clinical trials for FDA approval (Mann *et al.*, 2011) and is the current design used in the USA & Canada. This is different than the current design used outside of the USA and Canada, as of 1999, which has Calcium Phosphate on top of the Titanium plasma spray (referred to as double coat).

Due to the acquisition of Wright Medical by Stryker, the STAR implant had to be divested and so ownership will change.

Design Rationale

See Chapter on History of Ankle Replacements.

Additional Info

The walled talar implant restricts radiological analysis but Kofoed justified the reasons for the medial and lateral facets as follows:

- To cover the rough surfaces of the talar facets after gutter debridement.
- To preserve mobility as the facets assuming they are involved in disease process.
- To provide a broader surface area for talar component fixation. As the facets are covered in cartilage and normally articulate as part of the weight-bearing joint.

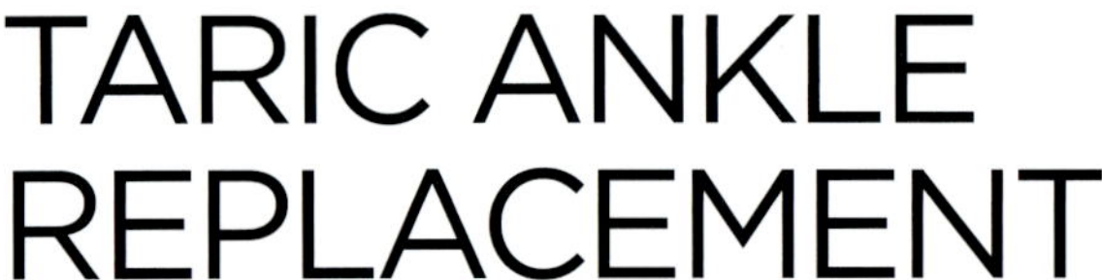

TARIC ANKLE REPLACEMENT

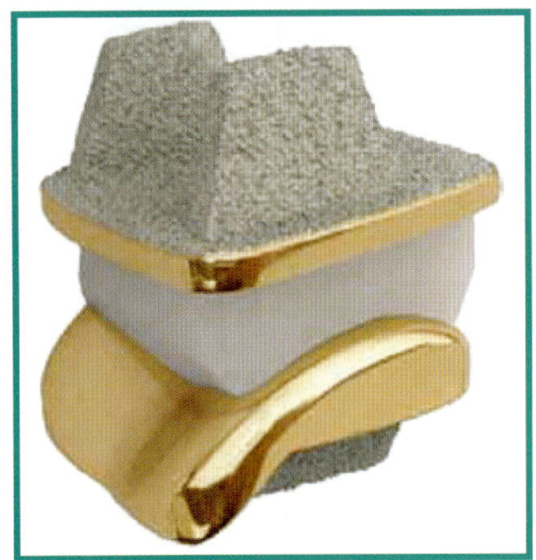

Photo of Taric Implant.

Manufacturer	Implantcast (Germany)
Inspiration behind name	
Surgeon inventor/designer(s)	Prof. Dr. Stefan Rehart, Frankfurt, Prof. Dr. Bernd Fink, Markgröningen, and Dr. Stephan Schill, Bad Aibling, Germany
FDA approved, date	Not FDA approved
CE mark, date	Assumed to be 2006
First operation date	2006
Number implanted to date	Unknown but small numbers
Generation	Third
Type	Mobile bearing

Evidence

No evidence available

	Material	Fixation	Sided
Tibial component	Two fins for primary fixation. Ti and HA coating allows a solid secondary fixation of the metal components to the bone.	Uncemented.	No
Talar component	Two fins for primary fixation. Ti and HA coating allows a solid secondary fixation of the metal components to the bone.	Uncemented.	No
Insert	Polyethylene.		

Design Rationale

Cementless Mobile bearing system. Two fins are configured for the primary fixation of the tibial and talar component. These fins clamp into the bone. The additional applied cpTi and HA coating allows a solid secondary fixation of the metal components to the bone.

Technique

Anterior approach. Instrumented technique.

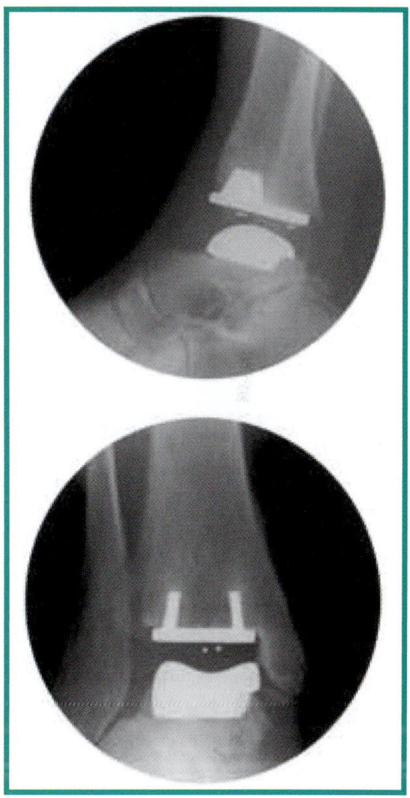

X-ray — AP and lateral view.

TNK ANKLE REPLACEMENT

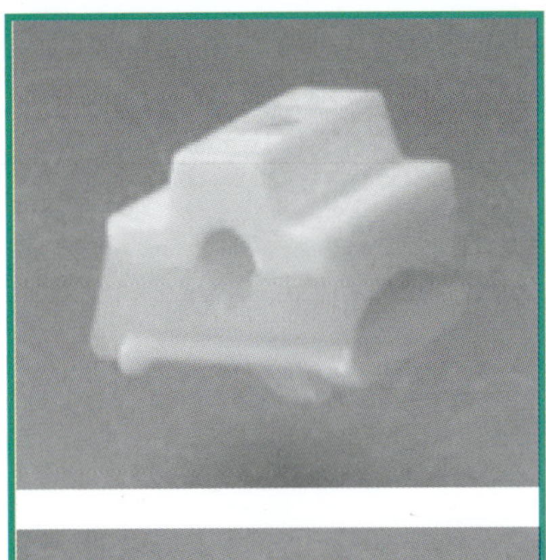

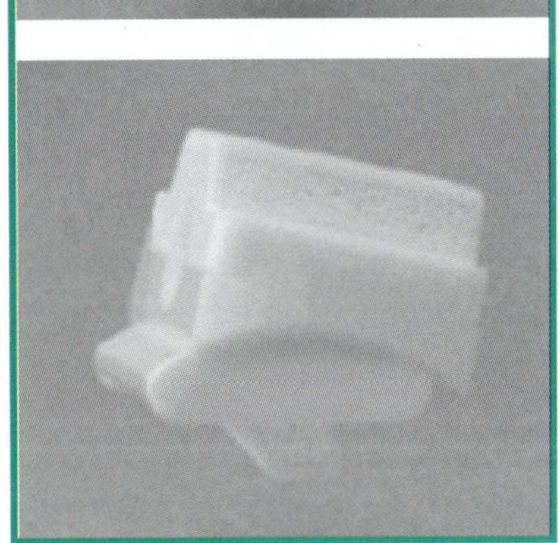

Manufacturer	Kyocera medical, Kyoto, Japan
Inspiration behind name	N/A
Surgeon designer(s)	Dr Yoshino Takakura
FDA approved, date	N/A
CE mark, date	Unknown
First operation date	1975
Number implanted to date	Unknown
Generation	Third
Type	Fixed bearing

Evidence	
Takakura (2008)	126 TNK ankles. Survival rate at 5.8 years 89%.
Tanaka and Takakura (2006)	Average 5 years follow-up of the third-generation TNK implant. 67 cases with average 62 months follow-up, with 96% survival.
Nishikawa *et al.* (2004)	27 rheumatoid cases followed up for a mean of 72 months, 89% survival. 75% rate of radiolucency observed, with tibial component migration in 13 cases, and talar collapse in 9.
Nagashima *et al.* (2004)	21 cases, of which 15 were hybrid implantations (talus cemented) with average follow-up 33.8 months in a rheumatoid population. 100% survival. 52% had significant radiolucent lines.
Shinomiya *et al.* (2003)	20 cementless replacements with a mean follow-up of 8 years. All patients showed functional improvement superior to those who underwent ankle arthrodesis in the same period. No revisions reported, although a radiolucent zone seen in 100% of cases.
Takakura *et al.* (2004) *Designer series*	This paper reviewed all three generations of implants. Significant loosening and subsidence was observed in the first generation. The second-generation implants were implanted in 60 ankles, of which 12 were cemented; however, loosening and subsidence again occurred in most within 5 years. The third generation was used in 70 ankles, with mean follow-up 5 years, with 3 cases revised.

History of Implant

It is currently the only total ankle prosthesis with alumina ceramic components.

The first generation was a cemented metal prosthesis, with the second generation being uncemented ceramic.

	Material	Fixation	Sided
Tibial component	Second and third generations alumina ceramic. New generation has processed microbeads made of alumina ceramic on surface in contact with the bone to aid osseointegration. AO screw is used to stabilise fixation if required.	Uncemented/cemented.	N/A
Talar component	Second and third generations alumina ceramic.	Uncemented/cemented.	N/A
Insert			

In 1988, Takakura *et al.*, reported a comparative study of 39 cemented metal and 30 uncemented ceramic TNK ankle two-component prostheses with high-density polyethylene fixed to the tibial component. The latter group were more satisfied which prompted further use of the implant.

In 1991, a third generation was introduced with the addition of a bead-formed alumina-coated with hydroxyapatite (HA).

Additional Info

The TNK ankle is similar to previous two-component prostheses that failed because of excessive shear forces and torque transfer to the implant–bone interface. Although reported failure rates are not discouraging, high loosening rates have been reported.

Osseointegration performance of HA-coated ceramic material is not known. As a result, high radiographic loosening rates in low demand (rheumatoid) patients have been reported.

Technique

Anterior approach to ankle.

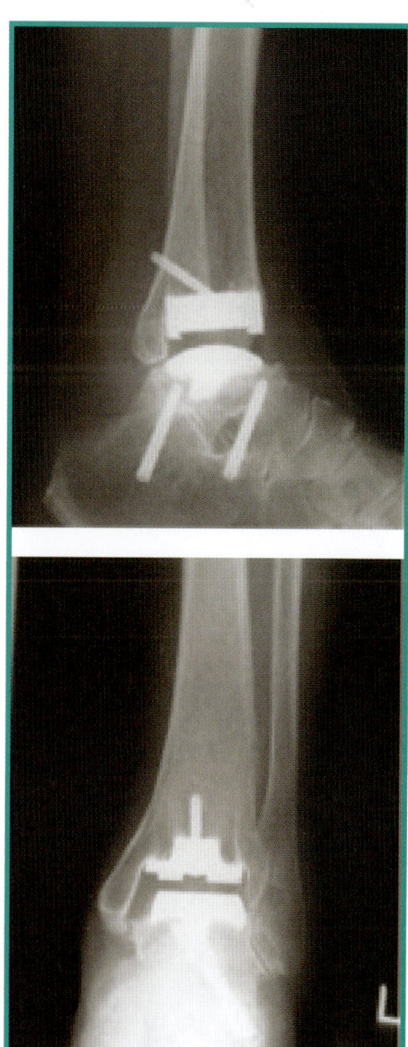

VANTAGE ANKLE REPLACEMENT

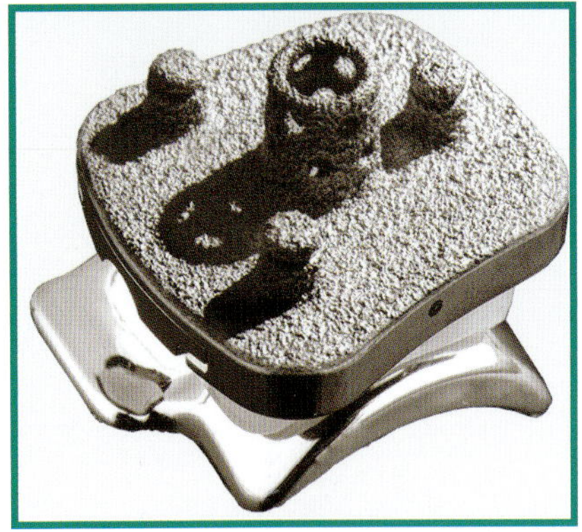

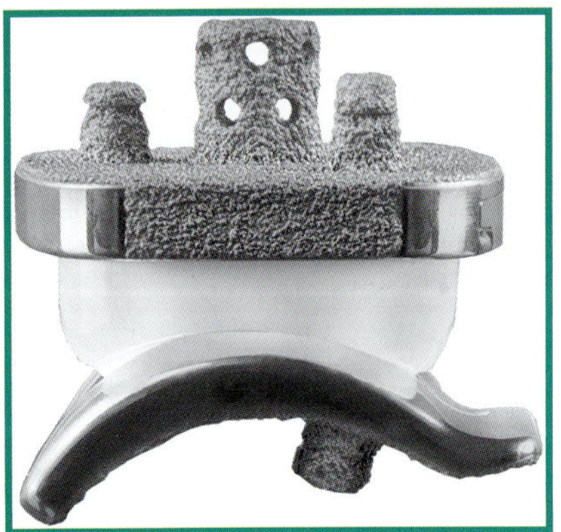

Photo — Oblique and lateral view.

Manufacturer	Exactech, Gainesville, FL, USA
Inspiration behind name	
Surgeon inventor/designer(s)	Victor Valderrabano, Basel, Switzerland; Dr Mark Easley, Dr James Nunley, and Dr James DeOrio, Durham, NC, USA
FDA approved, date	February 2016
CE mark, date	2017
First operation date	December 2017
Number implanted to date	Unknown
Generation	Third/fourth
Type	Mobile bearing (non-USA) and fixed bearing (USA)

Evidence

None yet available

	Material	Fixation	Sided
Tibial component	Stainless steel Nitronic 60.	Vertical cage pressfits for initial fixation. Peripheral pegs for rotational stability. In US, cemented fixation recommended in surgical technique.	Yes
Talar component	Stainless steel Nitronic 60.	Two pegs for press-fit stability. In US, cemented fixation recommended in surgical technique.	Yes
Insert	Bicondylar UHMWPE.	Fixed (USA) or Mobile (OUS).	

History of Implant

An international team comprised of European and US surgeons with intellectual property that differentiates itself from the market.

Design Rationale

Based on a CT reconstruction study of the healthy talus, the articular side of the talar component was said to be designed to allow for anatomic replication of the natural ankle biomechanics. The tibial component was developed to provide anatomic cortical coverage and account for fibular articulation. Two similar operative techniques are available for the mobile or fixed bearing implants.

Technique

Anterior approach.

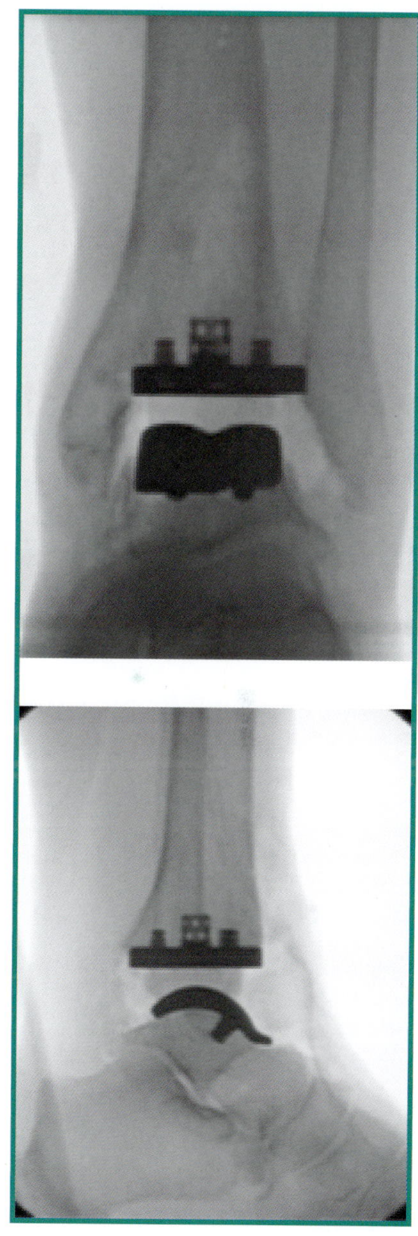

X-ray — AP and lateral view.

ZENITH ANKLE REPLACEMENT

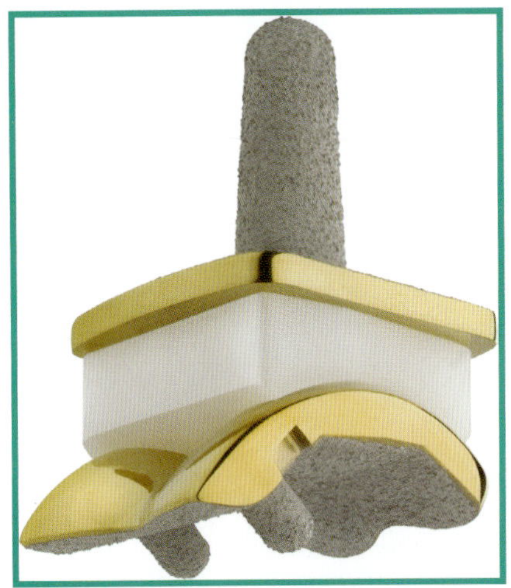

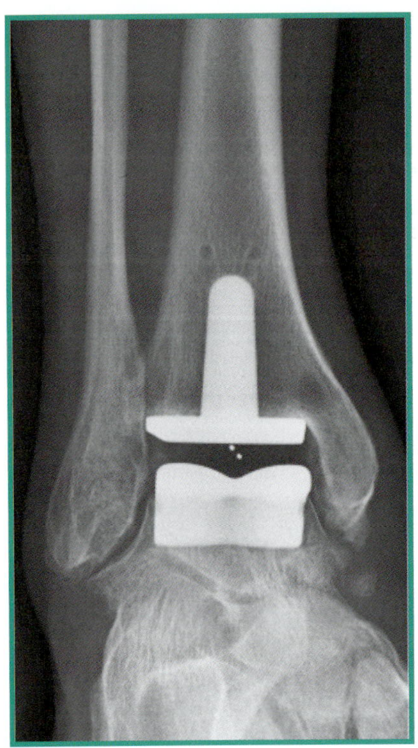

Manufacturer	Corin Group, Cirencester, UK
Inspiration behind name	N/A
Surgeon inventor/ designer(s)	Mr Ian Winson (Bristol, UK) and Herr Prof Dr med Jorg Jerosch, (Dusseldorf, Germany) amongst others
FDA approved, date	N/A
CE mark, date	2007
First operation date	2008
Number implanted to date	Unknown but more than 1000
Generation	Third
Type	Mobile bearing three-component total ankle replacement

Evidence	
Walter *et al.* (2015) **Designer series**	Mean follow-up was 50 months. Implant survival was 99.0% at 3 years and 93.8% at 7 years. Three cases underwent further surgery to address cysts, and 7 malleolar fractures were reported.
Mckenzie *et al.* (2012) **Designer series (EFORT 2012)**	Prospective follow-up of 81 ankles. 30 months survival of >95%.
Millar *et al.* (2012) (BOFAS)	50 patients with mean follow-up 30 months, 98% survival.

	Material	Fixation	Sided
Tibial component	Titanium alloy (Ti-6AL-4V). Articular surfaces have a ceramic titanium nitride (TiN) coating layer, which is aimed at reducing wear. It is a nickel-free implant.	Cementless, flat distal surface with central stem. Advanced biomimetic cementless technology coating incorporating titanium plasma spray with electrochemically applied calcium phosphate.	No
Talar component	Titanium alloy (Ti-6AL-4V). Articular surfaces have a ceramic titanium nitride (TiN) coating layer, which is aimed at reducing wear. Deep sulcus of talar component provides further stability for mobile insert.	Cementless. Two anterior pegs and three flat inferior surfaces with opening wedge effect for stability and maximum bone contact.	No
Insert	UHMWPE.		

History of Implant

This was developed based on the BP ankle by a team of design surgeons.

Design Rationale

Based on the Buechel–Pappas with a tibial stem.

Technique

Anterior approach, measured, minimal resection. Anterior tibial window may be required to allow tibial stem insertion.

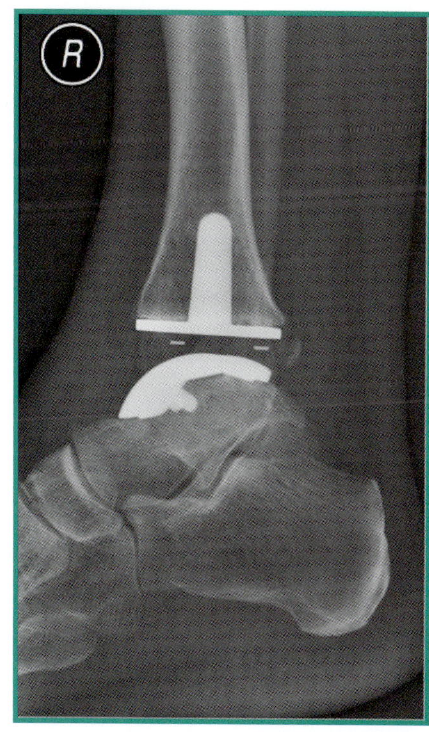

ZIMMER TRABECULAR METAL ANKLE REPLACEMENT

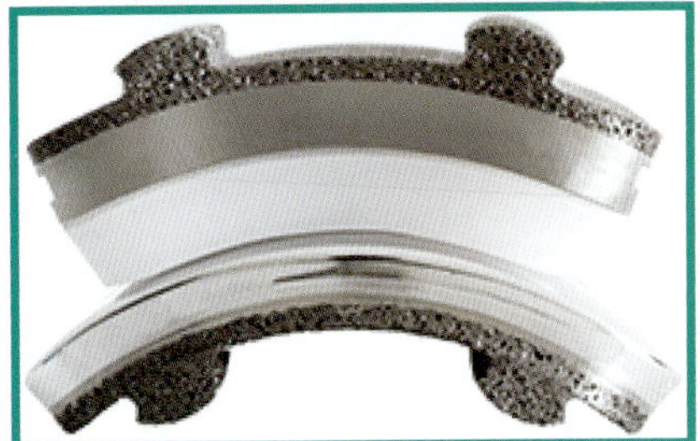

Image of Zimmer ankle.

Manufacturer	Zimmer-Biomet, Warsaw, IN, USA
Inspiration behind name	The name is a reflection of the primary material utilised to create the TM ankle
Surgeon inventor/ designer(s)	Lew Schon MD, Charlie Saltzman MD, Johnny Lau MD, Steve Herbst MD, Jonathan Deland MD, Christopher Chiodo MD
FDA approved, date	August 24, 2012
CE mark, date	November 10, 2012
First operation date	2012
Number implanted to date	Over 1000 worldwide
Generation	Third
Type	Two-piece semi-constrained bearing

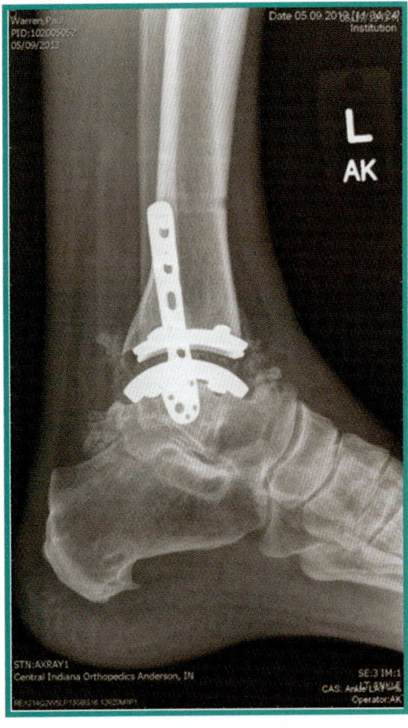

Lateral X-ray.

Evidence	
Bianchi *et al.* (2019)	Follow up of 30 implants with minimum follow up of 12 months. Most patients (91%) were satisfied. The rate of major complications requiring surgery was 23.3 % (7 patients), of which one had a perioperative dislocation of the ankle.
Barg *et al.* (2018)	55 ankles with implant survival of 93% at 24 months of follow-up. There were 3 revisions of a tibial component due to aseptic loosening. In 10 of the 55 cases (18%), a secondary procedure was performed during follow-up.
DeVries *et al.* (2017)	16 patients followed up for mean 25 months. 100% survival of implant. Three cases of delayed or non-union of the fibula (18.8%).
Barg and Saltzman (2017) (Abstract)	Implant survival 93% at 36 months. No delayed or non-union for fibula healing. Improvement in VAS scores at mean follow-up 26.6 months.
Usuelli *et al.* (2016)	67 patients with minimum follow-up 12 months. Improvement in pain and function scores.
Tan *et al.* (2016)	20 consecutive TARs with an average follow-up of 18 months. No fibular non-union or implant failure was found at 12 months postoperatively. One patient had asymptomatic mild tibial lucency. About 4 of 20 TARs underwent additional surgery for anterior impingement (one ankle), deep infection and symptomatic fibular hardware (one ankle), and symptomatic fibular hardware (two ankles).

	Material	Fixation	Sided
Tibial component	Made from Titanium® (Ti-6Al-4V) alloy diffusion bonded to a trabecular metal surface. The proximal surface includes two fixation rails to facilitate stability.	Cemented.	No
Talar component	Made from Zimaloy® (CoCrMo) alloy with a trabecular metal distal surface and a thin interlayer of commercially pure titanium. Larger sagittal radius of curvature laterally than medially. The distal surface includes two fixation rails to facilitate stability.	Cemented.	Yes
Insert	Made from Prolong® highly cross-linked polyethylene.		

History of Implant

The trabecular metal total ankle began as a marriage of two ideas between Drs Schon and Saltzman bringing together their concepts for a lateral approach and the utilisation of an external fixation frame to aid in restoring the ankle with an anatomic implant design.

Design Rationale

The transfibular approach is intended to maintain the integrity of the blood supply to the skin, potentially reducing wound healing complications. In many cases a separate medial incision is needed to deal with varus ankles.

Technique

Transfibular approach. Implant inserted using an alignment system. An additional medial incision may be required in cases of deformity.

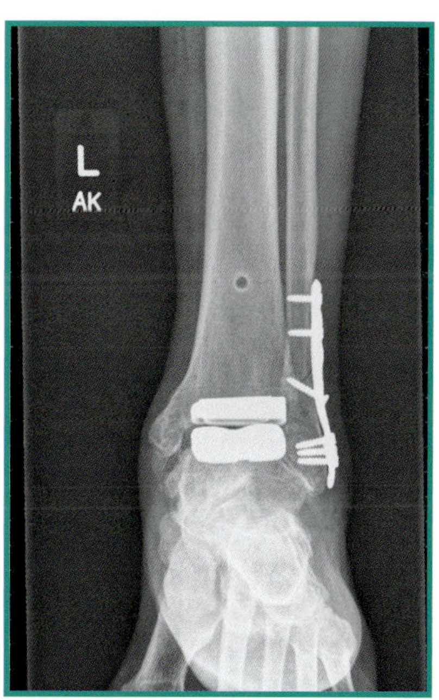

AP X-ray.

HISTORIC ANKLE REPLACEMENTS

This page was left blank intentionally

AGILITY ANKLE REPLACEMENT

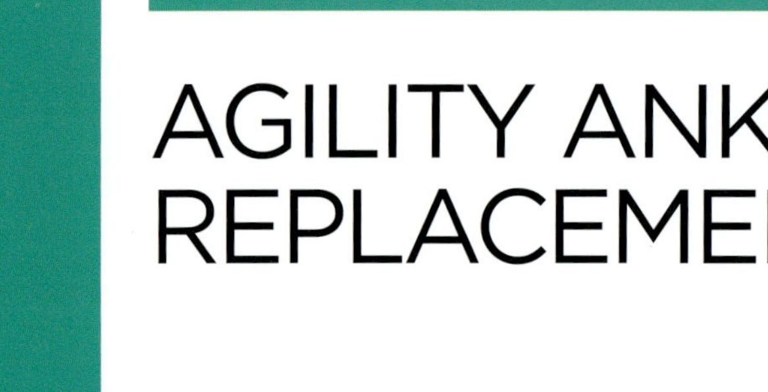

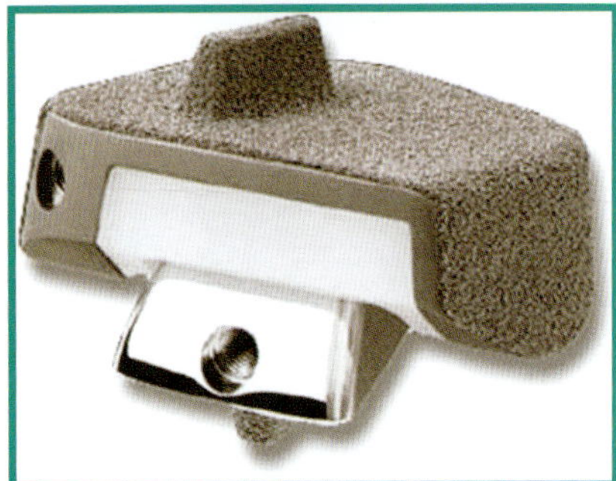

Manufacturer	DePuy, Warsaw, IN, USA
Inspiration behind name	The implant was named by the company
Surgeon inventor/ designer(s)	Frank Alvine
FDA approved, date	1992
CE mark, date	Unknown
First operation date	1984
Number implanted to date	Unknown
Generation	Second
Type	Fixed bearing, semiconstrained

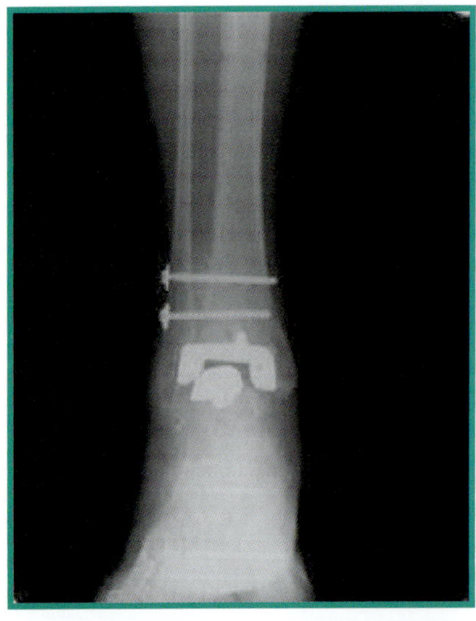

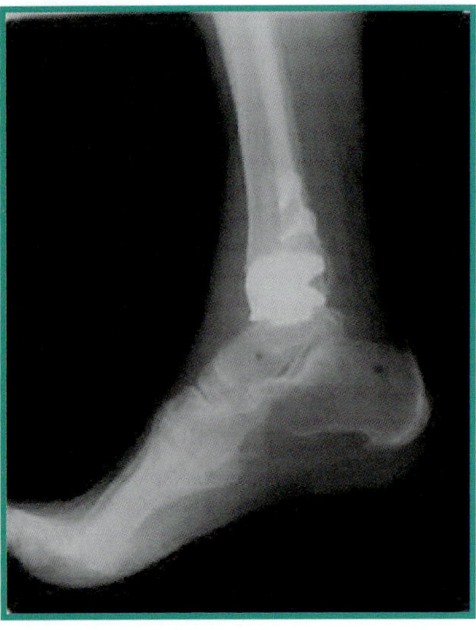

Evidence	
Raikin *et al.* (2017)	Review of prospectively collected data on 127 agility ankles. At average 9 years follow-up, survival was almost 80%, with satisfaction not correlating to the radiographic appearance of osteolysis. Age at the time of surgery and inflammatory/atraumatic arthritis were predictive of failure.
Lefrancois *et al.* (2017)	Mean improvement in total AOS score was 29.1, pain AOS score was 21.3, and disability AOS score was 17.3. Survival rates 77% at mean 6.1 years follow-up. Improvements in pain and function were comparable to Hintegra and STAR implants, and superior to mobility.
McInnes *et al.* (2014)	Cadaveric biomechanical study looking at bone–implant interface on loading. The agility exhibited greater relative motion than the STAR, suggesting that lack of primary stability may contribute to a higher aseptic loosening rate.
Roukis (2012)	Systematic review including 14 studies totalling 2312 agility ankle replacements, with an average follow-up of 22.8 months. There was 9.7% revision rate, of which the majority was for component revision (81%), then arthrodesis (15%) with a proportion requiring a below knee amputation (3.6%). Excluding inventor series doubled the revision rate.
Criswell *et al.* (2012)	65 implants were followed up over an average of 8 years (0.5–11). Survival of the implant was 61%. Of the 25 cases that retained their implant, 12 required second surgery, giving an overall reoperation rate of 68%.

Claridge and Sagherian (2009)	A review of 28 agility implants performed over 5 years. AOFAS score improved from 34.9 to 76.4. Complications occurred in 13 cases, the most common being wound healing issues, deep infection, and postoperative fracture.	
Kopp *et al.* (2006)	40 implants followed up for a mean of 44.5 months. AOFAS score improved from 33.6 to 83.3. 85% demonstrated radiographic lucency or lysis, with migration or subsidence of components in 45%. 37 of 38 patients were reported to be satisfied.	
Spirt *et al.* (2004)	Follow-up at average 33 months of 306 implants between 1995 and 2001. Survival rate at 5 years with reoperation at the end point was 56%, but for component revision was 80%.	
Knecht *et al.* (2004)	In total, 132 implants were followed up for an average of 9 years, with survival 89%. Radiographic assessment at minimum 2 years of 117 replacements revealed degeneration in the subtalar joint (19%), talonavicular joint (15%), and 8% had a syndesmosis non-union. There was evidence of peri-implant radiolucency in 76%.	
Pyevich *et al.* (1998)	Mean follow-up of 4.8 years of 100 implants. 55% of ankles were pain-free at this point. Delayed union of the syndesmosis 28% and non-union of the syndesmosis 9% were associated with the development of lysis around the tibial component.	

	Material	Fixation	Sided
Tibial component	Titanium with a sintered titanium bead surface. Articular surface of the tibial component is larger than that of the talar component.	Uncemented.	No
Talar component	Cobalt chromium with a sintered titanium bead surface.	Uncemented.	No
Insert	Polyethylene insert is locked into the tibial component.		

History of Implant

The Agility became the most widely used TAR in the United States in the 1990's since the introduction of the Agility LP ankle system which had a redesigned broad-based talar component and the ability to mix and match component sizes and a front loaded polyethylene insert for easier exchange. Since new implants came to the market in the last two decades, however, sales of the Agility have fallen.

Design Rationale

Arthrodesis of the tibiofibular syndesmosis is part of the design to allow greater transfer of weight to the fibula. This was achieved with screws or plating.

ALPHANORM

The Alphanorm TAR was developed by Professor Tilmann in Germany who has previous experience of using the TPR, BP prostheses and STAR (Tillman, 2003). The Alphanorm was first used in 1996. The Alphanorm is a non-constrained Buechel-Pappas type design with a 90° tibial stem without inclination. The components are made out of cobalt chrome alloy with a titanium coating. No published studies could be identified to assess outcomes.

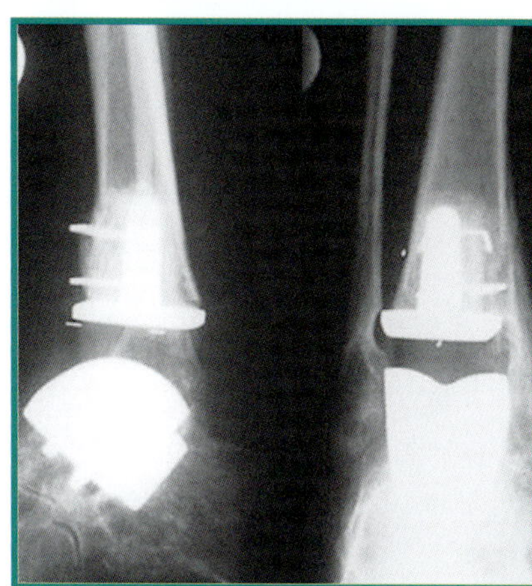

ANKLE EVOLUTIVE SYSTEM (AES)

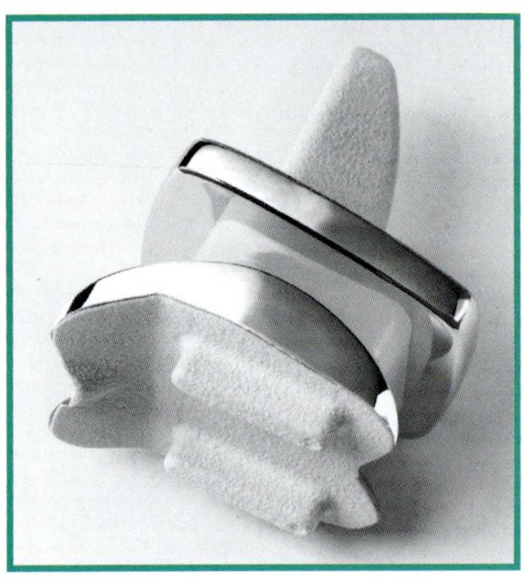

Photo of AES implant.

Manufacturer	Transysteme, France (Distributed by Biomet Merck, The Netherlands)
Inspiration behind name	Ankle Evolutive System (AES)
Surgeon designer(s)	Jo Asencio, Nimes France
FDA approved, date	N/A
CE mark, date	2009
First operation date	1999
Number implanted to date	Unknown — at least 600
Generation	Third
Type	Mobile bearing three-component design

Evidence	
Di Iorio *et al.* (2017)	At mean follow-up of 10 years, the mean AOFAS score was 75 points. About 15 TAR (20%) had reoperation for cyst curettage graft because of periprosthetic lesions. At last follow-up, 14 (19%) were revised to fusion.
Koivu *et al.* (2017)	This study reports results for 130 AES ankle replacements. 5-year survival was 87.3%. 10-year survival was 74.9%. Peri-implant osteolysis was found in 91 (70%) of ankles. The revision rate was 34% at median follow-up of 96 months.
Popelka *et al.* (2016)	15.3% of patients had cystic radiolucencies adjacent to tibial or talar implants at mean 6.1 years follow-up.
Besse *et al.* (2013)	Medium-term results for bone grafting to osteolytic lesions were poor. In 14 AES replacements, bone grafting led to 79% and 92% worse or unimproved clinical and radiological outcomes respectively. Revision with arthrodesis was recommended for progressive lesions.
Dalat *et al.* (2013)	Series of 84 implants followed up for 59.8 months. Of these, 25 underwent revision for osteolysis. Radiologically, all patients showed tibial and talar osteolytic lesions. All specimens showed macrophagic granulomatous inflammatory reactions in contact with a foreign body.
Kokkonen *et al.* (2011)	28 months follow-up of 38 implants. 2-year survival was 79% with an osteolysis rate of 74%.
Henricson *et al.* (2010)	93 implants were reviewed at average 3.5 years follow-up. They reported survivorship of 90% at 5 years with revision for any reason as an end point.
Rodriguez *et al.* (2010)	39.4 months follow-up of 21 cases with 2 revisions. AOFAS score improved from 52.2 to 86.6. 77% rate of osteolysis.

| | Morgan *et al.* (2010) | 57.8 months follow-up of 38 cases. Survival 94.7%. Nine had corrective surgery, and there were two revisions. Osteolysis present in 24%. |
| | Koivu *et al.* (2009) | 130 implants implanted over a 6-year period with minimum 1-year follow-up. Osteolytic lesions on plain films in 37%, with marked osteolysis in 21%. Revision rate 15.5%. |

	Material	Fixation	Sided
Tibial component	Cobalt chrome with HA coating. Modular stem. Tibial keel to improve component stability.	Uncemented.	No
Talar component	Cobalt chrome with HA coating. Symmetrical talar dome.	Uncemented.	No
Insert	UHMWPE.		

History of Implant

This implant was a development of the Buechel–Pappas-type stemmed tibial prosthesis but where the tibial stem had a curved sail-like shape.

Design Rationale

Buechel–Pappas-type prosthesis. Cobalt chromium three-component ankle prosthesis. Modular tibial stem allowing hemi replacement of medial tibiotalar and talofibular joints. Tibial stem anteriorly bowed. Modular talar facets covered.

Additional Info

A medical device warning was issued in 2012 by the MHRA due to high rates of osteolysis, and the product was withdrawn from the market shortly thereafter. Theories behind the high osteolysis rate include: polyethylene wear; third body wear from HA coating; and the interaction of metal particles from pathological stress shielding.

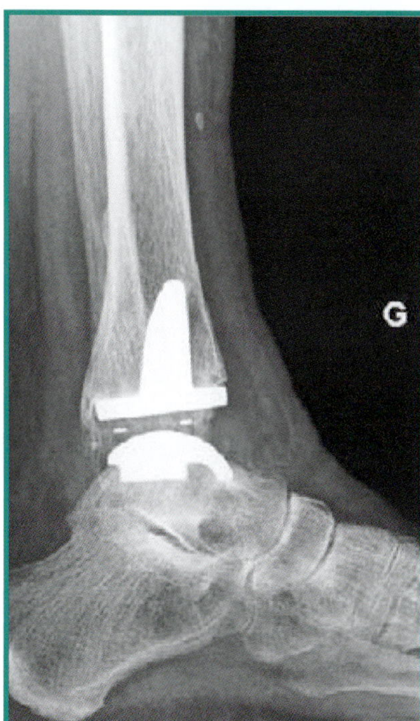

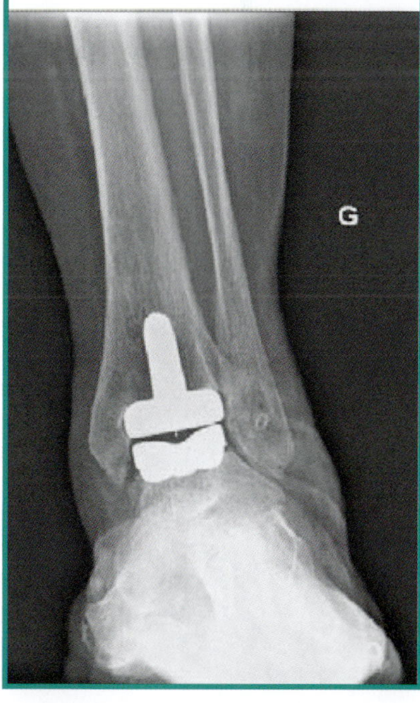

X-ray — AP and lateral view.

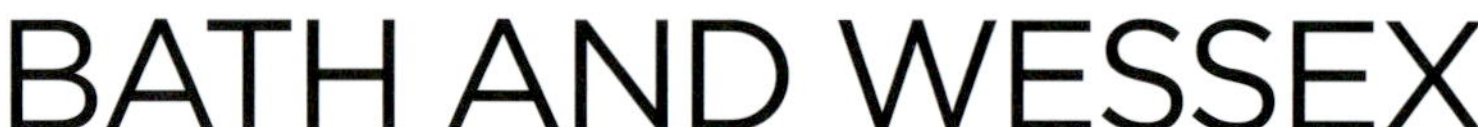

BATH AND WESSEX

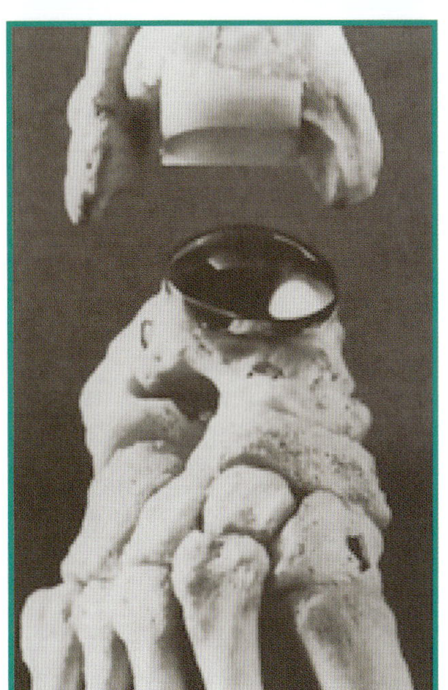

This implant was developed by John Kirkup who noted that children with congenital tarsal fusions developed a "ball and socket" ankle which provided polyaxial motion to compensate from stiff subtalar and midfoot motion. Whilst engaged in developing his own ankle, he noted that the Richard Smith ankle became available and so initially he started using this implant and reported on his first 24 cases (Kirkup, 1985). He felt he could improve on this design and hence developed his own two-component unconstrained cemented prosthesis with a polyethylene tibial component that was implanted from 1984 to 1996 (Marsh et al., 1987, Kirkup 1990). Survival in 72 implants was 83% and 66% at 5 and 10 years respectively (Carlsson et al., 2001).

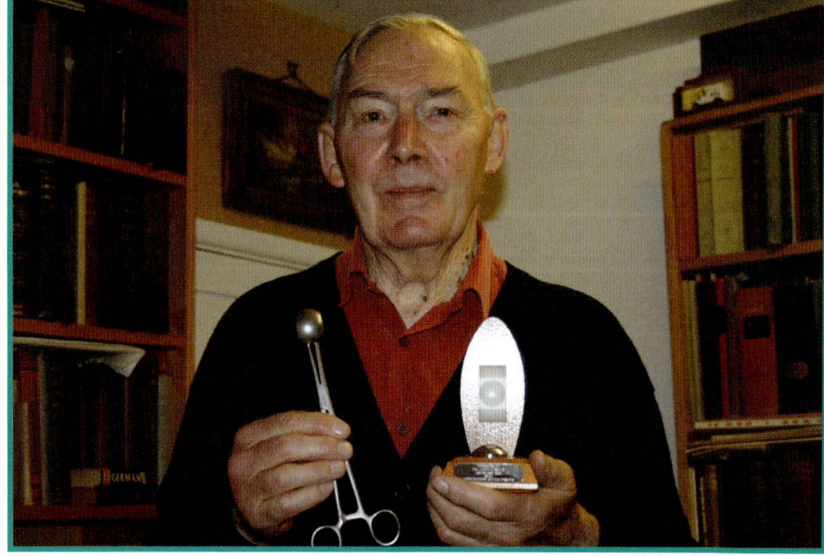

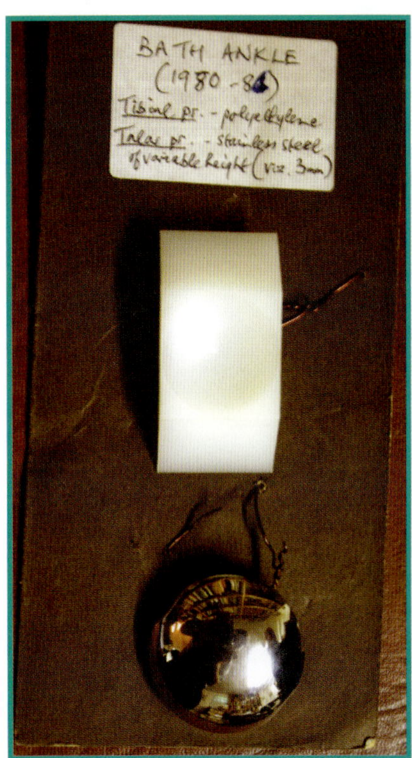

This page was left blank intentionally

BUECHEL–PAPPAS ANKLE REPLACEMENT

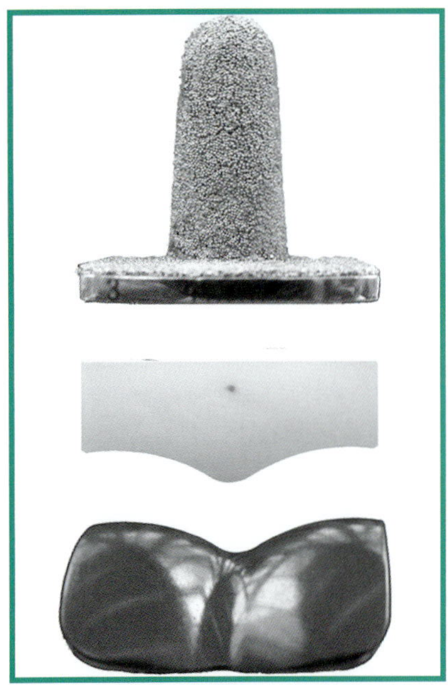

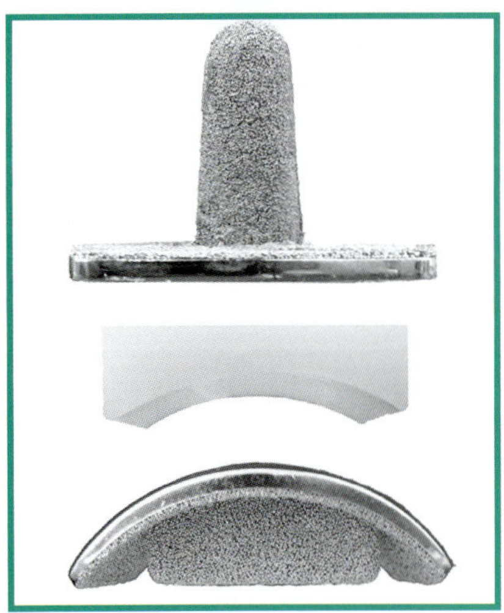

Manufacturer	Endotec (USA)
Inspiration behind name	Named after inventors
Surgeon inventor/designer(s)	Frederick Buechel (surgeon) and Michael Pappas (engineer)
FDA approved, date	The device never achieved FDA approval but several 510k applications were submitted. It was used on compassionate grounds as "surgeon specials" on a case by case basis
CE mark, date	Unknown
First operation date	1989
Number implanted to date	Unknown
Generation	Second
Type	Mobile bearing

Evidence	
Kraal *et al.* (2013)	A review of 93 implants, of which 74 were Buechel–Pappas (BP), the remaining LCS. At 15 years, 31 implants were assessed in surviving patients, with a cumulative failure rate of 20%, and an average AOFAS score of 80.4. In total, 23 cases required revision, with 3 implant exchanges, 3 bearing exchanges, and 17 arthrodeses.
Wood *et al.* (2009)	Randomised study of 200 ankle replacements. Compared BP and the Scandinavian Total Ankle Replacement (STAR). The 6-year survivorship of the BP design was 79% and of the STAR 95%. The factor that reached statistical significance for implant survival was the degree of preoperative coronal alignment.
Ali *et al.* (2007)	Follow-up of 35 implants with mean follow-up of 5 years, with 97% survival.
San Giovanni *et al.* (2006)	31 implants placed in a low demand rheumatoid group. At mean follow-up of 8.3 years, survivorship was 93%. They reported tibial or talar component subsidence in 18% of cases.
Doets *et al.* (2006)	93 total ankle arthroplasty (LCS in 19, BP in 74). Significant improvement in pain scores at 1 year. At 8 years follow-up, mean survival rate 84%.
Buechel *et al.* (2004) *Designer series*	Shallow sulcus design 40 implants, average follow-up 12 (range 2–20) years. The 20-year overall survivorship was 74.2%. Deep sulcus design — 75 implants, average follow-up 5 (range 2–12) years. The 12-year overall survivorship was 92.5%.

	Material	Fixation	Sided
Tibial component	Ti alloy. TiN (ultracoat) — ceramic coating. BioCoat — three layers porous coating. Stemmed with 7° anterior inclination — tibial window needs to be cut to allow implantation.	Uncemented.	No
Talar component	Ti alloy. TiN (ultracoat) — ceramic coating. BioCoat — three layers porous coating. Deep sulcus and dual fin fixation in mark 2 design.	Uncemented.	No
Insert	UHMWPE.		

History of Implant

Evolved from the LCS ankle replacement. It was the first reported three-component prosthesis with a Mobile bearing, and is the predecessor of many modern implants.

The design has been modified, with the initial "Mark 1" designed with removal of the anteroposterior constraint between the tibial and Mobile bearings resulting in a shallow sulcus prosthesis. The mark 2 was introduced after 1990 with a deeper sulcus on the talar component, two fins and a thicker meniscal component.

Design Rationale

Originally designed with a flat upper surface, with the conforming lower articular surface of the meniscus provides sliding and cylindrical motion on the bearing surfaces. There have been many design iterations, see Chapter 7.

Technique

Anterior approach. Instrumented technique.

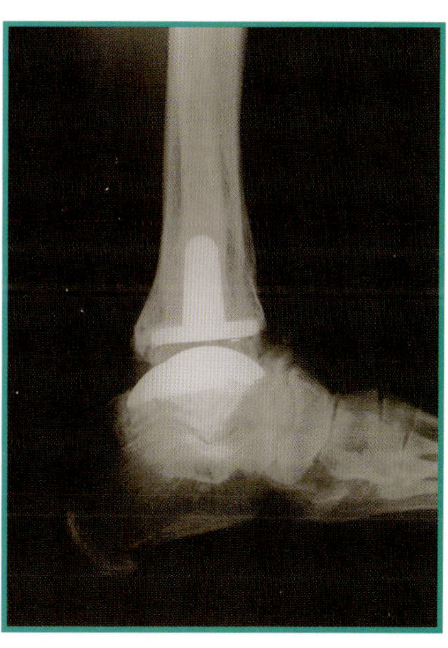

CCI ANKLE REPLACEMENT

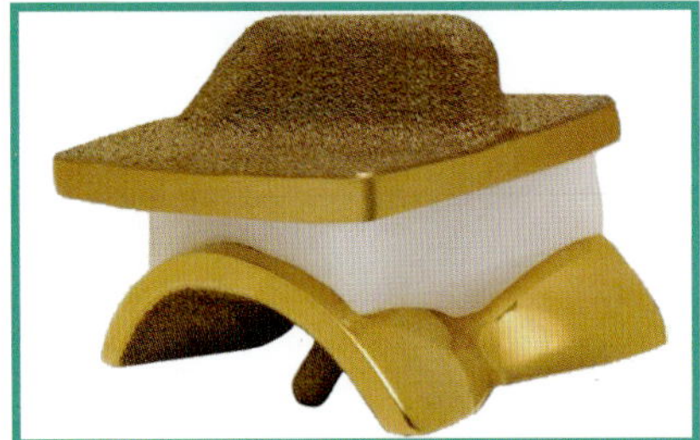

Manufacturer	Van Straten Medical — later sold to Wright Medical
Inspiration behind name	Ceramic-coated implant
Surgeon inventor/ designer(s)	Dr HC Doets, The Netherlands
FDA approved, date	N/A
CE mark, date	2003
First operation date	2003
Number implanted to date	Circa 2000
Generation	Third
Type	Mobile bearing three component design

Evidence	
Voesenek *et al.* (2017)	58 TAR followed up mean 21.6 months. High incidence of complications (37%) and re-operations (31%) when minor complications and reoperations are included. Nine malleolar fractures occurred in the group. 12 patients (21%) had either a component revision or a full revision to arthrodesis.
Nieuwe Weme *et al.* (2015)	90 TAR followed up with posttraumatic arthritis. 75 had CCI. 6-year survival rate 87%.

	Material	Fixation	Sided
Tibial component	Cobalt chrome. Trapezoidal design with fixation fin.	Uncemented. Titanium plasma spray surface structure with a Bonit® calcium phosphate coating on top.	No
Talar component	Cobalt chrome with two talar pegs. Three V-shaped surfaces build the implant–bone interface, allowing for instrument-guided bone cuts. The design of the talar component includes a deep sulcus.	Uncemented. Titanium plasma spray surface structure with a Bonit® calcium phosphate coating on top.	No
Insert	Polyethylene.		

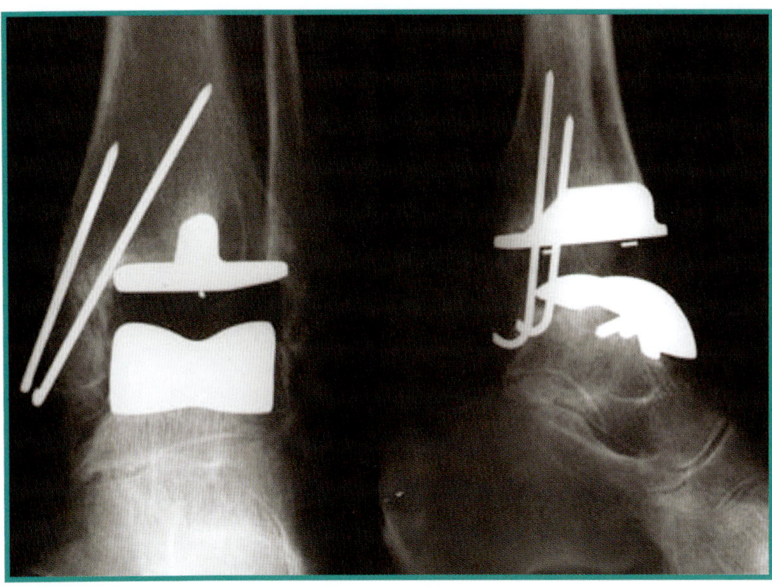

X-ray — AP and lateral view.

History of Implant
This implant was the idea of Kees Doets from Holland. He developed it Van Straten Medical, although after a few years they sold the *implant to Wright Medical who later chose to develop their own* ankle from scratch and the CCI was shelved.

Design Rationale
Symmetrical mobile bearing implant with minimal talar resection. Ceramic-coated implant with titanium nitride coating.

ECLIPSE

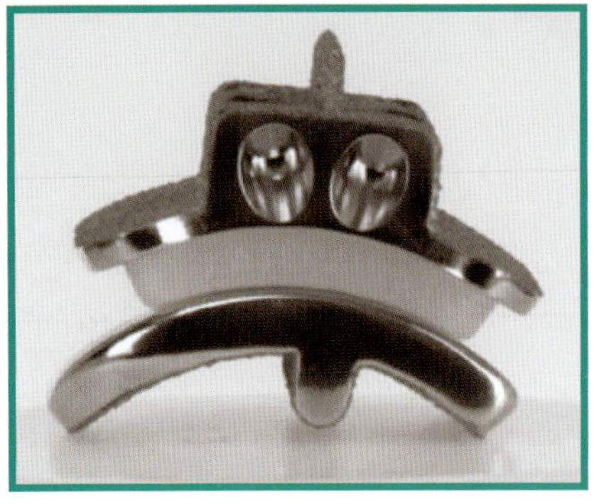

Introduced by Integra Life Sciences in 2006 on the basis of a 510k approval process as a class II device, this was a third-generation uncemented fixed-bearing two component design. Made from cobalt chrome with a titanium spray coat, it used an extra medullary jig with cylindrical cuts through a medial or lateral approach. Only a few were implanted prior to the product being shelved and there is no published outcome data.

This page was left blank intentionally

ESKA ANKLE REPLACEMENT

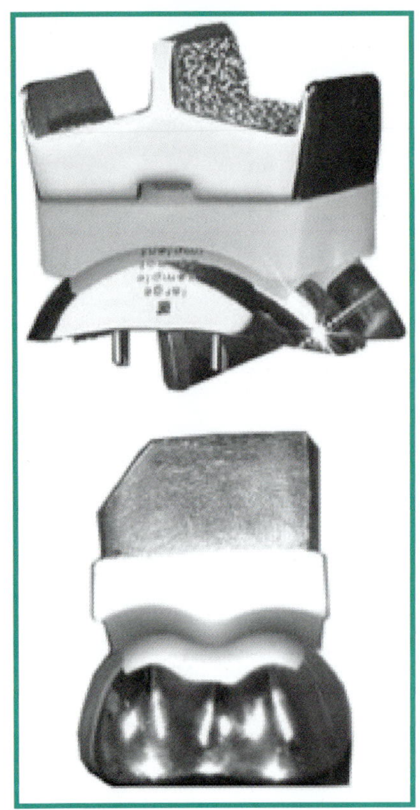

Manufacturer	**ESKA Orthodynamics, Germany**
Inspiration behind name	The name stems from the company ESKA
Surgeon inventor/ designer(s)	Dr Rudigier
FDA approved, date	N/A
CE mark, date	Unknown
First operation date	1990
Number implanted to date	Unknown
Generation	Third
Type	Non-constrained fixed-bearing two-component prosthesis

Evidence	
Rudigier *et al.* (2001, 2005) *Designer series*	At minimum 1-year follow-up, 40 cases showed survival 92.5%, with 2 implants revised for deep infection. Longer follow-up of a cohort of 159 implants, with increase in Kofoed score from 37.6 to 90.4. For those placed with 1–5 year follow-up, no implants failed. Those placed with 5–10 year follow-up, survival was 85%. For 12 implants with 10–15 year follow-up, survival was 67%.

	Material	Fixation	Sided
Tibial component	CoCr.	Uncemented with porous coated surface.	No
Talar component	CoCr.	Uncemented with porous coated surface. Shallow groove that is congruous to polyethylene bearing.	No
Insert	Polyethylene.	Fixed to tibial component.	

History of Implant

The cementless ESKA implant was developed between 1985 and 1989 and first implanted in 1990. The designer claimed it was developed as a consequence of the poor results of earlier cemented prostheses and used a lateral approach.

Design Rationale

Two-component cementless implantation with porous structured surface to aid osseointegration. Shear force and rotation force control by shape design, with ease of polyethylene replacement without disturbing prosthesis anchoring. Due to ridge shape and transverse anchoring peg, a lateral approach is used.

Additional Info

This implant was highly novel in that it used a lateral approach, a technique later adapted by the Zimmer ankle.

Technique

Lateral approach insertion with fibular osteotomy.

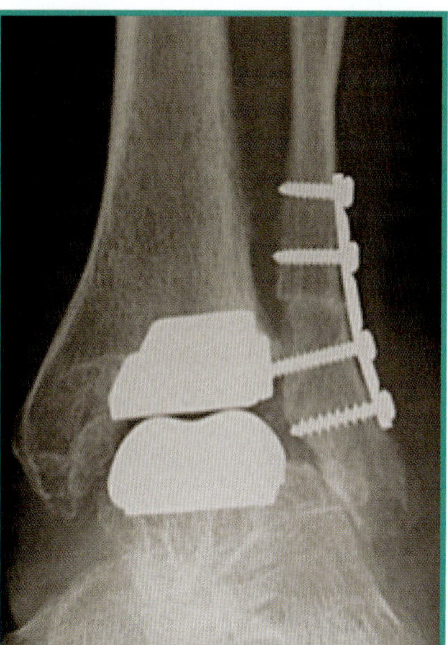

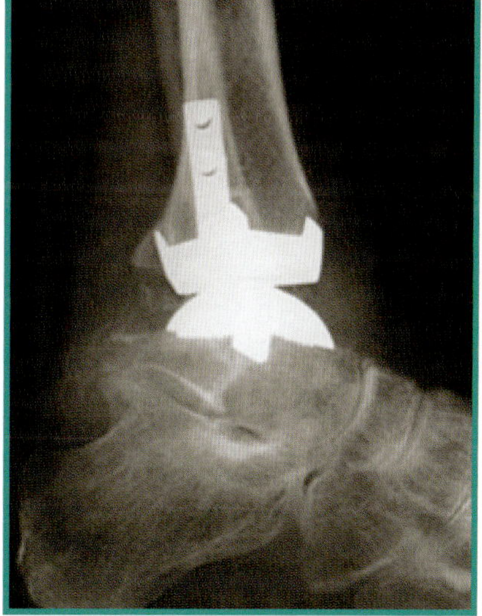

GERMAN ANKLE SYSTEM

The German Ankle System was designed by Martinus Richter in partnership with R-Innovation from Coburg in Germany. In 2007 Richter et al published data to suggest that their new three component mobile bearing design had improved kinematics in comparison to the Hintegra prosthesis. This was a conceptual design that never made it to the market due to intellectual property issues.

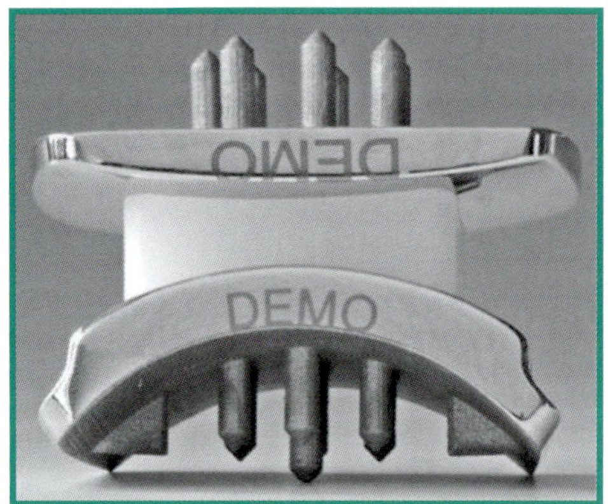

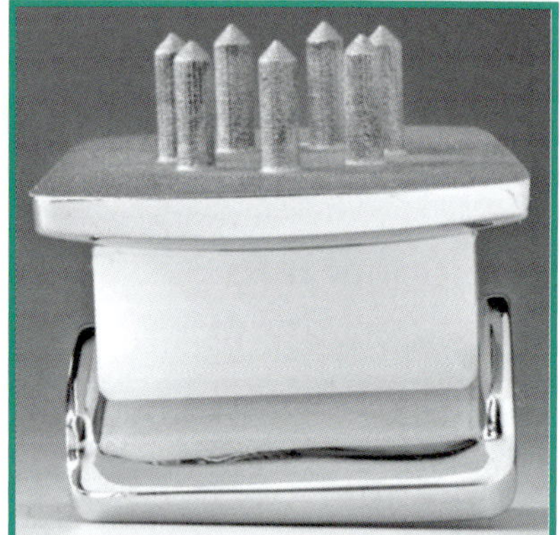

IMPERIAL COLLEGE OF LONDON HOSPITAL (ICLH)

Used from 1972 to 1981, this two-component constrained cemented prosthesis with a polyethylene tibial implant had elevated medial and lateral walls to limit coronal subluxation of the talus (Bolton-Maggs *et al.*, 1985; Freeman *et al.*, 1978; Kempson *et al.*, 1975). Satisfactory results were reported in 11 of 62 cases, with a 5.5 years revision rate of 47% (Bolton-Maggs *et al.*, 1985; Helm and Stevens, 1986).

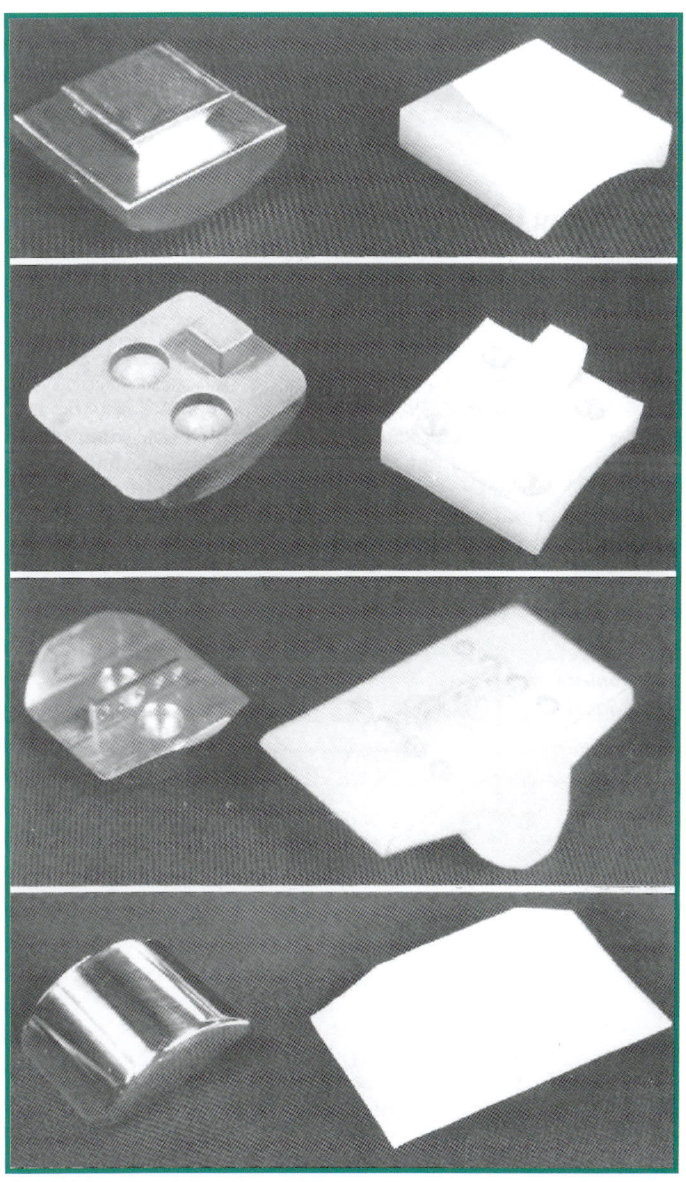

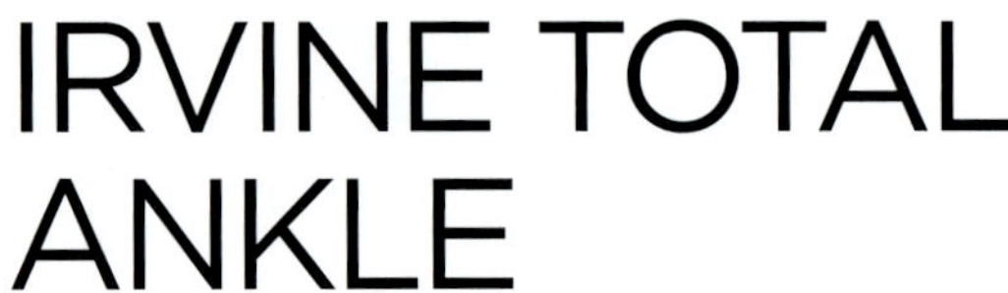

IRVINE TOTAL ANKLE

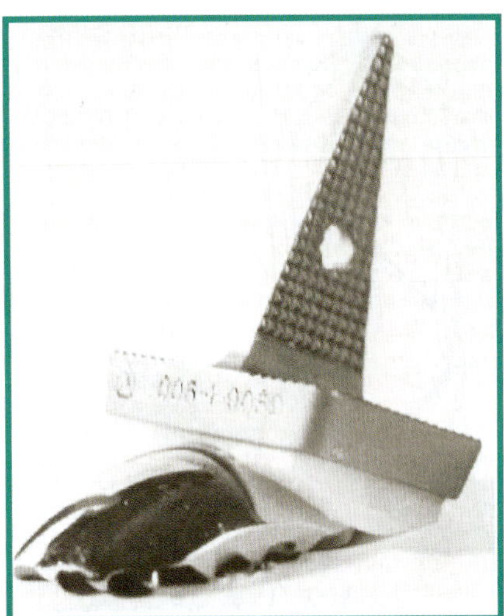

A Californian implant used in the 1970s. This was one of the early designs that aimed to recreate talar anatomy, but rotation of the components placed stress on the constraining ligaments. Early data documented two failures at 9 months for 28 implants, with no later data published (Waugh and Evanski, 1976).

LORD AND MAROTTE ANKLE

The first total ankle replacement was performed by Lord and Marotte in 1970 (Lord and Marotte, 1970). Like an inverted hip replacement, there was a long stemmed tibial component with a polyethylene component that was cemented into the calcaneus following removal of the talus. After 10 years, 7 of 25 procedures were considered to have a satisfactory outcome and the team concluded that a simple hinge prosthesis would be insufficient to mimic the normal ankle joint.

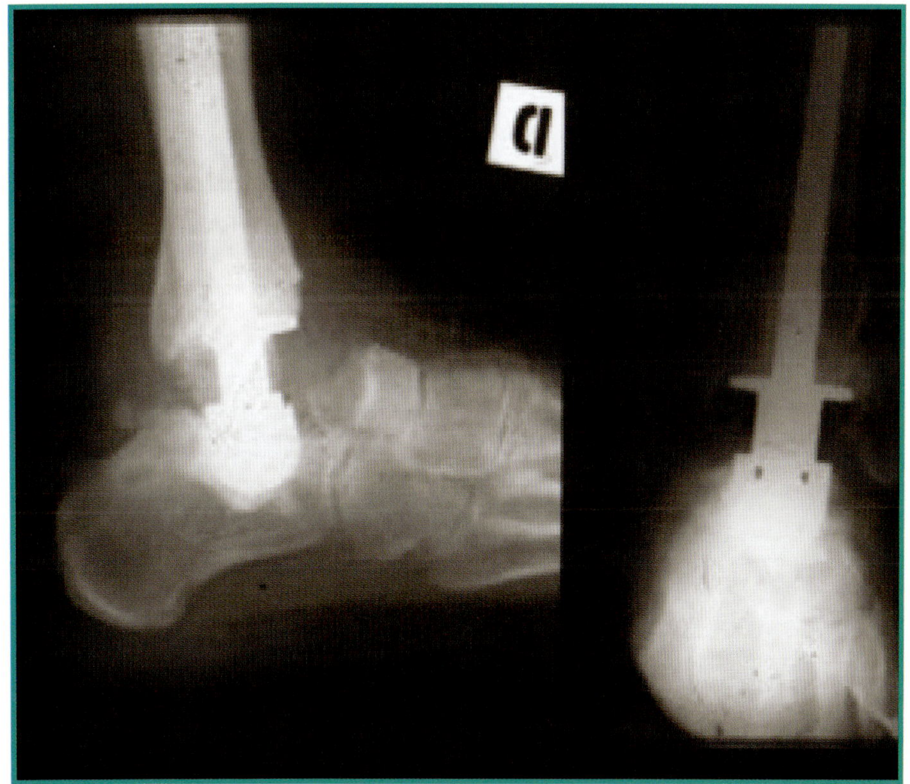

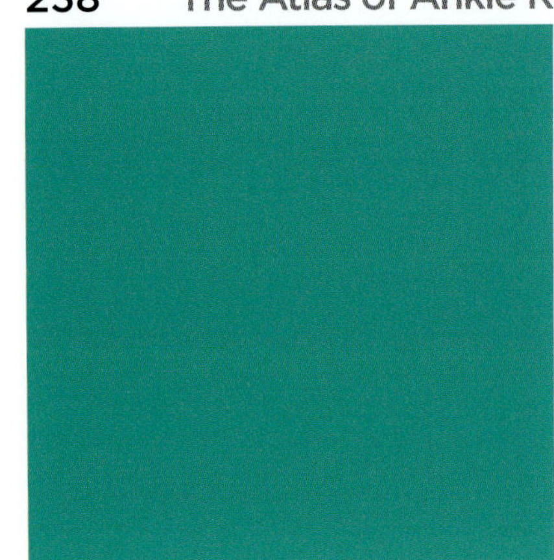

MAYO

Designed by the Mayo clinic in the 1970s, this was a highly congruous two-component constrained prosthesis. Both components were cemented, with the tibial component being made of polyethylene. Follow-up over a 12-year period of 204 implants showed 19% to have a good result, with 36% requiring removal. Implant survival at 5, 10, and 15 years was 79%, 65%, and 61% respectively (Kitaoka and Patzer, 1996).

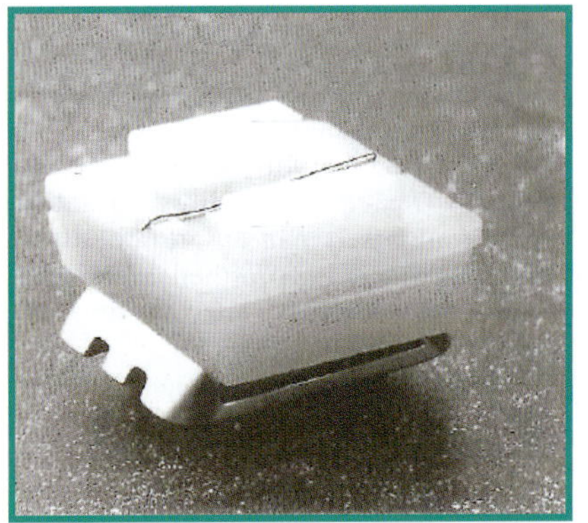

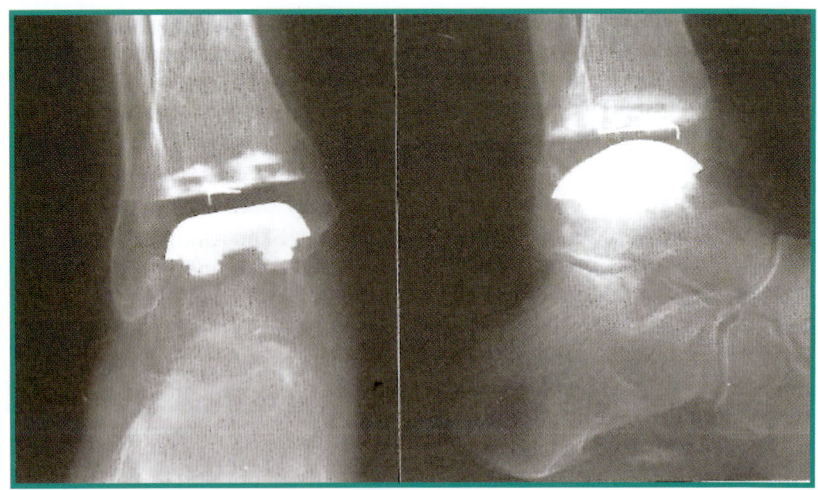

This page was left blank intentionally

MOBILITY ANKLE REPLACEMENT

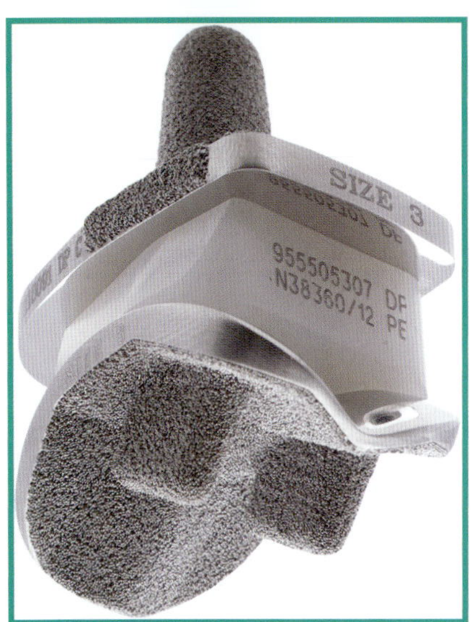

Photo of mobility implant.

Manufacturer	DePuy International, Leeds, UK
Inspiration behind name	To mobilise the ankle
Surgeon inventor/ designer(s)	Rippstein (Zurich, Switzerland), Wood (Wrightington, UK), Coetzee (Minnesota, USA)
FDA approved, date	N/A
CE mark, date	2002
First operation date	2003
Number implanted to date	More than 2000
Generation	Third
Type	Three-component unconstrained prosthesis

Evidence	
Lefrancois *et al.* (2017)	Prospective comparison of Hintegra, mobility, STAR, and agility. Inferior improvement with mobility TAR in pain and function compared with others. 19% were revised at mean follow-up 4.2 years.
Kerkhoff *et al.* (2016)	A series of 67 mobility TAR. Two intraoperative and 13 postoperative complications. Seven patients needed reoperation. Failure in three cases. Survival 95% at 61 months.
Daniels *et al.* (2014)	88 implants with average follow-up of 40 months. Cumulative survival at 4 years was 88.4%. Bone–implant interface abnormalities were reported in 43%, with the vast majority being located around the tibial plate.
Sproule *et al.* (2013)	40 months follow-up of 88 implants. Significant improvement in AOFAS, 88.4% survival at 4 years.
Muir, 2013	Average 4-year follow-up of 178 implants showed survival 94.4%. 18% had a poor outcome with persistent pain. Radiolucency in at least one zone in 29%.
Ahluwalia *et al.* (2013)	92.6% survival at 5 years.
Rippstein *et al.* (2011) *Designer series*	Average 36 months follow-up of 240 cases. There was improvement in AOFAS and VAS. Complications included intraoperative fracture (6%), delayed wound healing (2%), and late medial malleolar fractures (2%). Survival at 36 months was 97.9%, with reoperation necessary in 7.5% of cases.
Wood *et al.* (2010) *Designer series*	43 months follow-up of 100 implants showed survival of 93.6% at 4 years. Radiographic lucency present in 14 cases, which was greater than 10 mm wide in five ankles.

	Material	Fixation	Sided
Tibial component	Cobalt chromium.	Cementless, stemmed, coated with pure titanium-sintered metal beads (Porocoat®). Short conical tibial stem.	No
Talar component	Cobalt chromium.	Cementless, pegged, coated with pure titanium-sintered metal beads (Porocoat®). Superior dome of talus resurfaced while medial and lateral aspects of talus untreated. Central longitudinal fin.	No
Insert	Non-stearate containing UHMWPE.		

History of Implant

This implant became the most popular implant in Europe in or around 2011/12 and was the most frequently implanted in the UK. A US study was initiated around 2007 that was comparing the Mobility to the Agility but was abandoned due to poor recruitment. DePuy voluntarily withdrew the implant from the market in 2014.

Design Rationale

Tibial component is a long flat plate and rests on both the anterior and posterior cortices with a curved surface posteriorly to avoid impingement. Tibia has short conical stem which requires an anterior window. Talus has central longitudinal sulcus and two fins to enhance stability. Tibial side of the polyethylene insert is smaller than the tibial plate in order to avoid protrusion of the polyethylene insert medially or laterally.

Additional Info

Withdrawn from sales for commercial reasons from June 2014.

Technique

Measured, minimal resection; anterior approach.

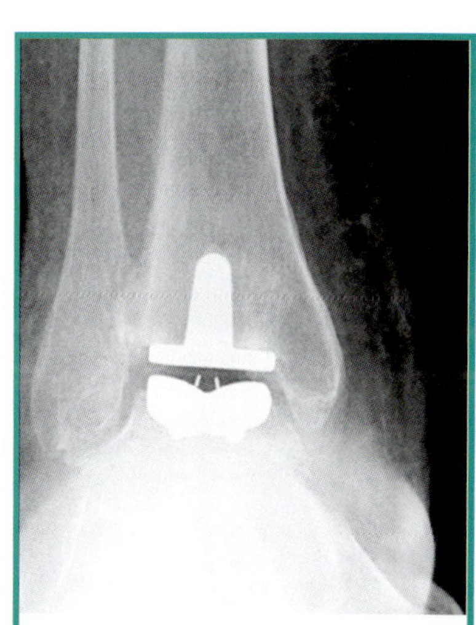

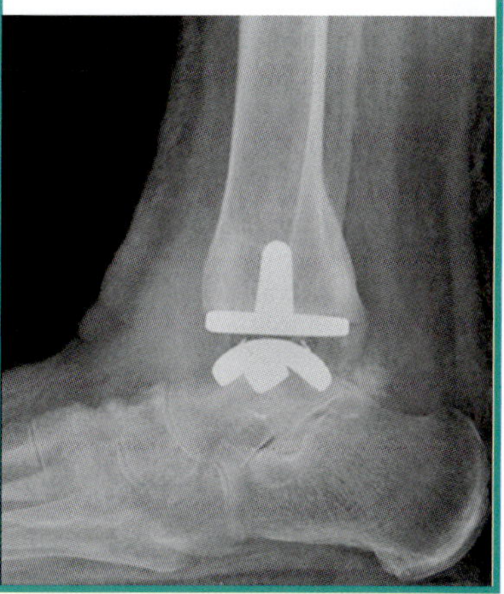

X-ray — AP and lateral view.

NEWTON ANKLE IMPLANT

Designed in Rutherford, NJ, USA, this was an incongruous surfaced two-component design. The polyethylene tibial component was a portion of a cylinder with the metallic talus being a portion of a sphere. Both components were cemented. Incongruency led to high polyethylene wear, with 34 out of 50 implants having 38% survival at 3-year follow-up (Newton, 1982).

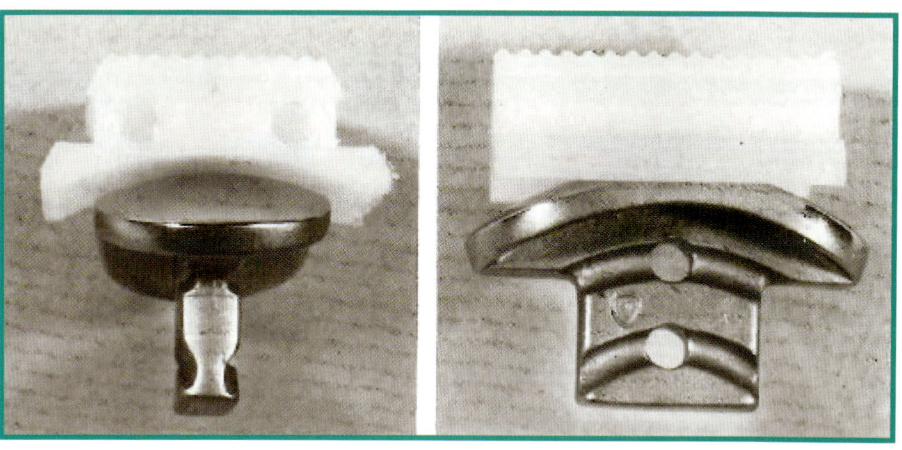

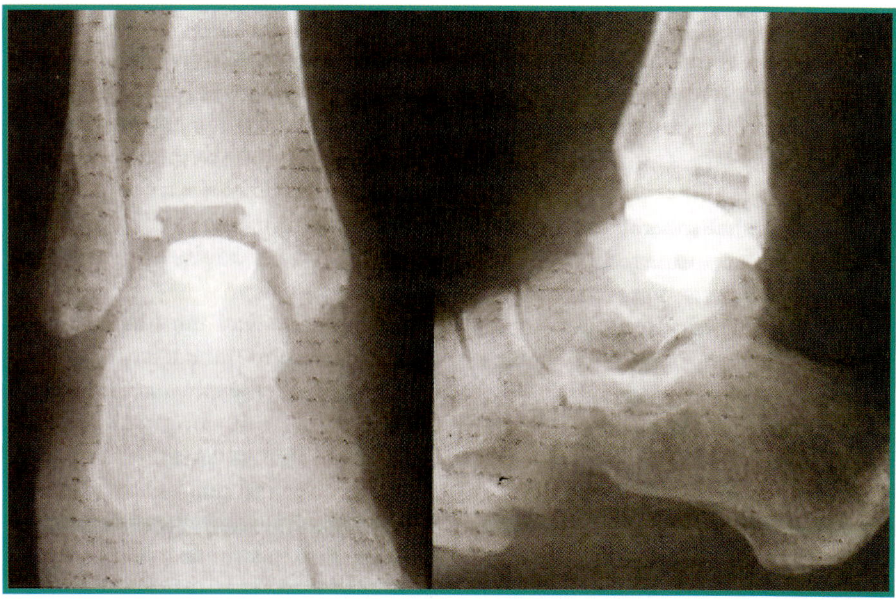

This page was left blank intentionally

RAMSES ANKLE REPLACEMENT

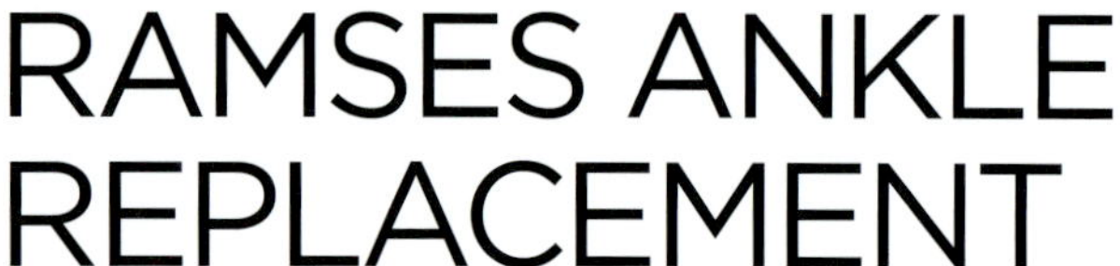

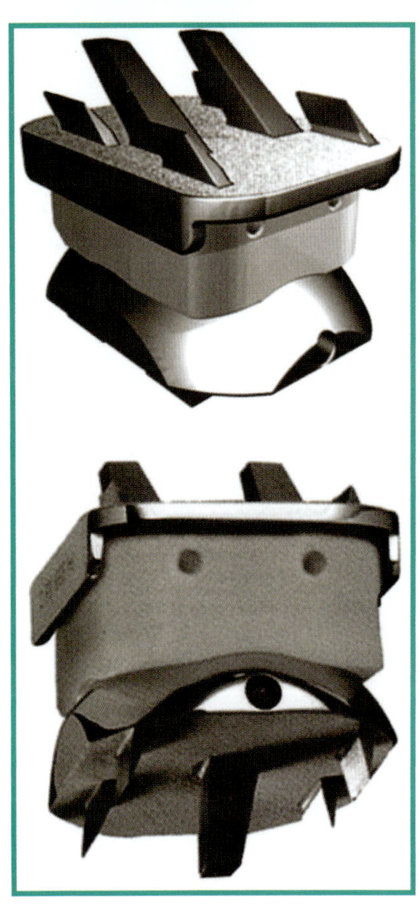

Manufacturer	Laboratoire Fournitures Hospitalieres, Heimsbrunn, France
Inspiration behind name	Unknown
Surgeon inventor/designer(s)	The Talus Group (France) which is a French group of foot and ankle surgeons: Diebold (Nancy); Mendolia (St. Martin Les Boulogne); Cermolacce (Marseille); Coillard (Lyon); De Lavigne (Merignac); Determe (Toulouse); Guillo (Merignac); Hummer (Nancy); Mouilleron (Arcachon); Laffenetre (Bordeaux); Peltre (Paris); Rocher (Bordeaux); Rougereau (Paris); Roussignol (Rouen)
FDA approved, date	N/A
CE mark, date	Unknown
First operation date	1989
Number implanted to date	Unknown
Generation	Third
Type	Three-component semi-constrained mobile bearing

Evidence	
Michael *et al.* (2008)	High revision rates of 18% and 34% at 2 and 10 years.
Mendolia *et al.* (2005) *Designer series*	After 10–14 years follow-up, 69 implants. Primary implant survival 82.6%, of which seven cases required arthrodesis, two had a bearing change, and three were revised.
Delagoutte (2002)	110 implants analysed across 22 hospitals, of which 66 were Ramses implants. Follow-up 3–37 months. There was no postoperative improvement in dorsiflexion, with revision required in two cases.

	Material	Fixation	Sided
Tibial component	Cobalt chrome. The tibial component has a flat glide plate with lateral edges to avoid mediolateral instability of polyethylene and malleolar impingement.	Uncemented.	N/A
Talar component	Cobalt chrome. Has a flat distal surface to facilitate the implantation. The articular surface (upper) is a double curve: anteroposterior for flexion extension with a long radius and mediolateral for valgus–varus with a smaller radius.	Uncemented.	N/A
Insert	High-density polyethylene, flat along its upper surface, and curved on its lower surface.		

History of Implant
From 1989 to 2000, all implants were cemented. After 2000 the implants were used uncemented.

Additional Info
Concerns are the wide talar bone resection, compromising future revision options, and the thin tibial loading platform (long-term fatigue possible).

In addition, frontal plane stability relies entirely on the medial and lateral ligamentous structures. This does not correspond to normal ankle biomechanics, where frontal plane stability relies mainly on joint congruency.

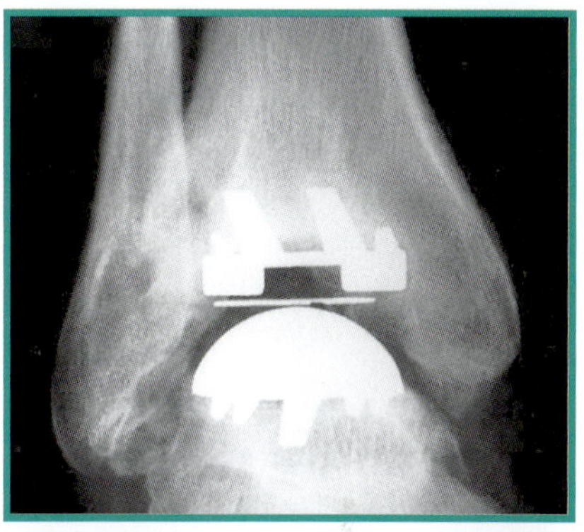

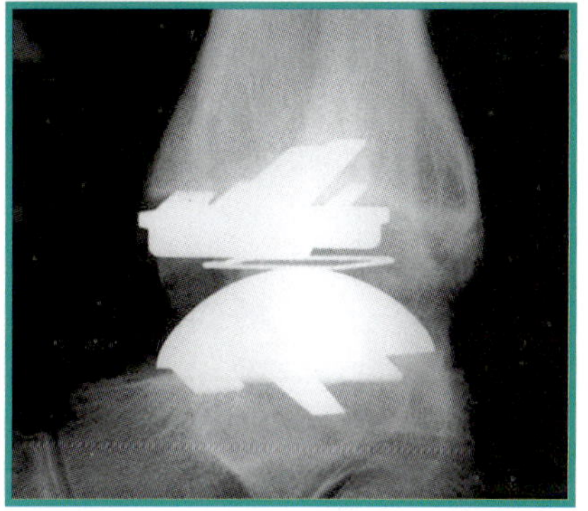

REBALANCE ANKLE REPLACEMENT

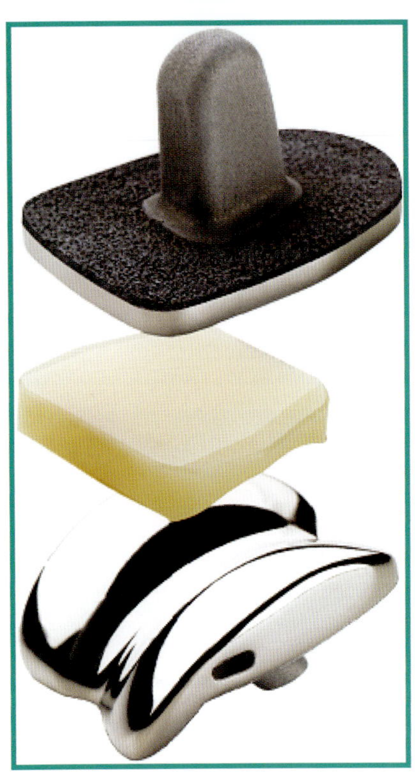

Photo of Rebalance.

Manufacturer	Zimmer Biomet
Inspiration behind name	The rebalance ankle is named after one of the primary design intents, rebalancing the arthritic ankle
Surgeon inventor/ designer(s)	Development team including Mr Nick Harris, Leeds, UK
FDA approved, date	Not FDA approved
CE mark, date	March 4, 2011
First operation date	2011
Number implanted to date	>300
Generation	Third
Type	Mobile bearing total ankle prosthesis

Evidence	
Harris *et al.* (2018)	2-year follow-up of 220 implants with 97% survival. Non-progressive radiolucent lines in nine cases, progressive in two cases. 29 patients had mean preoperative AOFAS of score 41 at 2 years was 75.5.

	Material	Fixation	Sided
Tibial component	CoCr with Macrobond and Bonemaster.	Uncemented.	N/A
Talar component	CoCr with Macrobond and Bonemaster.	Uncemented.	N/A
Insert	The polyethylene bearing is vitamin E infused polyethylene.		

History of Implant

The Rebalance ankle was designed at a time prior to Biomet's acquisition by Zimmer, but after the issues with the AES ankle that Biomet had been distributing before. Since the merger between Biomet and Zimmer, commercial focus however changed and interest in the Rebalance ankle subsided.

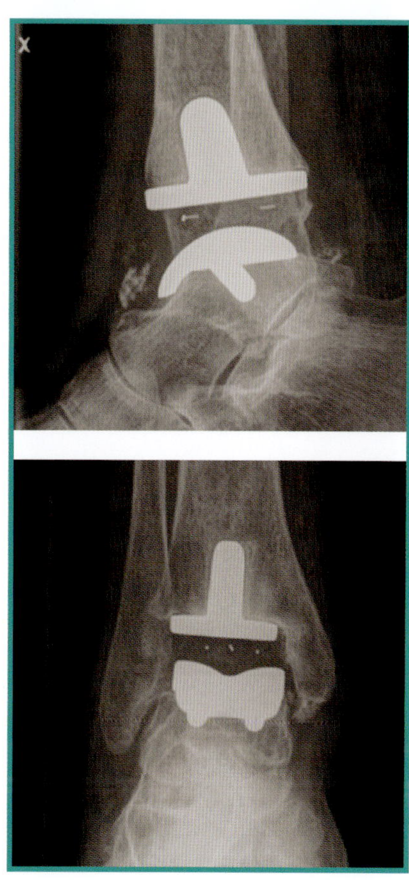

X-ray — AP and lateral view.

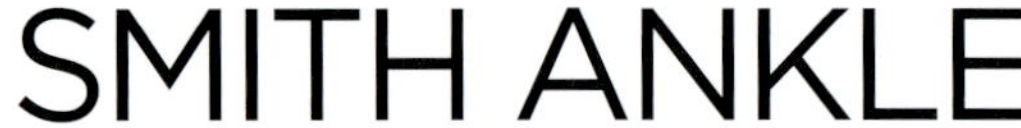

SMITH ANKLE

In most early designs of ankle replacement the polyethylene was used in the tibia and metal for the talus, but the Smith total ankle replacement reversed this and the implants were cemented. It was used between 1974–1979 and had a stainless steel tibial component. The single sized implant was an unconstrained ball in socket joint. Acceptable results for implants at the time were reported by Dini *et al.*, 1980 and Kirkup in 1985.

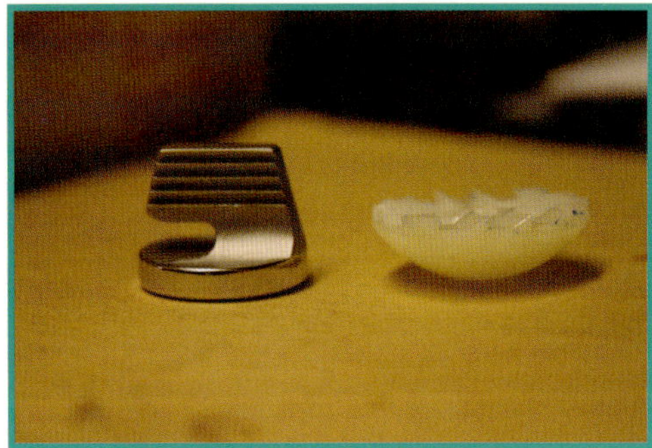

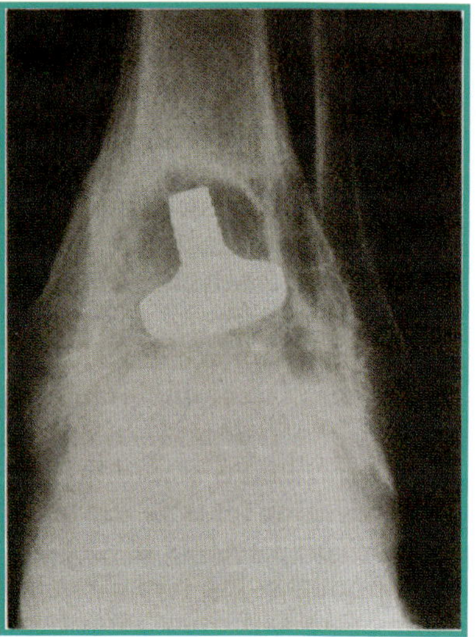

THOMPSON–RICHARD PROSTHESIS

Introduced in 1976, this was a two-component semi-constrained cemented implant. Medial and lateral lips on the polyethylene tibial component introduced constraint, but this caused shear forces to the bone cement interface (Wood *et al.*, 2000). Although survival in 27 ankles at 12 years was 87%, there was a high rate of radiolucency and patient dissatisfaction (Jensen and Kroner, 1992). The Norwegian joint registry reported 19% revision at 7.7 years (Tillmann *et al.*, 1998).

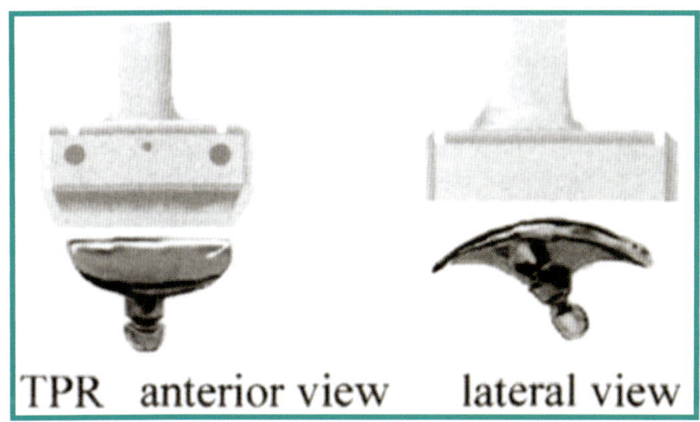

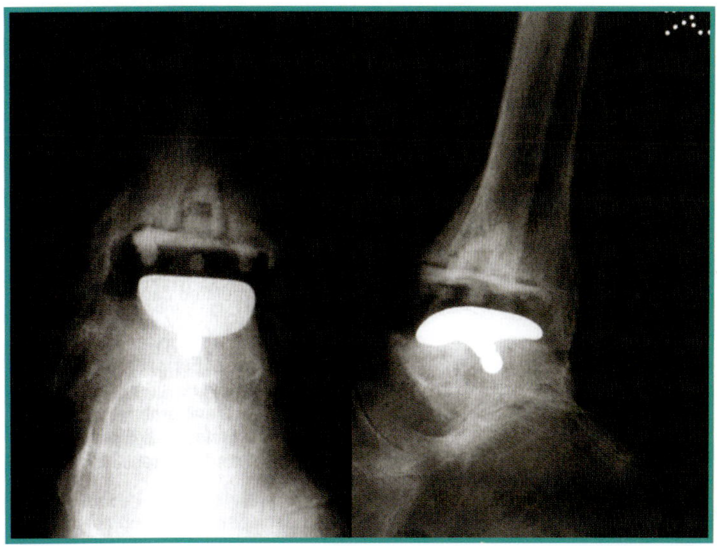

REFERENCES

Adams, S. B., Jr., Demetracopoulos, C. A., Queen, R. M., Easley, M. E., DeOrio, J. K. & Nunley, J. A. 2014. Early to mid-term results of fixed-bearing total ankle arthroplasty with a modular intramedullary tibial component. *J Bone Joint Surg Am*, 96, 1983–1989.

Ahluwalia, R. S., P. Cooke, M. Rogers & R. Sharp. 2013. Ankle replacement: A 14-year experience. *Orthop Proc*, 95-B(Suppl 21), 26.

Ali, M. S., Higgins, G. A. & Mohamed, M. 2007. Intermediate results of Buechel Pappas unconstrained uncemented total ankle replacement for osteoarthritis. *J Foot Ankle Surg*, 46, 16–20.

Bai, L. B., Lee, K. B., Song, E. K., Yoon, T. R. & Seon, J. K. 2010. Total ankle arthroplasty outcome comparison for post-traumatic and primary osteoarthritis. *Foot Ankle Int*, 31, 1048–1056.

Barg, A., Zwicky, L., Knupp, M., Henninger, H. B. & Hintermann, B. 2013. HINTEGRA total ankle replacement: Survivorship analysis in 684 patients. *J Bone Joint Surg Am*, 95, 1175–1183.

Barg, A. & Saltzman, C. 2017. Early clinical and radiographic outcomes of trabecular metal total ankle using transfibular approach. *Foot Ankle Surg,* 23(Suppl 1).

Barg, A., Bettin, C. C., Burstein, A. H., Saltzman, C. L. & Gililland, J. 2018. Early clinical and radiographic outcomes of trabecular metal total ankle replacement using a transfibular approach. *J Bone Joint Surg Am*, 100(6), 505–515. doi: 10.2106/JBJS.17.00018.

Barnett, C. H. & Napier, J. R. 1952. The axis of rotation at the ankle joint in man: Its influence upon the form of the talus and the mobility of the fibula. *J Anat*, 86(1), 1–9.

Berlet, G. C., Penner, M. J., Lancianese, S., Stemniski, P. M. & Obert, R. M. 2014. Total ankle arthroplasty accuracy and reproducibility using preoperative CT scan-derived, patient-specific guides. *Foot Ankle Int*, 35, 665–676.

Besse, J. L., Lienhart, C. & Fessy, M. H. 2013. Outcomes following cyst curettage and bone grafting for the management of periprosthetic cystic evolution after AES total ankle replacement. *Clin Podiatr Med Surg*, 30, 157–170.

Bianchi, A., Martinelli, N., Hosseinzadeh, M., Flore, J., Minoli, C., Malerba, F. & Galbusera, F. 2019. Early clinical and radiological evaluation in patients with total ankle replacement performed by lateral approach and peroneal osteotomy. *BMC Musculoskelet Disord*, 20(1), 132. doi: 10.1186/s12891-019-2503-6.

Bianchi, A., Martinelli, N., Sartorelli, E. & Malerba, F. 2012. The Bologna-Oxford total ankle replacement: A mid-term follow-up study. *J Bone Joint Surg Br*, 94, 793–798.

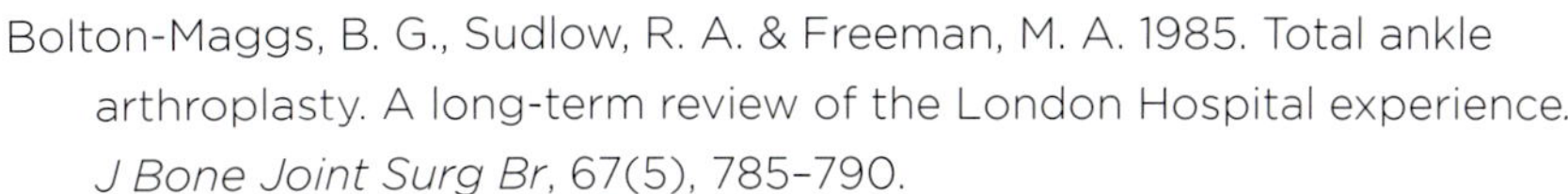

Bolton-Maggs, B. G., Sudlow, R. A. & Freeman, M. A. 1985. Total ankle arthroplasty. A long-term review of the London Hospital experience. *J Bone Joint Surg Br*, 67(5), 785–790.

Bonnin, M., Gaudot, F., Laurent, J. R., Ellis, S., Colombier, J. A. & Judet, T. 2011. The Salto total ankle arthroplasty: Survivorship and analysis of failures at 7 to 11 years. *Clin Orthop Relat Res*, 469, 225–236.

Brigido, S. A., Galli, M. M., Bleazey, S. T. & Protzman, N. M. 2014. Modular stem fixed-bearing total ankle replacement: Prospective results of 23 consecutive cases with 3-year follow-up. *J Foot Ankle Surg*, 53, 692–699.

Brigido, S. A., Wobst, G. M., Galli, M. M., Bleazey, S. T. & Protzman, N. M. 2015. Evaluating component migration after modular stem fixed-bearing total ankle replacement. *J Foot Ankle Surg*, 54, 326–331.

Brunner, S., Barg, A., Knupp, M., Zwicky, M., Kapron, A. L., Valderrabano, V. & Hintermann, B. 2013. The Scandinavian total ankle replacement: Long-term, eleven to fifteen-year, survivorship analysis of the prosthesis in seventy-two consecutive patients. *J Bone Joint Surg Am*, 95, 711–718.

Buechel, F. F., Pappas, M. J. & Lorio, L. J. 1988. New Jersey Low Contact Stress total ankle replacement: Biomechanical rationale and review of 23 cementless cases. *Foot Ankle*, 8, 279–290.

Buechel, F. F. & Pappas, M. J. 1992. Survivorship and clinical evaluation of cementless, meniscal-bearing total ankle replacements. *Semin Arthroplasty*, 3(1), 43–50.

Buechel, F. F. Sr., Buechel, F. F. Jr. & Pappas, M. J. 2003. Ten-year evaluation of cementless Buechel-Pappas meniscal bearing total ankle replacement. *Foot Ankle Int*, 24, 462–472.

Buechel, F. F. Sr., Buechel, F. F. Jr. & Pappas, M. J. 2004. Twenty-year evaluation of cementless mobile-bearing total ankle replacements. *Clin Orthop Rel Res*, 424, 19–26.

Carlsson, Å. S., Henricson, A., Linder, L., Nilsson, J. Å. & Redlund-Johnell, I. 2001. A 10-year survival analysis of 69 Bath and Wessex ankle replacements. *Foot Ankle Surg*, 7(1), 39–44.

Chao, J., Choi, J. H., Grear, B. J., Tenenbaum, S. Bariteau, J. T. & Brodsky J. W. 2015. Early radiographic and clinical results of Salto total ankle arthroplasty as a fixed-bearing device. *Foot Ankle Surg*, 21, 91–96.

Claridge, R. J. & Sagherian, B. H. 2009. Intermediate term outcome of the agility total ankle arthroplasty. *Foot Ankle Int*, 30, 824–835.

Cody, E. A., Taylor, M. A., Nunley, J. A., II, Parekh, S. G. & DeOrio, J. K. 2019. Increased early revision rate with the INFINITY total ankle prosthesis. *Foot Ankle Int*, 40(1), 9–17. doi: 10.1177/1071100718794933. Epub 2018 Sep 3.

Coetzee, J. C., Petersen, D. & Stone, R. M. 2017. Comparison of three total ankle replacement systems done at a single facility. *Foot Ankle Spec*, 10, 20-25.

Criswell, B. J., Douglas, K., Naik, R. & Thomson, A. B. 2012. High revision and reoperation rates using the Agility Total Ankle System. *Clin Orthop Relat Res*, 470, 1980-1986.

Daigre, J., Berlet, G., Van Dyke, B., Peterson, K. S. & Santrock, R. 2017. Accuracy and reproducibility using patient-specific instrumentation in total ankle arthroplasty. *Foot Ankle Int*, 38, 412–418.

Dalat, F., Barnoud, R., Fessy, M. H., Besse, J. L. & Afcp French Association of Foot Surgery. 2013. Histologic study of periprosthetic osteolytic lesions after AES total ankle replacement. A 22 case series. *Orthop Traumatol Surg Res*, 99, S285–S295.

Daniels, T. R., Younger, A. S., Penner, M., Wing, K., Dryden, P. J., Wong, H. & Glazebrook, M. 2014. Intermediate-term results of total ankle replacement and ankle arthrodesis: A COFAS multicenter study. *J Bone Joint Surg Am*, 96, 135–142.

Daniels, T. R., Mayich, D. J. & Penner, M. J. 2015. Intermediate to long-term outcomes of total ankle replacement with the Scandinavian Total Ankle Replacement (STAR). *J Bone Joint Surg Am*, 97, 895–903.

Daniels T. R., Kayum, S. & Khan, R. M. 2019. Two-year outcomes of total ankle replacement with the Cadence Total Ankle Replacement System. *Foot & Ankle Ortho*, 2019, 4(4). DOI: 10.1177/2473011419S00156.

Delagoutte, J. 2002. Retrospective analysis of 110 ankle prostheses. *Eur J Orthop Surg Traumatol*, 12, 198–205.

Deleu, P. A., Devos Bevernage, B., Gombault, V., Maldague, P. & Leemrijse, T. 2015. Intermediate-term results of mobile-bearing total ankle replacement. *Foot Ankle Int*, 36, 518–530.

DeVries, J. G., Scott, R. T., Berlet, G. C., Hyer, C. F., Lee, T. H. & DeOrio, J. K. 2013. Agility to INBONE: Anterior and posterior approaches to the difficult revision total ankle replacement. *Clin Podiatr Med Surg*, 30, 81–96.

DeVries, J. G., T. A. Derksen, B. M. Scharer & R. Limoni. 2017. Perioperative complications and initial alignment of lateral approach total ankle arthroplasty. *J Foot Ankle Surg*, 56, 996–1000.

Di Lorio, A., Derksen, T. A., Scharer, B. M. & Limoni, R. 2017. The AES total ankle arthroplasty analysis of failures and survivorship at ten years. *Int Orthop*, 41, 2525-2533.

Dini, A. A. & Bassett, F. H. 1980. Evaluation of the early result of Smith total ankle replacement. *Clin Orthop Relat Res*, 146, 228-230.

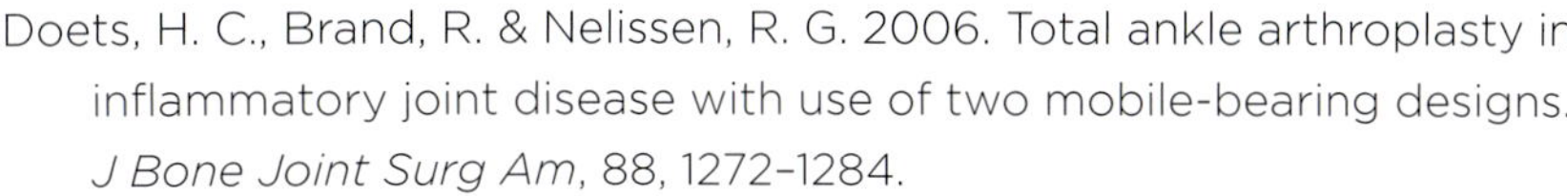

Doets, H. C., Brand, R. & Nelissen, R. G. 2006. Total ankle arthroplasty in inflammatory joint disease with use of two mobile-bearing designs. *J Bone Joint Surg Am*, 88, 1272–1284.

Freeman, M. A. R., Kempson, G. E., Tuke, M. A. & Samuelson, K. M. 1978. Total replacement of the ankle with the ICLH prosthesis. *Int Orthop, 2*(4), 327–331.

Frigg, A., Germann, U., Huber, M. & Horisberger, M. 2017. Survival of the Scandinavian Total Ankle Replacement (STAR): Results of ten to nineteen years follow-up. *Int Orthop*, 41, 2075–2082.

Gaudot, F., Colombier, J. A., Bonnin, M. & Judet, T. 2014. A controlled, comparative study of a fixed-bearing versus mobile-bearing ankle arthroplasty. *Foot Ankle Int*, 35, 131–140.

Giannini, S., Romagnoli, M., O'Connor, J. J., Malerba, F. & Leardini, A. 2010. Total ankle replacement compatible with ligament function produces mobility, good clinical scores, and low complication rates: An early clinical assessment. *Clin Orthop Relat Res*, 468, 2746–2753.

Giannini, S., Romagnoli, M., O'Connor, J. J., Catani, F., Nogarin, L., Magnan, B., Malerba, F., Massari, L., Guelfi, M., Milano, L., Volpe, A., Rebeccato, A. & Leardini, A. 2011. Early clinical results of the BOX ankle replacement are satisfactory: A multicenter feasibility study of 158 ankles. *J Foot Ankle Surg*, 50, 641–647.

Giannini, S., Romagnoli, M., Barbadoro, P., Marcheggiani Muccioli, G. M., Cadossi, M., Grassi, A. & Zaffagnini, S. 2017. Results at a minimum follow-up of 5 years of a ligaments-compatible total ankle replacement design. *Foot Ankle Surg*, 23, 116–121.

Harris, N., Hendricson, A., Rydholm, U., Knutson, K. & Popelka, S. 2018. The early multicentre results of the Rebalance total ankle replacement. *Orthop Proc*, 96-B, (Suppl 17).

Harston, A., Lazarides, A. L., Adams, Jr. S. B., DeOrio, J. K., Easley, M. E. & Nunley, II. J. A. 2017. Midterm outcomes of a fixed-bearing total ankle arthroplasty with deformity analysis. *Foot Ankle Int*, 38, 1295–1300.

Haytmanek Jr, T. C., Gross, C., Easley, M. E. & Nunley, J. A. 2015. Radiographic Outcomes of a Mobile-Bearing Total Ankle Replacement, FAI, 36(9), 1038–1044.

Helm, R. & Stevens, J. 1986. Long-term results of total ankle replacement. *J Arthroplast*, 1(4), 271–277.

Henricson, A., Knutson, K., Lindahl, J. & Rydholm, U. 2010. The AES total ankle replacement: A mid-term analysis of 93 cases. *Foot Ankle Surg*, 16, 61–64.

Hernandez, J. L., Laffenêtre, O., Toullec, E., Darcel, V. & Chauveaux, D., 2014. AKILE™ total ankle arthroplasty: Clinical and CT scan analysis of periprosthetic cysts. Orthopaedics & Traumatology: Surgery & Research, 100(8), 907–915.

Hintermann, B., Valderrabano, V., Dereymaeker, G. & Dick, W. 2004. The HINTEGRA ankle: Rationale and short-term results of 122 consecutive ankles. *Clin Orthop Relat Res*, 57–68.

Hintermann, B., Valderrabano, V., Knupp, M. & Horisberger, M. 2006. The HINTEGRA ankle: Short-and mid-term results. *Der Orthopade*, 35(5), 533–545.

Hintermann, B., Zwicky, L., Knupp, M., Henninger, H. B. & Barg, A. 2013. HINTEGRA revision arthroplasty for failed total ankle prostheses. *J Bone Joint Surg Am*, 95, 1166–1174.

Hofmann, K. J., Shabin, Z. M., Ferkel, E., Jockel, J. & Slovenkai, M. P. 2016. Salto talaris total ankle arthroplasty: Clinical results at a mean of 5.2 years in 78 patients treated by a single surgeon. *J Bone Joint Surg Am*, 98, 2036–2046.

Hsu, A. R., Davis, W. H., Cohen, B. E., Jones, C. P., Ellington, J. K. & Anderson, R. B. 2015. Radiographic outcomes of preoperative CT scan-derived patient-specific total ankle arthroplasty. *Foot Ankle Int*, 36, 1163–1169.

Hvid, I., Rasmussen, O., Jensen, N. C. & Nielsen, S. 1985. *Trabecular Bone Strength Profiles at the Ankle Joint*. Clinical Orthopedics, 199, 306–312.

Inman, V. T. *The Joints of the Ankle*. Williams & Wilkins, Baltimore, 1976.

Jastifer, J. R. & M. J. Coughlin. 2015. Long-term follow-up of mobile bearing total ankle arthroplasty in the United States. *Foot Ankle Int*, 36, 143–150.

Jensen, N. C. & Kroner, K. 1992. Total ankle joint replacement: A clinical follow up. *Orthopedics*, 15(2), 236–239.

Jung, H. G., Shin, M. H., Lee, S. H., Eom, J. S. & Lee, D. O. 2015. Comparison of the outcomes between two 3-component total ankle implants. *Foot Ankle Int*, 36, 656–663.

Karantana, A., Hobson, S. & Dhar, S. 2010. The Scandinavian total ankle replacement: Survivorship at 5 and 8 years comparable to other series. *Clin Orthop Relat Res*, 468, 951–957.

Kempson, G. E., Freeman, M. A. & Tuke, M. A. 1975. Engineering considerations in the design of an ankle joint. *Biomed Eng*, 10(5), 166–171, 80.

Kerkhoff, Y. R., Kosse, N. M. & Louwerens, J. W. 2016a. Short term results of the Mobility Total Ankle System: Clinical and radiographic outcome. *Foot Ankle Surg*, 22, 152–157.

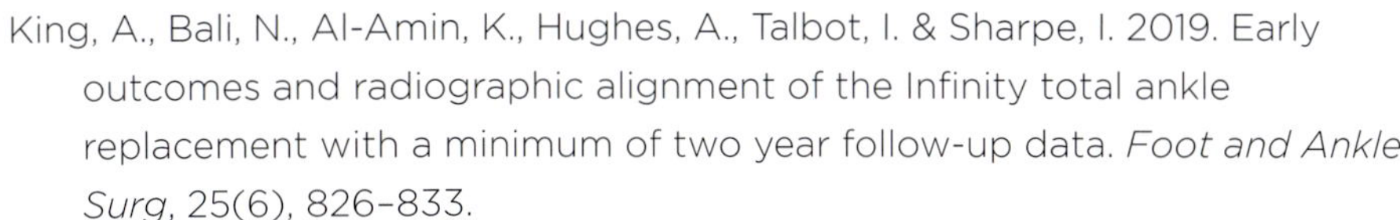

King, A., Bali, N., Al-Amin, K., Hughes, A., Talbot, I. & Sharpe, I. 2019. Early outcomes and radiographic alignment of the Infinity total ankle replacement with a minimum of two year follow-up data. *Foot and Ankle Surg*, 25(6), 826–833.

Kirkup, J. 1990. Rheumatoid arthritis and ankle surgery. *Ann Rheumatic Diseases*, 49, 837–844.

Kirkup, K. 1985. Richard Smith ankle arthroplasty. *J R Soc Med*, 78(4), 301–304.

Kitaoka, H. B. & Patzer, G. L. 1996. Clinical results of the Mayo total ankle arthroplasty. *J Bone Joint Surg Am*, 78(11), 1658–1664.

Knecht, S. I., Estin, M., Callaghan, J. J., Zimmerman, M. B., Alliman, K. J., Alvine, F. G. & Saltzman, C. L. 2004. The agility total ankle arthroplasty. Seven to sixteen-year follow-up. *J Bone Joint Surg Am*, 86-a, 1161–1171.

Kofoed, H. 1995. Cylindrical cemented ankle arthroplasty: A prospective series with long-term follow-up. *Foot Ankle Int*, 16, 474–479.

Kofoed, H. 2004. Scandinavian Total Ankle Replacement (STAR). *Clin Orthop Relat Res*, 424, 73–79.

Koivu, H., Kohonen, I., Sipola, E., Alanen, K., Vahlberg, T. & Tiusanen, H. 2009. Severe periprosthetic osteolytic lesions after the Ankle Evolutive System total ankle replacement. *J Bone Joint Surg Br*, 91, 907–914.

Koivu, H., Kohonen, I., Mattila, K., Loyttyniemi, E. & Tiusanen, H. 2017a. Long-term results of Scandinavian Total Ankle Replacement. *Foot Ankle Int*, 38, 723–731.

Kokkonen, A., Ikavalko, M., Tiihonen, R., Kautiainen, H. & Belt, E. A. 2011. High rate of osteolytic lesions in medium-term followup after the AES total ankle replacement. *Foot Ankle Int*, 32, 168–175.

Kopp, F. J., Patel, M. M., Deland, J. T. & O'Malley, M. J. 2006. Total ankle arthroplasty with the agility prosthesis: Clinical and radiographic evaluation. *Foot Ankle Int*, 27, 97–103.

Kraal, T., van der Heide, H. J., van Poppel, B. J., Fiocco, M., Nelissen, R. G. & Doets, H. C. 2013. Long-term follow-up of mobile-bearing total ankle replacement in patients with inflammatory joint disease. *Bone Joint J*, 95-b, 1656–1661.

Lefrancois, T., Younger, A., Wing, K., Penner, M. J., Dryden, P., Wong, H., Daniels, T. & Glazebrook, M. 2017. A prospective study of four total ankle arthroplasty implants by non-designer investigators. *J Bone Joint Surg Am*, 99, 342–348.

Lewis, Jr. J. S., Green, C. L., Adams, Jr. S. B., Easley, M. E., DeOrio, J. K. & Nunley, J. A. 2015. Comparison of first- and second-generation fixed-bearing total ankle arthroplasty using a modular intramedullary tibial component. *Foot Ankle Int*, 36, 881–890.

Lord, G. & Marotte, J. H. 1973. Prothese total de cheville: Technique et premier resultats. *Rev Chir Orthop Reparatrice Appar Mot,* 59, 139–151.

MacBarb, R. F., Lindsey, D. P., Bahney, C. S., Woods, S. A., Wolfe, M. L. & Yerby, S. A. 2017. Fortifying the Bone-Implant Interface Part 1: An In Vitro Evaluation of 3D Printed and TPS Porous Surfaces. *Int J Spine Surg,* 11, 15.

Mann, J. A., Mann, R. A. & Horton, E. 2011. STAR ankle: Long-term results. *Foot Ankle Int,* 32, S473–S484.

Marsh, C., Kirkup, J. & Regan. M. 1987. The Bath and Wessex ankle arthroplasty. *JBJS-Br* and *Br Ed Soc Bone Joint Surg.*

Mckenzie, J., Martin, B., Hughes, A. & Winson, I. 2012. *The Zenith: A New Total Ankle Replacement — First report of early survivorship and radiographic assessment of alignment.* In Presented at EFORT, Berlin.

McInnes, K. A., Younger, A. S. & Oxland, T. R. 2014. Initial instability in total ankle replacement: A cadaveric biomechanical investigation of the STAR and agility prostheses. *J Bone Joint Surg Am,* 96, e147.

Mendolia, G., Coillard, J. Y., Cermolacce, C. & Determe, P. 2005. Long-term (10 to 14 years) results of the Ramses total ankle arthroplasty. *Tech Foot & Ankle,* 4, 160–173.

Michael, J. M., Golshani, A., Gargac, S. & Goswami, T. 2008. Biomechanics of the ankle joint and clinical outcomes of total ankle replacement. *J Mech Behav Biomed Mater,* 1, 276–294.

Millar, T. & Garg, S. 2012. The Zenith total ankle replacement — early results of the first 50 cases in a non-inventor series. In *British Orthopaedic Foot & Ankle Society Annual Scientific Meeting.*

Morgan, S. S., Brooke, B. & Harris, N. J. 2010. Total ankle replacement by the Ankle Evolution System: Medium-term outcome. *J Bone Joint Surg Br,* 92, 61–65.

Muir, D., Aoina, J., Hong, T. & Mason, R. 2013. The outcome of the Mobility total ankle replacement at a mean of four years: Can poor outcomes be predicted from pre-and post-operative analysis?. *The Bone & Joint J,* 95(10), 1366–1371.

Myerson, M., Clancy, J., Paxson, B., Obert, R., Anderle, M., Brinker, L. & Daniel Lee, M. 2019. *Bi-Radial Curvature Morphology of the Healthy Talus.* In: Chicago, IL: American Orthopaedic Foot & Ankle Society Annual Meeting (e-poster).

Nagashima, M., Takahashi, H., Kakumoto, S., Miyamoto, Y. & Yoshino, S. 2004. Total ankle arthroplasty for deformity of the foot in patients with rheumatoid arthritis using the TNK ankle system: Clinical results of 21 cases. *Mod Rheumatol,* 14, 48–53.

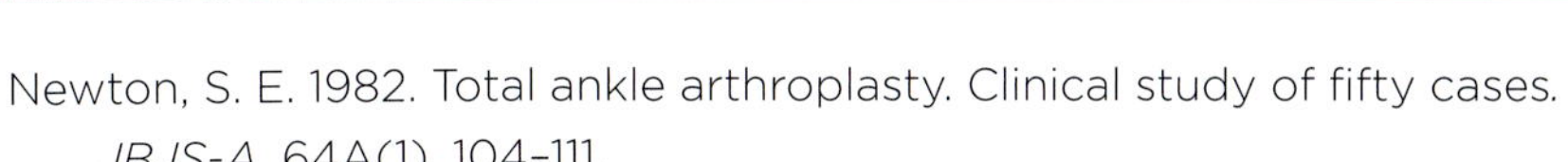

Newton, S. E. 1982. Total ankle arthroplasty. Clinical study of fifty cases. *JBJS-A*, 64A(1), 104–111.

Nieuwe Weme, R. A., van Solinge, G., Doornberg, J. N., Sierevelt, I., Haverkamp, D. & Doets, H. C. 2015. Total ankle replacement for posttraumatic arthritis. Similar outcome in postfracture and instability arthritis: A comparison of 90 ankles. *Acta Orthop,* 86, 401–406.

Nishikawa, M., Tomita, T., Fujii, M., Watanabe, T., Hashimoto, J., Sugamoto, K., Ochi, T. & Yoshikawa, H. 2004. Total ankle replacement in rheumatoid arthritis. *Int Orthop*, 28, 123–126.

Nodzo, S. R., Miladore, M. P., Kaplan, N. B. & Ritter, C. A. 2014. Short to midterm clinical and radiographic outcomes of the Salto total ankle prosthesis. *Foot Ankle Int*, 35, 22–29.

Oliver, S. M., Coetzee, J. C., Nilsson, L. J., Samuelson, K. M., Stone, R. M., Fritz, J. E. & Giveans, M. R. 2016. Early patient satisfaction results on a modern generation fixed-bearing total ankle arthroplasty. *Foot Ankle Int*, 37, 938–943.

Palanca, A., Mann, R. A., Mann, J. A. & Haskell, A. 2018. Scandinavian Total Ankle Replacement: 15-year follow-up. *Foot Ankle Int*, 39, 135–142.

Popelka, S., A. Sosna, P. Vavrik, D. Jahoda, V. Bartak & I. Landor. 2016. Eleven-year experience with total ankle arthroplasty. *Acta Chir Orthop Traumatol Cech*, 83, 74–83.

Pyevich, M. T., Saltzman, C. L., Callaghan, J. J. & Alvine, F. G. 1998. Total ankle arthroplasty: A unique design. Two to twelve-year follow-up. *J Bone Joint Surg Am*, 80, 1410–1420.

Raikin, S. M., Sandrowski, K., Kane, J. M., Beck, D. & Winters, B. S. 2017. Midterm outcome of the agility total ankle arthroplasty. *Foot Ankle Int*, 38, 662–670.

Richter, M., Zech, S., Westphal, R., Klimesch, Y. & Gosling, T. 2007. Robotic cadaver testing of a new total ankle prosthesis model (German Ankle System). *Foot & Ankle Int*, 28(12), 1276–1286.

Rodriguez, D., Bevernage, B. D., Maldague, P., Deleu, P. A., Tribak, K. & Leemrijse, T. 2010. Medium term follow-up of the AES ankle prosthesis: High rate of asymptomatic osteolysis. *Foot Ankle Surg*, 16, 54–60.

Roukis, T. S. 2012. Incidence of revision after primary implantation of the agility total ankle replacement system: A systematic review. *J Foot Ankle Surg*, 51, 198–204.

Rudigier, J. F. M. 2005. Ankle replacement by the cementless ESKA endoprosthesis. *Tech Foot Ankle Surg*, 4, 125–136.

Rudigier, J., Grundei, H. & Menzinger, F. 2001. Prosthetic replacement of the ankle in posttraumatic arthrosis 10-year experience with the cementless ESKA ankle prosthesis. *Eur J of Trauma*, 27(2), 66–74.

Saito, G. H., Sanders, A. E., de Cesar Netto, C., O'Malley, M. J., Ellis, S. J. & Demetracopoulos, C. A. 2018. Short-term complications, reoperations, and radiographic outcomes of a new fixed-bearing total ankle arthroplasty. *Foot Ankle Int*, 39(7), 787–794. doi: 10.1177/1071100718764107. Epub 2018 Mar 28.

San Giovanni, T. P., Keblish, D. J., Thomas, W. H. & Wilson, M. G. 2006. Eight-year results of a minimally constrained total ankle arthroplasty. *Foot Ankle Int*, 27, 418–426.

Schenk, K., Lieske, S., John, M., Franke, K., Mouly, S., Lizee, E. & Neumann, W. 2011. Prospective study of a cementless, mobile-bearing, third generation total ankle prosthesis. *Foot Ankle Int*, 32, 755–763.

Schimmel, J. J., Walschot, L. H. & Louwerens, J. W. 2014. Comparison of the short-term results of the first and last 50 Scandinavian total ankle replacements: Assessment of the learning curve in a consecutive series. *Foot Ankle Int*, 35, 326–333.

Schuberth, J. M., McCourt, M. J. & Christensen, J. C. 2011. Interval changes in postoperative range of motion of Salto-Talaris total ankle replacement. *J Foot Ankle Surg*, 50, 562–565.

Schweitzer, K. M., Adams, S. B., Viens, N. A., Queen, R. M., Easley, M. E., Deorio, J. K. & Nunley, J. A. 2013. Early prospective clinical results of a modern fixed-bearing total ankle arthroplasty. *J Bone Joint Surg Am*, 95, 1002–1011.

Siegler, S., Toy, J., Seale, D. & Pedowitz, D. 2013. New observations on the morphology of the talar dome and its relationship to ankle kinematics. *Clinical Biomechanics*, 29(1).

Shinomiya, F., Okada, M., Hamada, Y., Fujimura, T. & Hamada, D. 2003. Indications of total ankle arthroplasty for rheumatoid arthritis: Evaluation at 5 years or more after the operation. *Mod Rheumatol*, 13, 153–159.

Spirt, A. A., Assal, M. & Hansen, S. T. 2004. Complications and failure after total ankle arthroplasty. *J Bone Joint Surg Am*, 86-a, 1172–1178.

Sproule, J. A., Chin, T., Amin, A., Daniels, T., Younger, A. S., Boyd, G. & Glazebrook, M. A. 2013. Clinical and radiographic outcomes of the mobility total ankle arthroplasty system: Early results from a prospective multicenter study. *Foot Ankle Int*, 34, 491–497.

Stewart, M. G., Green, C. L., Adams, Jr. S. B., DeOrio, J. K. & Easley, M. E. 2017. Midterm results of the Salto Talaris total ankle arthroplasty. *Foot Ankle Int*, 38, 1215–1221.

Takakura, Y., Tanaka, Y., Kumai, T., Sugimoto, K. & Ohgushi, H. 2004. Ankle arthroplasty using three generations of metal and ceramic prostheses. *Clin Orthop Relat Res,* 424, 130–136.

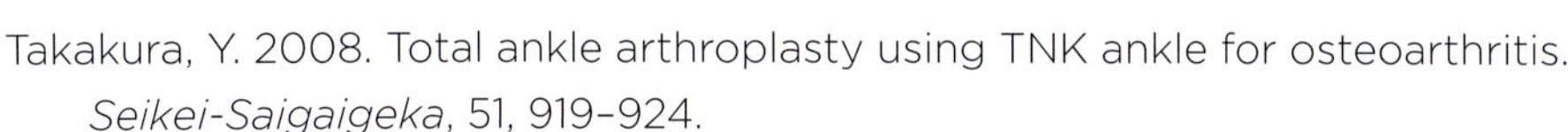

Takakura, Y. 2008. Total ankle arthroplasty using TNK ankle for osteoarthritis. *Seikei-Saigaigeka*, 51, 919–924.

Tan, E. W., Maccario, C., Talusan, P. G. & Schon, L. C. 2016. Early complications and secondary procedures in transfibular total ankle replacement. *Foot Ankle Int*, 37, 835–841.

Tanaka, Y. & Takakura, Y. 2006. The TNK ankle: Short- and mid-term results. *Orthop*, 35, 546–551.

Tillmann, K. Schirp, M., Schaar, B. & Fink, B. 1998. Cemented and uncemented ankle endoprosthesis: clinical and pedobarographic results. In H. Kofoed (ed.), *Current Status of Ankle Arthroplasty*, Springer, Berlin, pp. 22–25.

Tillmann, K. 2003. Endoprostheses of the ankle joint. Indications, development, current status and trends. *Orthopade*, 32, 179–186.

Usuelli, F. G., Indino, C., Maccario, C., Manzi, L. & Salini, V. 2016. Total ankle replacement through a lateral approach: Surgical tips. *SICOT J*, 2, 38.

Voesenek, J. A., Arts, J. J. & Hermus, J. P. S. 2017. The CCI mobile-bearing ankle replacement: A short-term clinical and radiographic assessment. *Orthop Proc*, 99-B(Suppl 1), 62.

Walter, R., Harries, W., Hepple, S. & Winson, I. 2015. The zenith total ankle replacement: Early to mid-term results in 155 cases. *Orthop Proc*, 97-B(Suppl 14), 15.

Wan, D. D., Choi, W. J., Shim, D. W., Hwang, Y., Park, Y. J. & Lee, J. W. 2018. Short-term clinical and radiographic results of the salto mobile total ankle prosthesis. *Foot Ankle Int*, 39, 155–165.

Waugh, T. R. & Evanski, P. M. 1976. Irvine ankle arthroplasty: Prosthetic design and surgical technique. *Clin Orthop Rel Res*, 114, 180–184.

Williams, J. R., Wegner, N. J., Sangeorzan, B. J. & Brage, M. E. 2015. Intraoperative and perioperative complications during revision arthroplasty for salvage of a failed total ankle arthroplasty. *Foot Ankle Int*, 36, 135–142.

Wood, P. L. R., Clough, T. M. & Jari, S. 2000. Clinical comparison of two total ankle replacements. *Foot Ankle Int*, 21(7), 546–550.

Wood, P. L. & Deakin, S. 2003. Total ankle replacement. The results in 200 ankles. *J Bone Joint Surg Br*, 85, 334–341.

Wood, P. L., Prem, H. & Sutton, C. 2008. Total ankle replacement: Medium-term results in 200 Scandinavian total ankle replacements. *J Bone Joint Surg Br*, 90, 605–609.

Wood, P. L., Sutton, C., Mishra, V. & Suneja, R. 2009. A randomised, controlled trial of two mobile-bearing total ankle replacements. *J Bone Joint Surg Br*, 91, 69–74.

Wood, P. L., Karski, M. T. & Watmough, P. 2010. Total ankle replacement: The results of 100 mobility total ankle replacements. *J Bone Joint Surg Br*, 92, 958–962.

Yang, H. Y., Wang, S. H. & Lee, K. B. 2019. The HINTEGRA total ankle arthroplasty: functional outcomes and implant survivorship in 210 osteoarthritic ankles at a mean of 6.4 years. *Bone Joint J,* 101-B(6), 695–701.

Yoon, H. S., Lee, J., Choi, W. J. & Lee, J. W. 2014. Periprosthetic osteolysis after total ankle arthroplasty. *Foot Ankle Int*, 35, 14–21.

OUTCOMES OF TOTAL ANKLE REPLACEMENT

A. Henricson

Summary

Most reports of results of total ankle replacement (TAR) are presented as survival rates. Survival at 5 years varies between 70% and 100%. The few available long-term studies report 10–19-year survival rates of 73–91% of the STAR design (Palanca *et al.*, 2018; Frigg *et al.*, 2017).

Systematic reviews have found an estimated overall 10-year survival rate of 89% with an annual failure rate of up to 1.9% per annum. They have also shown an increased range of motion and improved clinical outcomes (Zaidi *et al.*, 2013). No differences of the various scoring systems or in ROM between different designs have been found. Residual pain was common, but the patients were satisfied with the procedure in 79–97%. No superiority of any design could be detected.

National ankle registries, which are able to collect a higher number of patients, report survival rates at 5 years of 81–88% and estimated 10-year survival of 69–82% in relation to third generation TARs and gender or diagnosis did not appear to influence outcome.

The importance of learning curve has been emphasised.

Deformity at the ankle or in the adjacent joints can be difficult to handle and is one of the main reasons for failure. The results of TAR have so far not reached the results of total hip or knee arthroplasty, and with current designs they may never do so.

OUTCOMES OF TAR

Three systematic reviews of outcomes of TAR are available in the literature. Stengel *et al.* (2005) included 1107 third-generation TARs and concluded that TAR improves pain and joint mobility. The weighted 5-year survival rate averaged 90.6%. They compared the STAR prosthesis with the other designs namely ESKA, Ramses, LCS, and BP. There were no differences in rating with different scoring systems or any difference in ROM. A trend of lower deep infection rate with the STAR was noticed (Stengel *et al.*, 2005).

The review by Gougoulias *et al.* (2009) includes 1105 TARs, 304 being second generation (Agility and TNK) and 801 third-generation (STAR, BP, HINTEGRA, Salto, and Mobility) prostheses. They found an overall revision rate of 10%. Residual pain was common, in up to 60%, but the patients were to a high extent satisfied with the procedure (79–97%). Any superiority of any of the prosthetic designs could not be detected.

Zaidi *et al.* (2013) has produced the largest and most comprehensive systematic review and meta-analysis of TAR. Fifty-six papers with 2942 TARs of the second and third generation were included. The overall estimated 10-year survivorship was 89%. The AOFAS score was increased significantly at 7–10 years and ROM improved significantly. Radiolucencies were identified in up to 24% after 4.4 years (Zaidi *et al.*, 2013).

Comparing different reports of specific ankle replacements is a difficult task, mainly due to the variations of definition of revision of TAR. Indeed, the lack of consistency in definition of revision, accounts for why past revision rates and survival curves have differed so widely.

In a review, Henricson *et al.* (2011a) found several different definitions of revision and proposed a comprehensive definition — removal or exchange of one or more of the prosthetic components with the exception of incidental exchange of the polyethylene insert (Figure 1). This definition is used by the Swedish national ankle register and also by the UK National Joint Registry (NJR) for ankle replacements (Henricson *et al.*, 2011a).

Removal or exchange of one or more of the prosthetic components with the exception of incidental exchange of the polyethylene insert.

Figure 1. *Definition of revision of TAR.*

The level of evidence in reports of outcome of TAR is low. Most studies (70%) are Level IV (Zaidi *et al.*, 2013) and there are no Level I studies. Using the Cochrane Collaboration methodology there are intrinsic biases in all of reviewed papers by Zaidi *et al.* (2013).

The most studied TARs are the STAR and the BP prostheses. The designers have reported outstanding results in long-term follow-up studies (Kofoed, 2004; Buechel Sr *et al.*, 2004). With the STAR prosthesis independent and very experienced surgeons have shown that it is possible to achieve excellent 5-year results (Carlsson, 2006; Wood *et al.*, 2009; Mann *et al.*, 2011), but there is a deterioration at 10 years (Wood *et al.*, 2008; Brunner *et al.*, 2013; Nunley *et al.*, 2012; Daniels *et al.*, 2015) (Table 1). Two recent studies have demonstrated

Table 1. STAR survival summary.

Study	Number of cases	Follow-up (years)	5-year survival (%)	10-year survival (%)
Anderson *et al.* (2003)	51	4.3	70	
Kofoed (2004)	25	9.4	100	95 (12 years)
Carlsson (2006)	52	3.6	98	
Wood *et al.* (2008)	200	7.3	93	80
Wood *et al.* (2009)	100	4.5	95	
Karantana *et al.* (2010)	52	6.7	90	84 (8 years)
Mann *et al.* (2011)	84	9.1	96	90
Nunley *et al.* (2012)	82	5	93	86 (9 years)
Brunner *et al.* (2013)	77	12.4	92	71
Daniels *et al.* (2015)	11	9	89	66
Frigg *et al.* (2017)	46	19		94

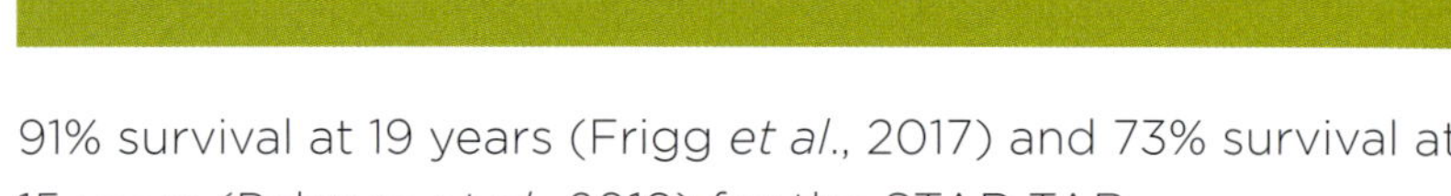

91% survival at 19 years (Frigg *et al.*, 2017) and 73% survival at 15 years (Palanca *et al.*, 2018) for the STAR TAR.

San Giovanni *et al.* (2006) and Doets *et al.* (2006), also independent, reached excellent 5-year results and preserved those at 10 years with the BP prosthesis (Table 2).

The Agility was until recently one of the most commonly used ankle prosthesis in USA, but seldom used in Europe. Knecht *et al.* (2004) in a large series (137 pts) with 9-years follow-up, reported superior results with a 5-year survival of 96% and a 10-year survival of 92%. However, they did not include two exchanges of polyethylene due to fracture and wear as revisions. On the other hand Spirt *et al.* (2004) found a 5-year survival rate of 80%, Hurowitz *et al.* (2007) a 6-year survival of 67%, and Criswell *et al.* (2012) a 62% survival at 10 years with the Agility design. Raikin *et al.* (2017) showed 80% survival at 9 years with patients functioning well despite radiographic outcomes.

There are only two follow-up studies concerning the AES prosthesis. Morgan *et al.* (2010) found a 6-year survival of 95% in 38 patients, while Henricson *et al.* (2010) in a somewhat larger study of 93 implants reported 90% survival rate at 5 years. Despite promising

Table 2. Survival rates of BP.

Study	Number of cases	Follow-up (years)	5-year survival (%)	10-year survival (%)
Buechel *et al.* (2004)	75	5	96	92 (12 yrs)
San Giovanni *et al.* (2006)	28	8.3	93	93
Doets *et al.* (2006)	74	7.6	89	89
Ali *et al.* (2007)	35	5	97	
Wood *et al.* (2009)	200	6	79	

published mid-term results, the AES was withdrawn by the manufacturer in 2012 due to reports of high incidence of osteolysis (Koivu *et al.*, 2009; Besse *et al.*, 2010). Di Iorio *et al.* showed a 10-year survival rate of 68% (Di Iorio *et al.*, 2017).

In a large series of the HINTEGRA prosthesis (722 ankles) by Barg *et al.* (2013) a 5-year survival of 94% and a 10-year survival of 84% has been reported (Barg *et al.*, 2013). Le Francois *et al.* (2017) showed mean improvements in total AOS scores. Survival rates and improvements in pain and function were comparable to Agility and STAR implants, and superior to Mobility. Survival rate was 92% at mean 3.5 years (Le Francois *et al.*, 2017). Deleu *et al.* (2015) demonstrated survival 90% at mean 45 month follow-up, with asymptomatic osteolysis in 48% (Deleu *et al.*, 2015). Yoon *et al.* (2014) followed up 99 ankle replacements for a mean of 40.8 months: In 37% of TAR there was radiologic evidence of osteolysis which was asymptomatic, with 10% developing progressive bone loss (Yoon *et al.*, 2014).

The European Salto prosthesis, a three component mobile bearing implant, differs from the US fixed bearing equivalent entitled the Salto Talaris. Bonnin *et al.* (2011), has reported 9-year follow-up of 98 cases of the Salto and found 19 patients with tibial or talar bone cysts-8 were bone grafted and three went on to arthrodesis. No component loosening was detected. The 10-year survival rate was 85%. Schenk *et al.* (2011) reported a 5-year survival of 87% in 218 patients. Wan *et al.* (2018) demonstrated survival of 94.9% at 35.9 months. There were significant improvements in pain, range of movement, and function (Wan *et al.*, 2018).

The Mobility (DePuy UK) prosthesis had 4-year survival rates published of 94% (Wood *et al.*, 2010) and of 98% (Rippstein *et al.*, 2011). Both these authors were principal designers. Independent researchers report 88% survival at 4 years (Sproule *et al.*, 2013). In a series of 67 Mobility TAR, there were two intra-operative and 13 postoperative complications at 61 months, with a survival of 91%. Seven patients needed reoperation (Kerkhoff *et al.*, 2016).

The Mobility prosthesis was, however, withdrawn voluntarily by the manufacturer in 2014.

Survival rates are commonly reported according to the Kaplan–Meier method. Based on annual revision rates Zaidi *et al.* (2013) estimated an overall 10-year survival of 89% (Table 3).

When considering survival rates of different prostheses one must firstly bear in mind the differences in definition of revision. Secondly there have been very few reports of the most widely used prostheses currently on the market and very few long-term studies. Thirdly there are few prospective studies and most are retrospective case series of low level evidence and with a high proportion of bias (Zaidi *et al.*, 2013). At present, no superiority of any ankle prosthesis can be found in the literature.

Table 3. Survival analysis of non-registry data (Zaidi *et al.*, 2013).

Study	Number of cases	Follow-up (years)	Number of revisions	Exposure time (years)	Annual failure rate	Estimated 10-year survival (%)
Ali *et al.* (2007)	34	5–13	1	168	0.006	0.94
Barg *et al.* (2011)	123	5–10	6	622	0.010	0.91
Bonnin *et al.* (2011)	96	9–11	12	802	0.015	0.86
Buechel *et al.* (2003)	50	5–10	2	282	0.007	0.93
Buechel *et al.* (2004)	75	5–12	6	905	0.007	0.94
Criswell *et al.* (2012)	42	8–11	16	296	0.054	0.58
Knecht *et al.* (2004)	96	9–16	14	820	0.017	0.84
Kofoed (2004)	25	9–12	1	238	0.004	0.96
Mann *et al.* (2011)	84	9–11	9	860	0.010	0.90
San Giovanni *et al.* (2006)	30	8–12	2	240	0.008	0.92
Wood *et al.* (2008)	200	7–13	24	1144	0.021	0.81
Total	855				0.012	0.89

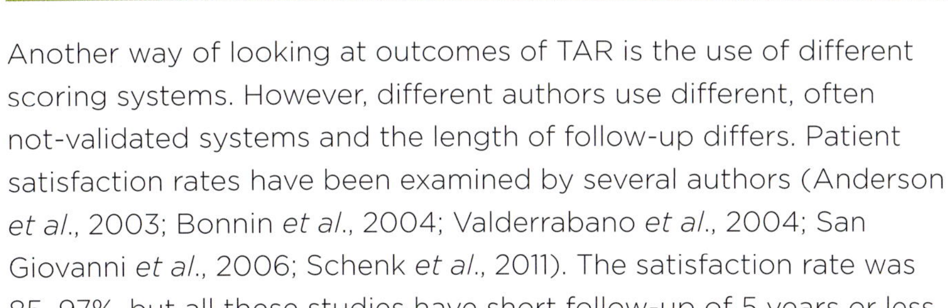

Another way of looking at outcomes of TAR is the use of different scoring systems. However, different authors use different, often not-validated systems and the length of follow-up differs. Patient satisfaction rates have been examined by several authors (Anderson *et al.*, 2003; Bonnin *et al.*, 2004; Valderrabano *et al.*, 2004; San Giovanni *et al.*, 2006; Schenk *et al.*, 2011). The satisfaction rate was 85–97%, but all these studies have short follow-up of 5 years or less.

The most generally used scoring system of clinical outcome of TAR is the AOFAS score. In their review, Zaidi *et al.* (2013) found that the AOFAS score increased significantly at 10 years and furthermore the VAS scores increased significantly at 5 years. Nonetheless, the AOFAS is no longer recommended to be used as a score for TAR, since it has not been validated (Pinsker and Daniels, 2011).

Sporting activity after TAR has been reported by Valderrabano *et al.* (2006), Naal *et al.* (2009), and Bonnin *et al.* (2009). More than half of the patients were physically active after surgery and the portion active patients had increased significantly. The most common activities were swimming, biking, hiking, and fitness training. All studies were short-term. In a systematic review Hörterer *et al.* (2015) found no evidence that sporting activity may be associated with higher increased failure rate of TAR. However, these authors strongly advised against participation in high impact sports.

The range of motion, especially the dorsiflexion, is important for walking ability. Zaidi *et al.* (2013) in their review found increased range of motion, statistically significant in dorsiflexion.

Radiolucencies have been reported around 24% of the tibial component and 1.7% of the talar component (Zaidi *et al.* 2013). Barely 10% of these patients were re-operated upon, or revised. Though the implication of these findings is not fully understood, it is a concern which calls for careful follow-up and some would argue preoperative CT or MRI scanning to determine whether there is progression of existing cysts or the development of new cysts postoperatively.

NATIONAL REGISTRIES

The advantage of national registries is the possibility to collect a larger number of procedures than any single surgeon or centrer can do. A registry also shows a truer impression of generalisable results in a country or region, rather than any individual's series since reports from low volume surgeons or centres are incorporated. The disadvantages of registries are many including lack of detailed clinical or radiological information; the possibility of incomplete reporting; and the capture of only hard end points, namely revision, meaning that the results of a painful TAR which has not yet been revised is not included.

Four national registries have published their results — namely the Swedish (Henricson *et al.*, 2007, 2011b), the Norwegian (Fevang *et al.*, 2007), the New Zealand (Hosman *et al.*, 2007; Tomlinson and Harrison, 2012), and the Finnish registries (Skytta *et al.*, 2010). The UK NJR publishes its results annually on line and in hard copy. Zaidi and Goldberg published a data-linkage study of the UK NJR data and Hospital Episodes Statistics (HES) database. TAR has a 30-day readmission rate of 2.2%, which is similar to that of knee replacement but lower than that of total hip replacement. About 6.6% of patients undergoing primary TAR require a reoperation within 12 months of the index procedure. Early revision rates are significantly higher in low-volume centres (Zaidi, 2016). Reporting rates, the male/female ratio and the diagnoses of the registries published in peer reviewed literature are given in Table 4.

Table 4. Data from the national registries.

	Reporting rate (%)	Male/ female (%)	Diagnoses (%)
Sweden	100	39/61	IJD 36, OA 24, PTA 34
Norway	not given	33/67	IJD 50, OA 20, PTA 23
New Zealand	78	61/39	IJD 12, OA 71, PTA 17
Finland	>95	40/60	IJD 49, OA 19, PTA 22

In the New Zealand registry, one fifth of the implanted ankles are missing — implying a possible impact on the survival rate from New Zealand (Hosman *et al.*, 2007).

The diagnoses are inflammatory joint disease (IJD) in 36–50% in the Scandinavian registries but only 12% in the New Zealand registry. The definitions of diagnoses might differ, especially for posttraumatic arthritis, but it is obvious that IJD as a reason for TAR is much more common in Scandinavia than in New Zealand. None of the registries could detect any difference of revision rate due to diagnoses.

The Swedish registry which has excellent compliance has shown an overall survival rate of 81% at 5 years and 69% at 10 years (Henricson *et al.*, 2011b). Forty-one percent of the prostheses were the STAR, the rest being BP, AES, HINTEGRA, Mobility, and CCI prostheses.

The Norwegian registry includes only one third-generation prosthesis, the STAR with 88% survival at 5 years (Fevang *et al.*, 2007).

In New Zealand the prevailing prostheses are the Mobility, the Salto, and the STAR. The 10-year survival rate is 82% (Tomlinson and Harrison, 2012).

Two of the third-generation implants were analysed in the Finnish register. The authors excluded designs that were implanted in a number less than 40. The 5-year survival rate was 83% with no difference between the STAR and the AES prostheses, respectively (Skytta *et al.*, 2010).

The Finnish and the New Zealand registries analysed the difference between high volume and low volume hospitals and found no difference in revision rates. The figures were however small. This is in contrast to the findings from the UK NJR which showed an increased odds of revision in those orthopaedic units preforming less than 20 ankle replacements per year (Zaidi and Goldberg, *et al.*, 2016).

The importance of learning curve is emphasised by the Swedish registry. When comparing the results of the three surgeons that had performed most ankle arthroplasties in Sweden, the 5-year survival rate of 70% for their 90 first cases was increased to 86% for their following 132 cases (Henricson *et al.*, 2007).

Lower age implied a higher revision rate in the Swedish registry, though only statistically significant for women below the age of 60 years with osteoarthritis (Henricson *et al.*, 2011b). Gender or age did not influence the results in the Norwegian, New Zealand, or Finnish registry.

The mean 5-year survival rate of these registries is 85%, which is in accordance with most single surgeons' or centres' reports (Table 5).

The Swedish experience of the STAR prosthesis was poor, showing a 10-year survival of 58%. When excluding the STAR prosthesis from the analysis the 10-year survival was 78% (Henricson *et al.*, 2011b).

Table 5. National registers.

	Number of TARs	Type of prosthesis	5-year survival (%)	10-year survival (%)
Norway (2007)	257	STAR	88	
New Zealand (2007, 2012)	202	Agility, STAR, Salto, Box, Ramses, Mobility	86	82
Finland (2010)	515	STAR, AES	83	
Sweden (2011)	780	STAR, AES, BP, HINTEGRA, Mobility, CCI	81	69 (78)

THE FUTURE FOR TAR

Aseptic loosening is the most common reason for revision in all these registries. The next most common reasons for revision are technical errors and instability.

The most common reason for revision and failure is aseptic loosening implying that fixation of components to bone is a key issue. New materials, e.g. porous metals, might in the future improve the strength of the bone–implant interface.

The second most common reason for failure is instability and malalignment leading to edge loading, subluxation or dislocation of the polyethylene insert. It is well known that preoperative varus/valgus position of the ankle or the hindfoot gives rise to a higher revision rate (Doets *et al.*, 2006; Henricson and Ågren, 2007; Wood *et al.*, 2008, 2009). It is crucial that surgeons performing TARs on one hand are familiar with different techniques to align the ankle and hindfoot and on the other hand have strict indications for the procedure.

In terms of health economics TAR compares favourably to ankle arthrodesis due to shorter immobilisation time, thus causing fewer consultations and visits to surgery. On the other hand secondary surgery, revisions as well as reoperations and additional procedures occur more frequently after TAR (Spirt *et al.*, 2004; Knecht *et al.*, 2004; Valderrabano *et al.*, 2004; Henricson *et al.*, 2010; Karantana *et al.*, 2010). Courville *et al.* (2011) has suggested that TAR might be more cost-effective treatment than ankle fusion, but much further work is to be done in this respect.

ALTERNATIVE TREATMENTS TO ANKLE REPLACEMENT

When evaluating outcomes of TAR it is necessary to consider the outcomes of the alternative treatments of ankle arthritis, the most obvious being debridement, arthrodesis, distraction arthroplasty, and total allograft replacement.

Arthrodesis of the ankle is the most used method of treatment of ankle arthritis. In a systematic review Haddad *et al.* (2007) found a non-union rate of 10%, while Anderson *et al.* (2005a) had 25% non-union. Infection rates of 0–12% have been reported (Anderson *et al.*, 2005b). Haddad *et al.* (2007) also found a below-knee-amputation rate of 5% following ankle arthrodesis. Long-term follow-up has shown that following ankle arthrodesis, radiographic subtalar and Chopart joint arthritis appear in more than half of the cases. Many patients also experience pain from prolonged standing and walking (Coester *et al.*, 2001; Muir *et al.*, 2002).

The reports of arthroscopic debridement of the ankle in arthritis are few including small groups of patients. Ogilvie-Harris and Sekyi-Otu *et al.* (1995) reported that arthroscopic debridement relieved the symptoms of two thirds of the patients for almost four years. Hassouna *et al.* (2007) found that more than one-quarter of the patients needed major ankle surgery within 5 years of debridement. With such sparse supporting evidence, the authors recommends that this technique is reserved for synovectomy, loose bodies, soft-tissue impingement, and osteophytes.

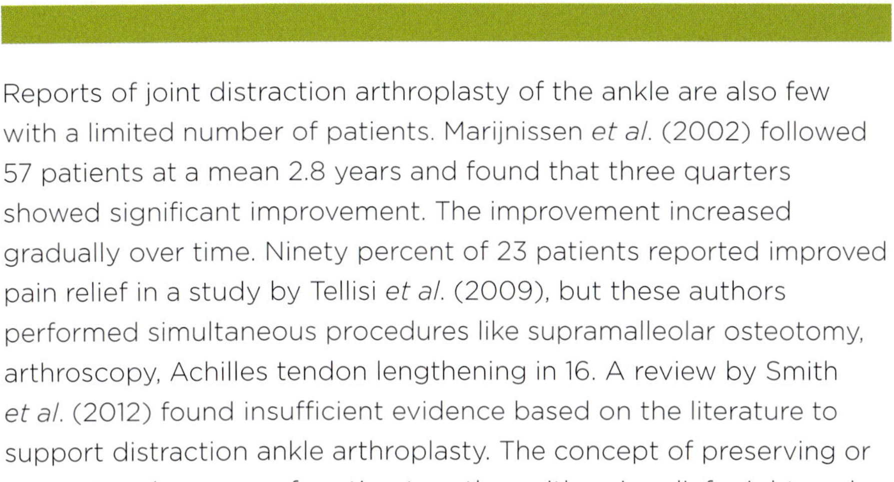

Reports of joint distraction arthroplasty of the ankle are also few with a limited number of patients. Marijnissen *et al.* (2002) followed 57 patients at a mean 2.8 years and found that three quarters showed significant improvement. The improvement increased gradually over time. Ninety percent of 23 patients reported improved pain relief in a study by Tellisi *et al.* (2009), but these authors performed simultaneous procedures like supramalleolar osteotomy, arthroscopy, Achilles tendon lengthening in 16. A review by Smith *et al.* (2012) found insufficient evidence based on the literature to support distraction ankle arthroplasty. The concept of preserving or increasing the range of motion together with pain relief might push the TAR forward, but the evidence is sparse.

Two recent reports of total ankle allograft replacement show conflicting results. Lee (2008) found no complications and good clinical results after 1 year, while Jeng *et al.* (2008) had an extremely high rate of failures with 2 years follow-up. No prospective studies concerning these alternative methods are available, all reports are Level III–IV studies. The need for further studies is obvious.

COMPARISON OF ANKLE REPLACEMENT AND ARTHRODESIS

Saltzman *et al.* (2009), in a prospective non-randomised (Level III) study compared the STAR prostheses with ankle fusion. In the short-term, the need for secondary surgery was more common in the arthroplasty group. Pain relief was equal in both groups but the arthroplasty group had better function.

The need for secondary procedures was also found to be more frequent for TAR patients in a smaller retroprospective study with 4 years follow-up (Saltzman *et al.*, 2010). In this study, with a dropout rate of 12 and 21%, respectively, the TAR group had better pain relief than the fusion group.

Compared to ankle fusion, TAR has been shown to lead to improved gait patterns (Hahn *et al.*, 2012); better quality of life (Esparragoza *et al.*, 2011), and to be more cost effective (Courville *et al.*, 2011).

Reviewing articles on outcomes of TAR and ankle arthrodesis up to 2005 Haddad *et al.* (2007) compared outcomes. They studied results from different scoring and rating systems as well as survival rates and revision rates. Though the results were in a slight favour of TAR, the differences were small and a significant heterogeneity was detected in most of the studies. There are studies which suggest some advantages to TAR, such as range of movement and biomechanics, but the studies are few, mostly short-term and non-randomised (DiGiovanni and Guss, 2017; Morash *et al.*, 2017; Krause and Schmid, 2012).

A prospective multicentre study by the Canadian Orthopaedic Foot & Ankle Society (COFAS) looking at 890 patients with ankle arthritis, was presented at IFFAS in Lisbon in 2017 and showed equivalent results of TAR and ankle arthrodesis at 5.5 years for non-complex patients (COFAS Types 1 & 2). They also showed that for complex patients (COFAS Types 3 & 4), TAR leads to significantly better outcomes over ankle arthrodesis. Their cohorts were prospective but not randomised and hence are subject to selection bias. They also identified that reoperation rates (non-revision) are significantly higher for TAR than AF overall (21% vs 14%) (Penner *et al.*, 2018).

A multicentre prospective randomised study comparing Total Ankle Replacement Versus ankle Arthrodesis (TARVA) is currently underway in the United Kingdom (Goldberg *et al.*, 2016).

CONCLUSIONS

The scientific evidence of TAR is weak, since most published studies are Level IV (case series) studies. Comparative studies of TAR and ankle arthrodesis show a trend towards better outcomes for TAR, especially in complex patients, but in the main the numbers are small, the follow-up times short, and the study designs heterogeneous.

Recent studies of TAR have 5-year survival rates of 90% or more, and the few long-term studies from independent researchers show 10-year survival rates of 78–93%.

The need for secondary surgery (reoperation other than revision) is greater for TAR than for ankle fusion. However, patient's satisfaction rates are good with figures of 85–97%.

Development of prosthetic designs, instrumentation and above all the skill and experience of foot and ankle surgeons will no doubt improve the results in the future. The need for longer and larger studies of the outcome of TAR is obvious.

REFERENCES

Ali, M. S., Higgins, G. H., Mohammed, M. 2007. Intermediate results of Buechel-Pappas unconstrained uncemented total ankle replacement for osteoarthritis. *J Foot Ankle Surgery*, 46, 16–20.

Anderson, T., Maxander, P., Rydholm, U., Besjakov, J. & Carlsson, A. 2005a. Ankle arthrodesis by compression screws in rheumatoid arthritis: Primary nonunion in 9/35 patients. *Acta Orthop*, 76, 884–890.

Anderson, T., Montgomery, F. & Carlsson, A. 2003. Uncemented Star total ankle prostheses. Three to eight-year follow-up of fifty-one consecutive ankles. *J Bone Joint Surg Am*, 85-A, 1321–1329.

Anderson, T., Rydholm, U., Besjakov, J., Montgomery, F. & Carlsson, A. 2005b. Tibiotalocalcaneal fusion using retrograde intramedullary nails as salvage procedure for failed total ankle prosthesis in rheumatoid arthritis: A report of sixteen cases. *Foot Ankle Surg*, 11, 143–147.

Barg, A., Elsner, A., Anderson, E. A. & Hintermann, B. 2011. The effect of three component total ankle replacement malalignment on clinical outcome, pain relief and functional outcome in 317 consecutive patients. *J Bone Joint Surg Am*, 93, 1969–1978.

Barg, A., Zwicky, L., Knupp, M., Henninger, H. B. & Hintermann, B. 2013. Hintegra total ankle replacement: Survivorship analysis in 684 patients. *J Bone Joint Surg Am*, 95, 1175–1183.

Besse, J. L., Colombier, J. A., Asencio, J., Bonnin, M., Gaudot, F., Jarde, O., Judet, T., Maestro, M., Lemrijse, T., Leonardi, C., Toullec, E. & L'afcp 2010. Total ankle arthroplasty in France. *Orthop Traumatol Surg Res*, 96, 291–303.

Bonnin, M., Gaudot, F., Laurent, J. R., Ellis, S., Colombier, J. A. & Judet, T. 2011. The salto total ankle arthroplasty: Survivorship and analysis of failures at 7 to 11 years. *Clin Orthop Relat Res*, 469, 225–236.

Bonnin, M., Judet, T., Colombier, J. A., Buscayret, F., Graveleau, N. & Piriou, P. 2004. Midterm results of the salto total ankle prosthesis. *Clin Orthop Relat Res*, 6–18.

Bonnin, M. P., Laurent, J. R. & Casillas, M. 2009. Ankle function and sports activity after total ankle arthroplasty. *Foot Ankle Int*, 30, 933–944.

Brunner, S., Barg, A., Knupp, M., Zwicky, L., Kapron, A. L., Valderrabano, V. & Hintermann, B. 2013. The Scandinavian total ankle replacement: Long-term, eleven to fifteen-year, survivorship analysis of the prosthesis in seventy-two consecutive patients. *J Bone Joint Surg Am*, 95, 711–718.

Buechel Sr, F. F., Buechel Jr, F. F. & Pappas, M. J. 2003. Ten-year evolution of cementless Buechel-Pappas meniscal bearing total ankle replacement. *Foot Ankle Int*, 24, 462–472.

Carlsson, A. 2006. Single- and double-coated Star total ankle replacements: A clinical and radiographic follow-up study of 109 cases. *Orthopade*, 35, 527–532.

Coester, L. M., Saltzman, C. L., Leupold, J. & Pontarelli, W. 2001. Long-term results following ankle arthrodesis for post-traumatic arthritis. *J Bone Joint Surg Am*, 83-A, 219–228.

Courville, X. F., Hecht, P. J. & Tosteson, A. N. 2011. Is total ankle arthroplasty a cost-effective alternative to ankle fusion? *Clin Orthop Relat Res*, 469, 1721–1727.

Criswell, B. J., Douglas, K., Naik, R. & Thomson, A. B. 2012. High revision and reoperation rates using the agility total ankle system. *Clin Orthop Relat Res*, 470, 1980–1986.

Daniels, T. R., Mayich, D. J. & Penner, M. J. 2015. Intermediate to long-term outcomes of total ankle replacement with the Scandinavian total ankle replacement (Star). *J Bone Joint Surg Am*, 97, 895–903.

Deleu, P. A., Devos Bevernage, B., Gombault, V., Maldague, P. & Leemrijse, T. 2015. Intermediate-term results of mobile-bearing total ankle replacement. *Foot Ankle Int*, 36, 518–530.

Di Iorio, A., Viste, A., Fessy, M. H. & Besse, J. L. 2017. The AES total ankle arthroplasty analysis of failures and survivorship at ten years. *Int Orthop*, 41, 2525–2533.

Digiovanni, C. W. & Guss, D. 2017. Ankle replacement or ankle fusion: Who reigns supreme?: commentary on an article by Marisa R. Benich, Bs, *et al.*: "Comparison of treatment outcomes of arthrodesis and two generations of ankle replacement implants". *J Bone Joint Surg Am*, 99, E115.

Doets, H. C., Brand, R. & Nelissen, R. G. 2006. Total ankle arthroplasty in inflammatory joint disease with use of two mobile-bearing designs. *J Bone Joint Surg Am*, 88, 1272–1284.

Esparragoza, L., Vidal, C. & Vaquero, J. 2011. Comparative study of the quality of life between arthrodesis and total arthroplasty substitution of the ankle. *J Foot Ankle Surg*, 50, 383–387.

Fevang, B. T., Lie, S. A., Havelin, L. I., Brun, J. G., Skredderstuen, A. & Furnes, O. 2007. 257 Ankle arthroplasties performed in norway between 1994 and 2005. *Acta Orthop*, 78, 575–583.

Frigg, A., Germann, U., Huber, M. & Horisberger, M. 2017. Survival of the Scandinavian total ankle replacement (Star): Results of ten to nineteen years follow-up. *Int Orthop*, 41, 2075–2082.

Goldberg, A. J., Zaidi, R., Thomson, C., Dore, C. J., Skene, S. S., Cro, S., Round, J., Molloy, A., Davies, M., Karski, M., Kim, L., Cooke, P. & GROUP, T. S. 2016.

Total ankle replacement versus arthrodesis (TARVA): Protocol for a multicentre randomised controlled trial. *BMJ Open*, 6, e012716.

Gougoulias, N. E., Khanna, A. & Maffulli, N. 2009. How successful are current ankle replacements? A systematic review of the literature. *Clin Orthop Relat Res*, 468, 199–208.

Haddad, S. L., Coetzee, J. C., Estok, R., Fahrbach, K., Banel, D. & Nalysnyk, L. 2007. Intermediate and long-term outcomes of total ankle arthroplasty and ankle arthrodesis. A systematic review of the literature. *J Bone Joint Surg Am*, 89, 1899–1905.

Hahn, M. E., Wright, E. S., Segal, A. D., Orendurff, M. S., Ledoux, W. R. & Sangeorzan, B. J. 2012. Comparative gait analysis of ankle arthrodesis and arthroplasty: Initial findings of a prospective study. *Foot Ankle Int*, 33, 282–289.

Hassouna, H., Kumar, S. & Bendall, S. 2007. Arthroscopic ankle debridement: 5-year survival analysis. *Acta Orthop Belg*, 73, 737–740.

Henricson, A. & Ågren, P.-H. 2007. Secondary surgery after total ankle replacement: The influence of preoperative hindfoot alignment. *Foot Ankle Surg*, 13, 41–44.

Henricson, A., Carlsson, A. & Rydholm, U. 2011a. What Is a revision of total ankle replacement? *Foot Ankle Surg*, 17, 99–102.

Henricson, A., Knutson, K., Lindahl, J. & Rydholm, U. 2010. The AES total ankle replacement: A mid-term analysis of 93 cases. *Foot Ankle Surg*, 16, 61–64.

Henricson, A., Nilsson, J. A. & Carlsson, A. 2011b. 10-Year survival of total ankle arthroplasties: A report on 780 cases from the Swedish ankle register. *Acta Orthop*, 82, 655–659.

Henricson, A., Skoog, A. & Carlsson, A. 2007. The Swedish ankle arthroplasty register: An analysis of 531 arthroplasties between 1993 and 2005. *Acta Orthop*, 78, 569–574.

Hörterer, H., Miltner, O., Müller-Rath, R., Phisitkul, P. & Barg, A. 2015. Sports activity in patients with total ankle replacement. *Sports Orthop Traumatol*, 31, 34–40.

Hosman, A. H., Mason, R. B., Hobbs, T. & Rothwell, A. G. 2007. A New Zealand national joint registry review of 202 total ankle replacements followed for up to 6 years. *Acta Orthop*, 78, 584–591.

Hurowitz, E. J., Gould, J. S., Fleisig, G. S. & Fowler, R. 2007. Outcome analysis of agility total ankle replacement with prior adjunctive procedures: Two to six year followup. *Foot Ankle Int*, 28, 308–312.

Jeng, C. L., Kadakia, A., White, K. L. & Myerson, M. S. 2008. Fresh osteochondral total ankle allograft transplantation for the treatment of ankle arthritis. *Foot Ankle Int*, 29, 554–560.

Karantana, A., Hobson, S. & Dhar, S. 2010. The Scandinavian total ankle replacement: Survivorship at 5 and 8 years comparable to other series. *Clin Orthop Relat Res*, 468, 951–957.

Kerkhoff, Y. R., Kosse, N. M. & Louwerens, J. W. 2016. Short term results of the mobility total ankle system: Clinical and radiographic outcome. *Foot Ankle Surg*, 22, 152–157.

Knecht, S. I., Estin, M., Callaghan, J. J., Zimmerman, M. B., Alliman, K. J., Alvine, F. G. & Saltzman, C. L. 2004. The agility total ankle arthroplasty. Seven to sixteen-year follow-up. *J Bone Joint Surg Am*, 86-A, 1161–1171.

Kofoed, H. 2004. Scandinavian total ankle replacement (Star). *Clin Orthop Relat Res*, 73–79.

Koivu, H., Kohonen, I., Sipola, E., Alanen, K., Vahlberg, T. & Tiusanen, H. 2009. Severe periprosthetic osteolytic lesions after the ankle evolutive system total ankle replacement. *J Bone Joint Surg Br*, 91, 907–914.

Krause, F. G. & Schmid, T. 2012. Ankle arthrodesis versus total ankle replacement: How do i decide? *Foot Ankle Clin*, 17, 529–543.

Lee, D. K. 2008. Ankle arthroplasty alternatives with allograft and external fixation: Preliminary clinical outcome. *J Foot Ankle Surg*, 47, 447–452.

Le Francois, T., Younger, A., Wing, K., Penner, M. J., Dryden, P., Wong, H., Daniels, T. & Glazebrook, M. 2017. A prospective study of four total ankle arthroplasty implants by non-designer investigators. *J Bone Joint Surg Am*, 99, 342–348.

Mann, J. A., Mann, R. A. & Horton, E. 2011. Star ankle: Long-term results. *Foot Ankle Int*, 32, S473–S484.

Marijnissen, A. C., Van Roermund, P. M., Van Melkebeek, J., Schenk, W., Verbout, A. J., Bijlsma, J. W. & Lafeber, F. P. 2002. Clinical benefit of joint distraction in the treatment of severe osteoarthritis of the ankle: Proof of concept in an open prospective study and in a randomized controlled study. *Arthritis Rheum*, 46, 2893–2902.

Morash, J., Walton, D. M. & Glazebrook, M. 2017. Ankle arthrodesis versus total ankle arthroplasty. *Foot Ankle Clin*, 22, 251–266.

Morgan, S. S., Brooke, B. & Harris, N. J. 2010. Total ankle replacement by the ankle evolution system: Medium-term outcome. *J Bone Joint Surg Br*, 92, 61–65.

Muir, D. C., Amendola, A. & Saltzman, C. L. 2002. Long-term outcome of ankle arthrodesis. *Foot Ankle Clin*, 7, 703–708.

Naal, F. D., Impellizzeri, F. M., Loibl, M., Huber, M. & Rippstein, P. F. 2009. Habitual physical activity and sports participation after total ankle arthroplasty. *Am J Sports Med*, 37, 95–102.

Nunley, J. A., Caputo, A. M., Easley, M. E. & Cook, C. 2012. Intermediate to long-term outcomes of the Star total ankle replacement: The patient perspective. *J Bone Joint Surg Am*, 94, 43–48.

Ogilvie-Harris, D. J. & Sekyi-Otu, A. 1995. Arthroscopic debridement for the osteoarthritic ankle. *Arthroscopy*, 11, 433–436.

Palanca, A., Mann, R. A., Mann, J. A. & Haskell, A. 2018. Scandinavian total ankle replacement: 15-year follow-up. *Foot Ankle Int*, 39, 135–142.

Penner, M. J., Wing, K., Glazebrook, M. & Daniels, T. 2018. The effect of deformity and hindfoot arthritis on midterm outcomes of ankle replacement and fusion: A prospective COFAS multi-centre study of 890 patients. *Foot Ankle Orthop*, 3, S107–S108.

Pinsker, E. & Daniels, T. R. 2011. Aofas position statement regarding the future of the Aofas clinical rating systems. *Foot Ankle Int*, 32, 841–842.

Raikin, S. M., Sandrowski, K., Kane, J. M., Beck, D. & Winters, B. S. 2017. Midterm outcome of the agility total ankle arthroplasty. *Foot Ankle Int*, 38, 662–670.

Rippstein, P. F., Huber, M., Coetzee, J. C. & Naal, F. D. 2011. Total ankle replacement with use of a new three-component implant. *J Bone Joint Surg Am*, 93, 1426–1435.

Saltzman, C. L., Kadoko, R. G. & Suh, J. S. 2010. Treatment of isolated ankle osteoarthritis with arthrodesis or the total ankle replacement: A comparison of early outcomes. *Clin Orthop Surg*, 2, 1–7.

Saltzman, C. L., Mann, R. A., Ahrens, J. E., Amendola, A., Anderson, R. B., Berlet, G. C., Brodsky, J. W., Chou, L. B., Clanton, T. O., Deland, J. T., Deorio, J. K., Horton, G. A., Lee, T. H., Mann, J. A., Nunley, J. A., Thordarson, D. B., Walling, A. K., Wapner, K. L. & Coughlin, M. J. 2009. Prospective controlled trial of Star Total ankle replacement versus ankle fusion: Initial results. *Foot Ankle Int*, 30, 579–596.

San Giovanni, T. P., Keblish, D. J., Thomas, W. H. & Wilson, M. G. 2006. Eight-year results of a minimally constrained total ankle arthroplasty. *Foot Ankle Int*, 27, 418–426.

Schenk, K., Lieske, S., John, M., Franke, K., Mouly, S., Lizee, E. & Neumann, W. 2011. Prospective study of a cementless, mobile-bearing, third generation total ankle prosthesis. *Foot Ankle Int*, 32, 755–763.

Skytta, E. T., Koivu, H., Eskelinen, A., Ikavalko, M., Paavolainen, P. & Remes, V. 2010. Total ankle replacement: A population-based study of 515 cases from the finnish arthroplasty register. *Acta Orthop*, 81, 114–118.

Smith, N. C., Beaman, D., Rozbruch, S. R. & Glazebrook, M. A. 2012. Evidence-based indications for distraction ankle arthroplasty. *Foot Ankle Int*, 33, 632–636.

Spirt, A. A., Assal, M. & Hansen, S. T., Jr. 2004. Complications and failure after total ankle arthroplasty. *J Bone Joint Surg Am*, 86-A, 1172–1178.

Sproule, J. A., Chin, T., Amin, A., Daniels, T., Younger, A. S., Boyd, G. & Glazebrook, M. A. 2013. Clinical and radiographic outcomes of the mobility total ankle arthroplasty system: Early results from a prospective multicenter study. *Foot Ankle Int*, 34, 491–497.

Stengel, D., Bauwens, K., Ekkernkamp, A. & Cramer, J. 2005. Efficacy of total ankle replacement with meniscal-bearing devices: A systematic review and meta-analysis. *Arch Orthop Trauma Surg*, 125, 109–119.

Tellisi, N., Fragomen, A. T., Kleinman, D., O'malley, M. J. & Rozbruch, S. R. 2009. Joint Preservation of the osteoarthritic ankle using distraction arthroplasty. *Foot Ankle Int*, 30, 318–325.

Tomlinson, M. & Harrison, M. 2012. The New Zealand Joint Registry: Report of 11-year data for ankle arthroplasty. *Foot Ankle Clin*, 17, 719–723.

Valderrabano, V., Hintermann, B. & Dick, W. 2004. Scandinavian total ankle replacement: A 3.7-year average followup of 65 patients. *Clin Orthop Relat Res*, 47–56.

Valderrabano, V., Pagenstert, G., Horisberger, M., Knupp, M. & Hintermann, B. 2006. Sports and recreation activity of ankle arthritis patients before and after total ankle replacement. *Am J Sports Med*, 34, 993–999.

Wan, D. D., Choi, W. J., Shim, D. W., Hwang, Y., Park, Y. J. & Lee, J. W. 2018. Short-term clinical and radiographic results of the Salto mobile total ankle prosthesis. *Foot Ankle Int*, 39, 155–165.

Wood, P. L., Karski, M. T. & Watmough, P. 2010. Total ankle replacement: The results of 100 mobility total ankle replacements. *J Bone Joint Surg Br*, 92, 958–962.

Wood, P. L., Prem, H. & Sutton, C. 2008. Total ankle replacement: Medium-term results in 200 Scandinavian total ankle replacements. *J Bone Joint Surg Br*, 90, 605–609.

Wood, P. L., Sutton, C., Mishra, V. & Suneja, R. 2009. A randomised, controlled trial of two mobile-bearing total ankle replacements. *J Bone Joint Surg Br*, 91, 69–74.

Yoon, H. S., Lee, J., Choi, W. J. & Lee, J. W. 2014. Periprosthetic osteolysis after total ankle arthroplasty. *Foot Ankle Int*, 35, 14–21.

Zaidi, R., Cro, S., Gurusamy, K., Siva, N., Macgregor, A., Henricson, A. & Goldberg, A. 2013. The outcome of total ankle replacement: A systematic review and meta-analysis. *Bone Joint J*, 95-B, 1500–1507.

Zaidi, R., Macgregor, A. J., Goldberg, A. 2016. Quality measures for total ankle replacement, 30-day readmission and reoperation rates within 1 year of surgery: A data linkage study using the NJR data set. *BMJ Open 2016*; 6:e011332. doi:10.1136 bmjopen-2016-011332.

SURGICAL TECHNIQUE

CHAPTER
10

A. Ramasamy, A.-A. Najefi, P. H. Cooke and A. J. Goldberg

Summary

The successful implantation of a total ankle replacement is a multistep process beginning with appropriate selection and preparation of the patient preoperatively. A key principle of successful surgery is obtaining anatomic alignment of the limb during weightbearing, including a plantar grade foot with balanced muscular forces across the foot and ankle throughout the gait cycle. Obtaining reproducible anatomic alignment while correcting coronal and sagittal plane deformity is critical to reduce the incidence of eccentric wear, component loosening, subsidence, and reoperation.

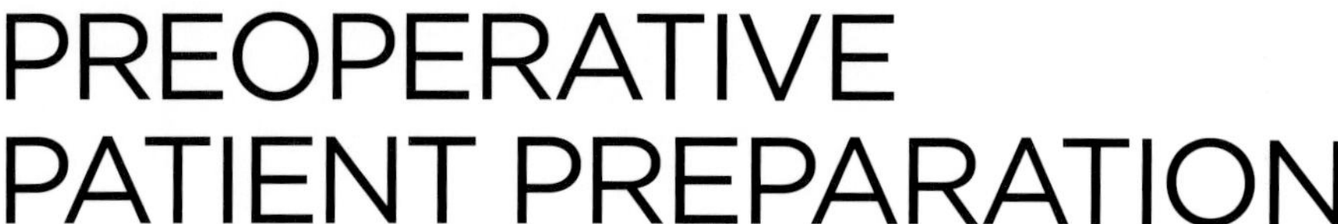

PREOPERATIVE PATIENT PREPARATION

Patients embarking on ankle replacement will usually be seen in a preadmission clinic where their general health will be checked as will their suitability for the anaesthetic. Ankle replacement is never an emergency procedure and there is ample opportunity to optimise the patient's general condition (e.g. diabetic control, hypertension, etc.) prior to surgery. Health-related factors, such as high body mass index (BMI), peripheral vascular disease, and diabetes should be considered carefully as these may be relative contra-indications to surgery.

A full history, including a comprehensive drug history is essential. Generally, patients must not stop steroid medication prior to surgery, and there is little point in stopping immunosuppressive drugs, such as methotrexate and leflunomide (because of the long half-life of the drugs and the adverse effects of stopping them). Indeed, it remains controversial as to whether to stop the modern disease modifying agents. Therefore, it is recommended that decisions on medication changes should be made within a multidisciplinary team setting involving the patient's rheumatologist. The leading patient factors that increase the risk of reoperation and revision are rheumatoid arthritis, preoperative deformity, and high ASA grade. In terms of hospital/surgeon factors, early revision rates are significantly higher in low-volume centres (Zaidi *et al.*, 2016).

Examination begins by assessment of the deformity and the affected leg should be compared to the other side. The patient should be observed walking into the clinic and the gait should be assessed. Ankle and foot alignment, joint range of motion, rotation of the limb, and leg length should be measured. Adjacent joints, such as the subtalar joint, knee, and hip joints, should be evaluated. The vascularity, sensation, and integrity of the skin, as well as the presence of previous scars must be documented. Where the quality of skin or the presence of previous surgical scars may compromise the surgical approach, advice may need to be sought from a plastic surgeon. All patients should be risk assessed for thromboembolic risk and been offered a discussion by the anaesthetist on perioperative anaesthetic blocks for postoperative pain management.

PREOPERATIVE PLANNING

Up to date, weightbearing mortise or anterior–posterior (AP) ankle views, as well as lateral radiographs of the ankle are essential to evaluate the amount of arthritis and any hindfoot deformity. In addition, dorso-plantar (DP) radiograph is also necessary to document any preexisting subtalar and talonavicular osteoarthritis (OA) before the surgery.

We recommend, the use of long-length alignment X-rays to assess the mechanical axis of the lower limb and the anatomical axis of the tibia. This allows the surgeon to plan prosthesis positioning in the coronal and sagittal planes.

Typically, measurements of lower limb alignment are performed using plain radiographs (Figure 1). On normal weightbearing AP radiographs, a vertical line that extends distally from the centre of the pubic symphysis is known as the vertical axis. This axis is used as a reference axis/line from which the other axes are determined. The mechanical axis is defined as a line from the centre of the proximal joint to the centre of the distal joint. In the lower limb, this is taken from the centre of the femoral head to the centre of the tibiotalar joint in the coronal plane. The mechanical axis of the tibia alone is from the centre of the knee joint to the centre of the tibiotalar joint. The medial angle formed by the mechanical axis of the femur and the mechanical axis of the tibia is called the hip–knee–ankle angle (HKA). This is usually slightly less than 180° in normal knees. The anatomical axis of the tibia is measured by drawing a line from the centre of the tibial diaphysis to the middle of the tibial metaphysis, approximately located 10 cm above the surface of the ankle joint. The anatomical axes can deviate markedly depending on femoral or tibial deformities from trauma or inherited conditions, or previous corrective or replacement surgery. In the majority of cases, anatomical axes of the tibia and mechanical axes of the tibia are similar. However, there is usually a difference between the tibial axis and the mechanical axis of the lower limb, which varies with deformity (Moreland *et al.*, 1987; Greisberg *et al.*, 2004; Trajkovski *et al.*, 2013). This needs to be considered and planned to ensure that the implant is positioned accurately. We would recommend alignment of the ankle replacement to the mechanical axis of the lower limb in the coronal plane.

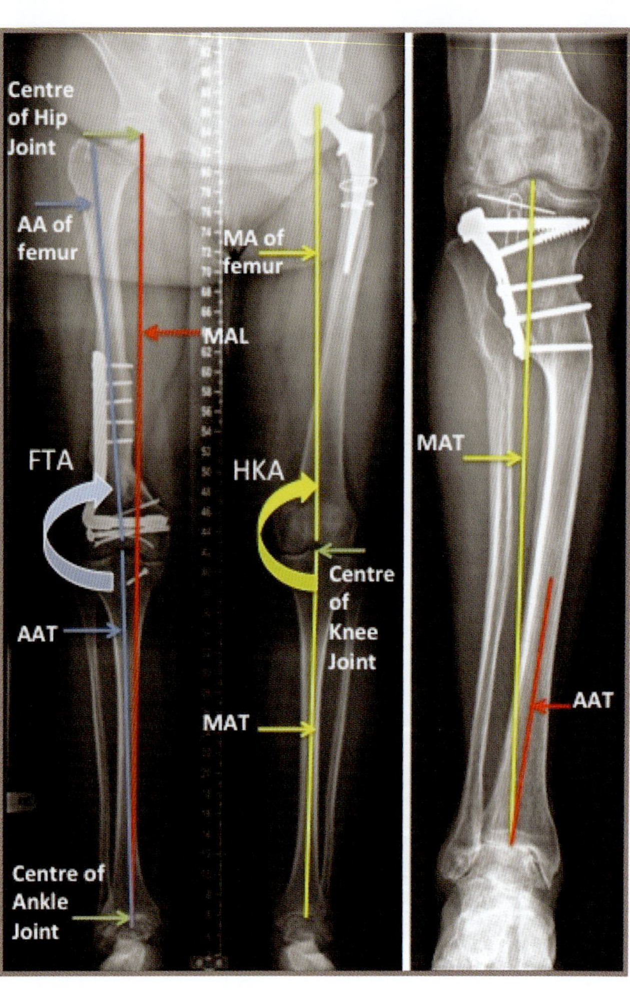

Figure 1. *Full length lower limb AP radiographs. On the left, the red line demonstrates the mechanical axis of the lower limb (MAL). In most circumstances the anatomical axis of the tibia (AAT) and the mechanical axis of the tibia (MAT) correspond with the MAT but differs where the MAT does not go through the centre of the knee. The femoro-tibial angle (FTA) and the hip knee angle (HKA) are also shown. The radiograph on the right demonstrates a malunited tibial plateau fracture that causes a large discrepancy between the MAT and AAT.*

Supplementary radiographic investigations such as CT or MRI may be particularly helpful to look for adjacent hindfoot or midfoot arthritis. The use of CT scans will inevitably give a more accurate outline of the anatomy and orientation of the femur and tibia, which will allow for more reliable templating. They will also enable the surgeon to be aware of any cysts that exist preoperatively. The rotational alignment of the lower limb (tibial tuberosity and transmalleolar axis) is something that two-dimensional radiographs cannot assess. It is also difficult to determine this accurately intraoperatively especially in cases of rotational malalignment (e.g. tibial deformity or malunion), which can affect the placement of extramedullary guides.

Preoperative MRI or CT may also be useful to investigate avascular necrosis in conditions, such as hemochromatosis or haemophilia and help assess sizing accurately in particularly small or large patients.

OPERATIVE TECHNIQUE

There are many important differences that set the ankle apart from other large joints, making prosthetic replacement more difficult. Access and exposure, especially to the talus, are limited, and unlike the hip and knee, the ankle cannot be dislocated in the course of operation. Furthermore, there is very little soft tissue coverage around the ankle. The talus is a small bone, and when resected, results in approximately one half of the surface area of that of the upper tibia at the knee.

Three challenges must be met to produce an acceptable result from an ankle replacement: (i) perfect alignment of the components, (ii) good soft tissue balance, and (iii) compatibility between the tibial and talar components. The surgeon seeks to produce an ankle replacement which is ideally aligned in the coronal, sagittal, and axial planes. The tibia is matched to the talus in rotation, with a joint line at the appropriate level. The soft tissues are balanced in flexion and extension, and tensioned sufficiently to produce stability, but without limiting the range of movement or producing excessive compression on the polyethylene. Inadequate correction of alignment in the coronal, sagittal, or axial planes will inevitably lead to failure of the ankle replacement.

Other Foot or Ankle Deformity

Coronal or sagittal plane deformity, previous surgery, or any degenerative change at the hip, femur, or tibia may influence the alignment of the ankle and foot. Therefore, it is recommended that these are corrected first. Fusion procedures to adjacent joints and supramalleolar osteotomies should be performed before any ankle replacement. Performing subtalar arthrodesis at the same time as ankle replacement may risk the blood supply to the talus and causes higher rates of instability and dislocation. Furthermore, any deformity distal to the ankle must also be noted. Issues include a cavus or planus deformity, degenerative changes in adjacent joints, or medial or lateral ligamentous laxity. Corrective procedures, such as a calcaneal osteotomy and dorsiflexion first ray osteotomy for a cavus foot, should be done before the ankle replacement. Performing an ankle replacement together with other corrective procedures lengthens tourniquet time and may cause wound problems due to multiple incisions.

Preparation

Full precautions should be taken to prevent prosthetic infection including thorough skin preparation, barrier occlusion of the operative site, and prophylactic antibiotics appropriate to the hospital — administered a few minutes prior to application of a tourniquet. Similarly, appropriate thromboprophylaxis is advised.

The leg should be positioned so the foot is pointing directly upwards (this is usually accomplished with a sandbag under the buttocks), and we find it helpful in maintaining this, as well as protecting the posterior structures during the operation by positioning the calf on a padded foam elevator with the heel dependent so that the talus is not pushed forwards (Figure 2).

Approach/Incision

For most prostheses, the surgical approach is via an anterior midline approach. The incision should be of adequate length to avoid excessive retraction. Full thickness flaps should be created and undermining avoided. The lateral skin has a relatively good and close blood supply, but the medial skin edges receive a more distant supply from branches of the posterior tibial artery. Hence special care must be taken of the wound edges, avoiding undercutting, and excessive traction. Ideally no self-retaining retractors should be used.

The medial branch of the superficial peroneal nerve is identified at the distal portion of the incision and sometimes has to be mobilised. We tend to place a coloured vascular loop around the nerve for identification and retraction (Figure 3). Deep dissection to the anterior tibia and talus is via the interval between the tibialis anterior and extensor hallucis longus (EHL) tendons — keeping

Figure 2. *An ankle replacement, foot holder, allowing the heel to hang free so as not to push the ankle forwards. During surgery the foot holder is covered in sterile coverings and lifts the foot above the contralateral ankle to enable lateral radiography.*

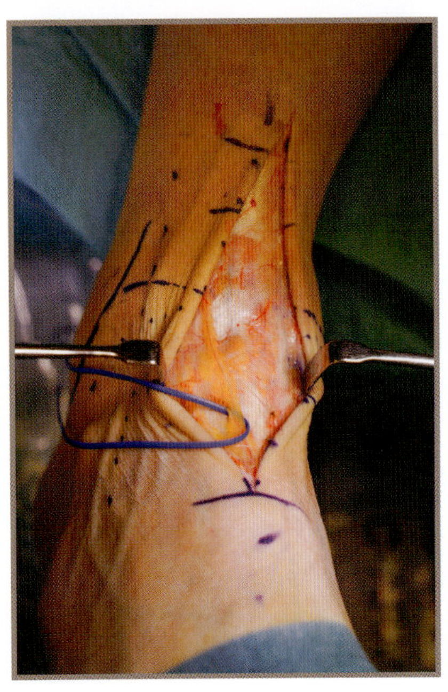

Figure 3. *Anterior approach to the ankle showing the medial branch of the superficial peroneal nerve identified with a coloured vascular loop for identification and retraction.*

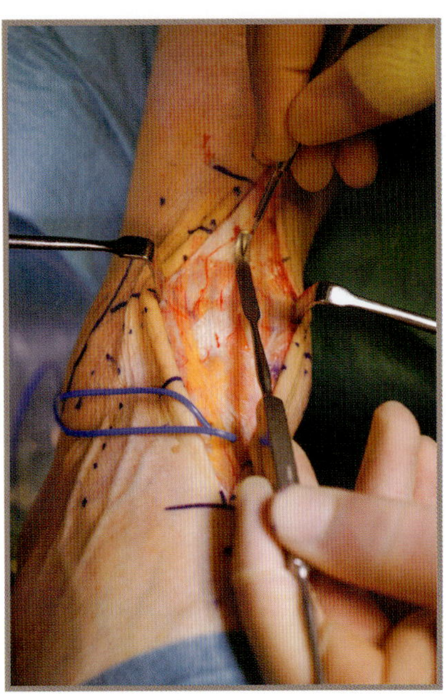

Figure 4. *A McDonald's elevator is placed inside the retinaculum to protect the tendon from the blade used for incision.*

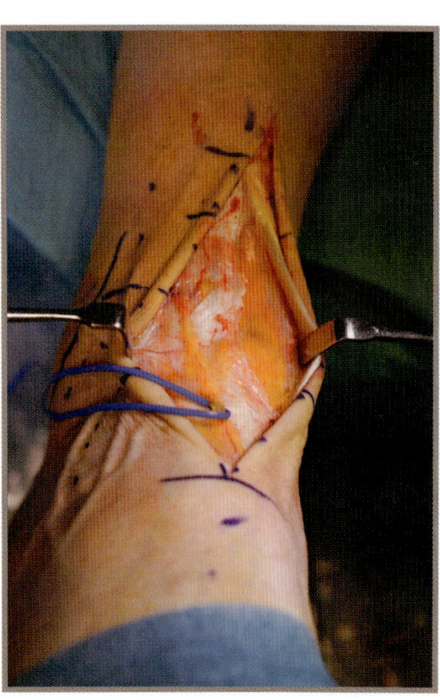

Figure 5. *The tibialis anterior tendon is retracted medially.*

the neurovascular bundle (anterior tibial artery and deep peroneal nerve) lateral and protected by the EHL. The extensor retinaculum is carefully incised using a blade and a McDonald elevator to protect the tibialis anterior tendon (Figure 4). The tendon is then retracted medially (Figure 5) and the capsule in the tendon bed is incised longitudinally (Figure 6) and elevated off the bone to gain good exposure from the medial to lateral gutters (Figure 7).

Surgical Technique

Details of surgical technique then vary with individual implants but the principles remain the same. Some implants start with the talus and some with the tibia. The crucial step is to ensure alignment in the sagittal and coronal planes and rotation in the axial plane. In

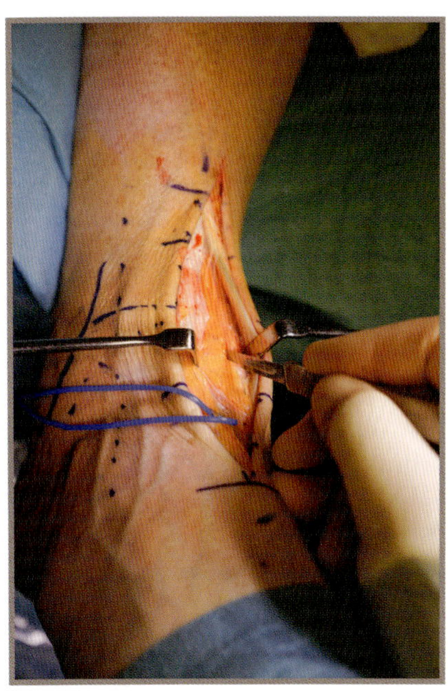

Figure 6. *The capsule in the base of the tibialis anterior tendon sheath is incised to access the anterior tibia.*

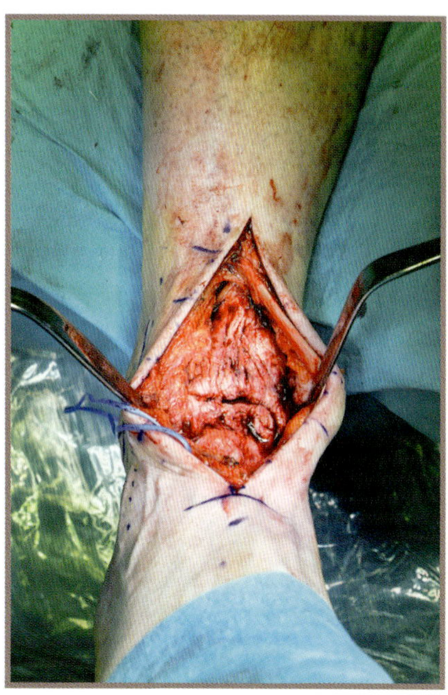

Figure 7. *Deep dissection through the capsule to expose the medial and lateral gutters of the tibiotalar joint.*

most fixed bearing implants, the setting of the first implant axial orientation dictates the rotation of the second. For example, if the tibia is positioned in internal rotation then the talus will also be internally rotated and medial impingement may result. In mobile bearing implants the two are disconnected but axial malalignment can lead to meniscal impingement on the gutters.

Soft tissues must be inspected. In varus malaligned cases, the medial structures will be tight and a medial release is likely to be required. This involves stripping the deltoid (both superficial and deep) from its tibial attachment so that the medial side can open. Remember that the deltoid has a broad attachment and this can be achieved with a blade or a periosteal elevator but remember that the neurovascular structures sit close postero-medially. In some cases a vertical sliding medial malleolar osteotomy or a flexor tendon z-lengthening is required.

Preliminary preparation by removal of anterior osteophytes allows accurate positioning of tibial or talar jigs. The tibia or talar flat cuts must be made to enable the correct alignment of the implant in the coronal plane. There are variations as to the exact angle the jigs will represent relative to the tibia and these are factored into the jig of each implant. Please reference the surgical technique of the implant you will be using.

Many surgeons excavate the medial and lateral gutters to remove a potential source of pain from impingement. This is a controversial area and some believe that gutter clearance is a proxy method for dealing with incorrect axial alignment of the implant components (Najefi *et al.*, 2019). If the gutters are being cleared, great care must be taken to protect the tendinous and neurovascular structures.

The tibial cut is made from front to back, coupled with a vertical cut medially and for some implants a vertical cut laterally. Care must be taken not to fracture or saw through the malleoli (and if fracture does occur it should be fixed immediately).

Depending upon the bone quality or the morphology of the medial malleolus, it may be prudent to prophylactically fix the malleolus prior to cutting the tibia. Also, care must be taken to protect the posterior structures — and here the positioning of the calf on an elevator with the foot dependent is a further safety factor. The tibial surface is then removed with care (the risk of medial malleolar fracture is 6% and lateral malleolar fracture is 1%; levering or toggling at the side of the fragments should be avoided).

Next, the talar superior surface is cut flat (note that in some designs the talus is cut first). It is important to note that when cutting the talus, the foot must be positioned exactly beneath the leg, and plantigrade with the foot at 90° to the tibia in all planes and the ligaments under physiological tension. Therefore, it is essential that any hindfoot deformity, whether by release or by osteotomy should be performed prior to this cut. The talar cut should be parallel to the floor (and the tibial cut) with a sufficient gap to allow implantation of the metal and plastic components.

A variety of secondary jigs are then used to prepare the rest of the tibia and talus to accept the implants, the technique of which differs with each implant. You should therefore, ensure you are fully trained on the prosthesis you have chosen to implant, but these steps usually involve a saw cut to the posterior chamfer as well as burrs or routers to prepare the anterior surface.

After preparation of the surfaces, trial implants are inserted and a check made of alignment. It is tempting to "overstuff" the joint by using too large a component, leading to an inability to dorsiflex the foot at this stage. This should be avoided.

Rotation of the implant must be assessed in relation to the transmalleolar axis and the tibial tuberosity. This can vary greatly between patients, and whereas some studies quote the mean to be around 20° of external tibial torsion, there can be variability of up to 80°. Medial impingement can occur due to the talus abutting against the medial malleolus on weightbearing. Some surgeons believe that gutter debridement is essential to prevent impingement, others believe that exposure of cancellous bone surfaces as opposed to the native articular surfaces is also contra-indicated. Ultimately, rotational alignment and the role of gutter clearance remains ill-understood and hence it is recommended that the surgeon thinks about rotation as much as coronal and sagittal alignment aiming to ensure appropriate dorsiflexion and plantarflexion without gutter impingement occurring.

A thorough lavage now takes place and surgical gloves are changed. The final components are now implanted and the range of movement and stability are once more checked. The wounds are then closed carefully in layers. Closure of the extensor retinaculum is essential to prevent bowstringing of tendons. The use of drains comes down to surgical preference, as does the form of immobilisation with either a cast or walker boot. The dressings should be well padded, and the foot must be in a neutral position.

Additional Procedures

The key to success of an ankle replacement is that there is a plantigrade balanced foot underneath it. This means that any hindfoot deformity or instability must be corrected.

Release of lateral osteophytes and removal of loose bodies should be performed and the lateral ligament tested. If there is lateral instability then this should be dealt with prior to closure. The options for stabilisation is either a direct Brostrom anatomical repair or the use of lateral tendon weaves, allograft reconstructions, or synthetic graft supports.

In cases of a cavovarus foot, where the heel is in significant varus (inversion at the subtalar joint) or the 1st ray is plantarflexed, then a heel shift and dorsiflexion osteotomy of the 1st ray must be considered, either in a staged procedure or at the same sitting as the replacement.

An Achilles tendon lengthening is required in about 15% of ankle replacements if an equinus persists after posterior release and no other cause can be identified.

Valgus ankles also require ligament balancing, although the deltoid rarely requires reconstruction. Medial displacement calcaneal osteotomies and tendon transfers may be required. In severe deformity with arthritic changes, a subtalar fusion, or a double or triple fusion may be required, again in a staged or combined procedure.

POSTOPERATIVE CARE

The principles of postoperative care and rehabilitation are of caring for the patient, their wound, and maximising outcome. During the postoperative period, high-risk patients (those with risk factors including previous embolic episodes, family history, overweight, and smokers) should receive appropriate prophylaxis against thromboembolism. Most hospitals will set down protocols and guidance in this regard and these should be adhered to. Invariably, this will include both chemical and mechanical modalities.

At the end of surgery, a cast is usually applied to maintain position and specifically not to allow the ankle to drift into equinus. The cast or splint should be split, or designed to allow for swelling.

There is wide variation in postoperative practice. Some surgeons practice day case surgery, whereas others keep their ankle replacements in for 3–5 days depending on co-morbidities. Some surgeons use drains routinely and others never. Some surgeons allow for out of cast motion to begin immediately, whereas others leave the wound undisturbed for 2 weeks prior to first inspection.

Weightbearing status again varies between surgeons and between cases. In most routine cases, where fixation appeared adequate and no soft tissue or additional bony surgery took place, then weightbearing can begin immediately in a cast or boot titrated to the patients pain levels.

In cases, where additional bony surgery or tendon surgery has occurred the surgeon may wish to keep the patient non-weightbearing for between 2 and 6 weeks.

Sutures or clips are removed at 10–14 days once the wound is dry. Immobilisation from there onwards is surgeon dependent based on wound healing and adjunct procedures, but most will mobilise weight bearing in a plaster or walker boot at 2 weeks. At 4-6 weeks after the surgery the patient can mobilise with a supramalleolar orthosis (SMO) during at risk activities.

Physiotherapy for proximal chain kinetics, and core stability can begin immediately (and be taught to the patient preoperatively) irrespective of the immobilisation of the ankle.

Conventional physiotherapy to the ankle; however, typically begins once the immobilisation is removed from the ankle. This should consist of a series of increasing intrinsic and extrinsic exercises, and range of movement work leading to a course of gait and proprioceptive reeducation.

It may take a year or longer before the final result of surgery is known. Some swelling and a need for support on rough and uneven ground may persist long term.

The Authors Preferred Protocol

We tend to use modern flexible casts with posterior reinforcement applied at the time of surgery, split and then retained throughout the postoperative period, reducing the need for cast changes (and cost). Whilst other groups have demonstrated the use of compression dressings and no casts we have found these to be labour intensive and only really work in the presence of good multidisciplinary support.

We do not tend to use intraoperative drains but have been trialling the use a negative pressure dressing applied at the end of surgery on the closed wound. This drains out any fluid that would otherwise seep out into the dressings through a continuous negative pressure of −125 mmHg for for 5 days before it is removed and a conventional dressing applied (Figures 8 and 9). The backslab is then reapplied to rest the wound until the 14 day point where the sutures are removed.

In simple cases, gentle movements of active and assisted dorsiflexion and inversion/eversion of the heel and rotation of the midfoot

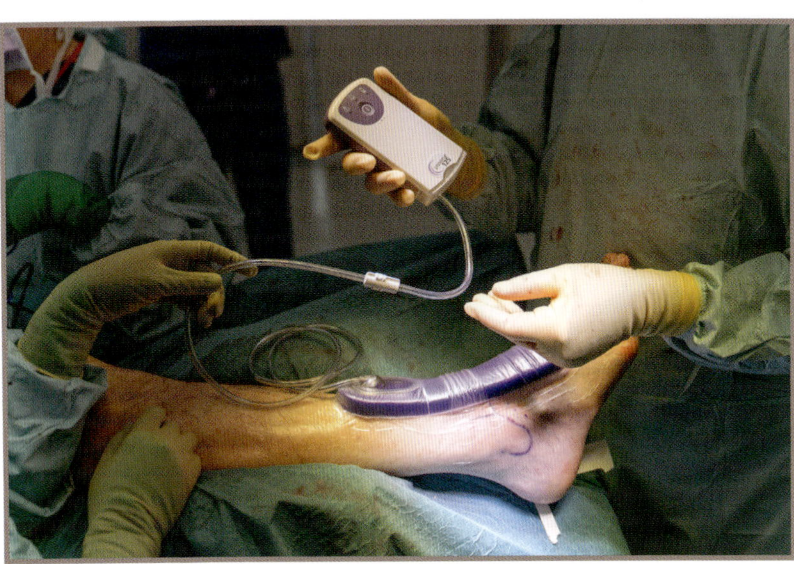

Figure 8. *The use of a PREVENA™ Incision Management System (3M, Saint Paul, Minnesota).*

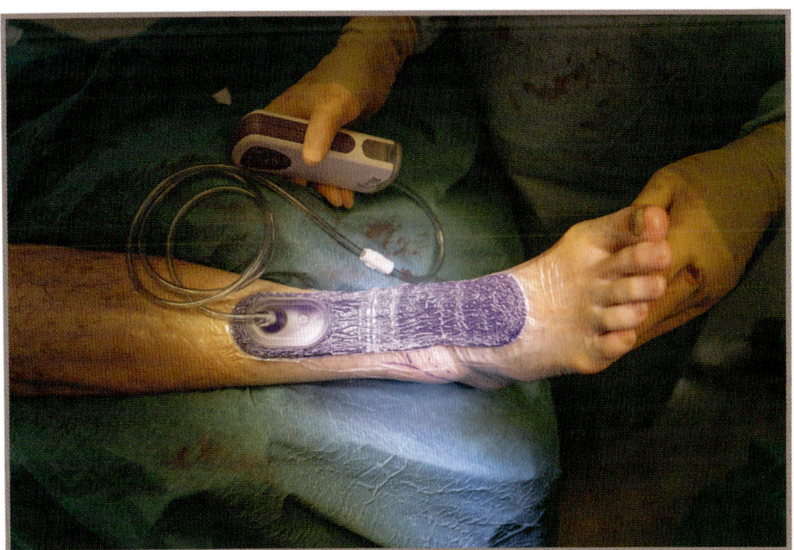

Figure 9. *Once the machine in Figure 8 is switched on the dressing is flat and then covered in a wool and plaster back-slab.*

(drawing circles with the foot) can be started at this point and a walker boot is applied for support during weight bearing for the first 6 weeks.

In cases where the fixation is in question or where other procedures have taken place, a cast may be continued for up to 6 weeks and weight bearing in the cast is dependent on those other surgeries. For example following a heel shift the patient is non weight bearing for 6 weeks.

All rehabilitation is a balance of keeping movement whilst ensuring optimum wound healing which is key to the success of the procedure.

The average stay in our institution is one night unless other co-morbidities and disabilities exist. The prerequisites for discharge are that the patient's pain is under control; and the patient is safe to manage at home.

REFERENCES

Greisberg, J., Hansen, S. T. & Digiovanni, C. 2004. Alignment and technique in total ankle arthroplasty. *Oper Tech Orthop*, 14(1), 21–30.

Moreland, J. R., Bassett, L. W., & Hanker, G. J. 1987. Radiographic analysis of the axial alignment of the lower extremity. *J Bone Joint Surg Am*, 69(5), 745–749.

Trajkovski, T., Pinsker, E., Cadden, A. & Daniels, T. 2013. Outcomes of ankle arthroplasty with preoperative coronal-plane varus deformity of 10° or greater. *J Bone Joint Surg Am,* 95(15), 1382–1388.

COMPLICATIONS IN TOTAL ANKLE REPLACEMENT

J. K. DeOrio and D. Latt

Summary

Ankle replacement surgery is one of the most fascinating, complicated, and satisfying operations we perform. Learning to achieve the best results while avoiding complications should be the goal of every surgeon performing ankle replacement. We hope that the information contained in this chapter that was gained through collective experience will help you in achieving this goal. Specifically, we will provide recommendations on techniques which will help you avoid and treat the complications of malalignment, fractures, infection, wound healing problems, component subsidence, heterotopic ossification, tendon and nerve injuries, stiffness, and impingement.

INTRODUCTION

Total ankle replacement (TAR) is a technically demanding procedure that has the potential to be associated with many complications. An unforeseen misadventure awaits the unsuspecting surgeon at every turn. It is only through rigorous attention to detail that one can hope to provide the patient with the benefits of pain relief and motion without encountering the complications that can lead to a suboptimal result. Recent literature has reported a plethora of complications. All of these potential complications, as well as some new ones, their presumed causes, and methods of avoidance will be discussed in this chapter. For the sake of clarity, the complications have been divided chronologically into intraoperative, early postoperative, and late postoperative.

INTRAOPERATIVE

The majority of complications occur either during operation or are a direct result of intraoperative decision making (DeOrio and Easley, 2008). A number of studies reported their intraoperative complications (Myerson and Mroczek, 2003; Wood *et al.*, 2008; Haskell and Mann, 2004; Lee *et al.*, 2008; Schuberth *et al.*, 2006; Schutte and Louwerens, 2008; Saltzman *et al.*, 2009). These studies represent 1124 arthroplasties. The intraoperative complications reported include: neurovascular or tendon injury, malleolar or distal tibia fracture, malleolar impingement, and malalignment or malpositioning of both the tibial and/or talar sides of the joint (Table 1).

Table 1. Intraoperative complications.

Complications are listed as a percentage of study population. Not all complications were discussed in all studies. Overall frequency was calculated by dividing the number of reported cases by the number of subjects in the studies that reported that complication. If a study did not report a complication, it was not included in the calculation.

Complication	Myerson (2003)	Haskell (2004)	Schuberth (2006)	Lee (2008)	Schutte (2008)	Wood (2008)	Saltzman (2009)	Total (no. cases)	Frequency (%)
Prosthesis	Agility	STAR	Agility	Hintegra	STAR	STAR	STAR		
Subjects	50	189	50	50	49	143	593	1124	
Injury to critical structures	4	5	0	5	1	—	—	15	2.9
Neurovascular	2	5	0	3	1	—	6	20	2.0
Tendon	2	—	0	2	0	—	—	4	2.7
Fracture (any)	—	—	—	—	—	—	—	—	11.2
Medial mal	6	—	13	—	6	—	—	25	16.8
Lateral mal	2	—	5	—	2	—	—	9	6.0
Unspecified mal	—	18	1	5	2	9	—	35	10.7
Distal tibia	—	—	—	—	3	—	—	3	6.1
Unspecified	—	—	—	—	—	—	13.5	72	13.5
Malleolar impingement	—	4	3	—	—	—		7	2.9
Malalignment/ Malposition								176	33.1
Tibial frontal	24	—	8	5	5	—		42	7.9
Tibial sagittal	16	—	—	2	9	58		85	16
Talus	25	—	—	7	12	—		44	8.3
Unspecified	—	5	—	—	—	—		5	0.9

Note: % of sample "—" indicates not reported.

Neurovascular and Tendon Injury

The reported incidence of significant neurovascular and tendon injury ranges from 2% to 9% (Lee *et al.*, 2008). This may represent reporting bias or injuries that were not clinically detected. In Table 1 you will note that we identified 20 patients with neurovascular injury and 4 patients with tendon injury which account for 2% and 2.7%, respectively, of cases in studies that reported these complications.

The superficial and deep peroneal nerves are at risk with the anterior approach to the ankle. Damage to these nerves can lead to painful neuromas, complex regional pain syndrome, or decreased sensation over the dorsum of the foot. The decrease or loss of sensation in the region of the navicular tuberosity, caused by stretching or transecting the sensory fibers of the medial branch of the superficial peroneal nerve as it crosses in front of the ankle, is quite common (approximately 20%), and is not considered to be a significant complication as it does not appear to affect either the patients perceived outcome or satisfaction with the procedure (Saltzman *et al.*, 2009).

The anterior neurovascular structures are best protected by careful dissection and retraction during approach to the ankle joint. The senior author (JKD), recommends identifying and then outlining the superficial peroneal nerve with a marker to prevent inadvertent transection (Figure 1). If it is inadvertently transected, it should be buried in a drill hole in bone to avoid the irritation that may occur in a more superficial location (Raikin and Myerson, 2006). The tibial nerve, the posterior tibial tendon and the flexor hallucis longus tendon (Figures 2 (a) and (b)) are at risk during resection of the tibial plafond. Injury is best avoided by angling the saw away from the posteromedial gutter and finishing the cuts with a reciprocating saw that allows the resected bone to be removed piecemeal under direct vision (Myerson and Mroczek, 2003). Additionally, the placement of a towel "bump" immediately behind the ankle should be avoided as this practice translates the tendon anteriorly into the vicinity of the saw blade when cutting the distal tibia. Moreover, caution should be exercised when using sharp osteotomes to remove bone posteriorly, for if they are placed too deeply they can injure the

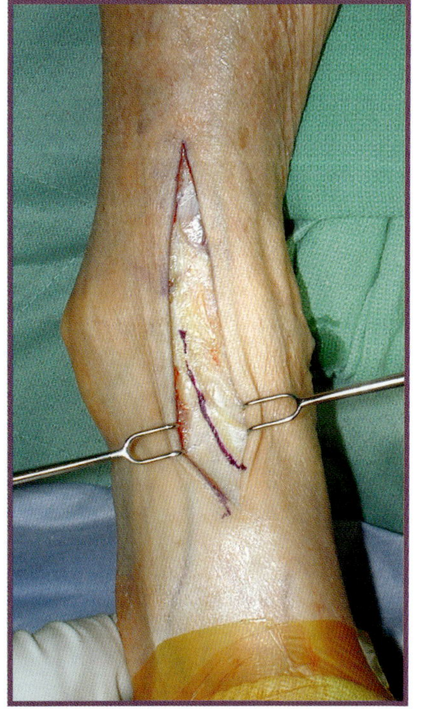

Figure 1. *Superficial peroneal nerve marked to alert the surgeon to its presence throughout the case.*

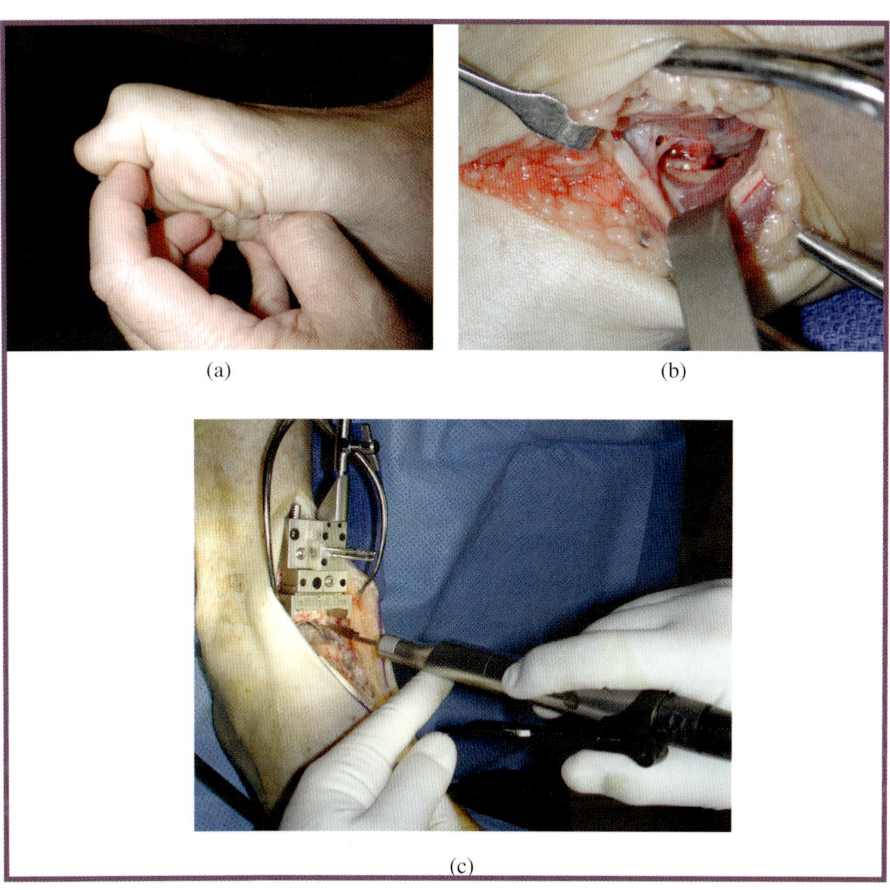

(a)   (b)

(c)

Figure 2. *(a) Flexor halucis longus entrapped 6 months after TAR. (b) This required subsequent intraoperative release. (c) Small reciprocating saw used to make fines cut in the bone to avoid soft tissue structures.*

posterior tibial nerve. It is better to use a reciprocating saw under direct vision, for it allows finer control with lower excursion. Figure 2 (c) shows how we approach posterior structures.

Fracture

Fractures discovered during surgery, or in the early postoperative period, are relatively common. They are reported to occur in 10–38%

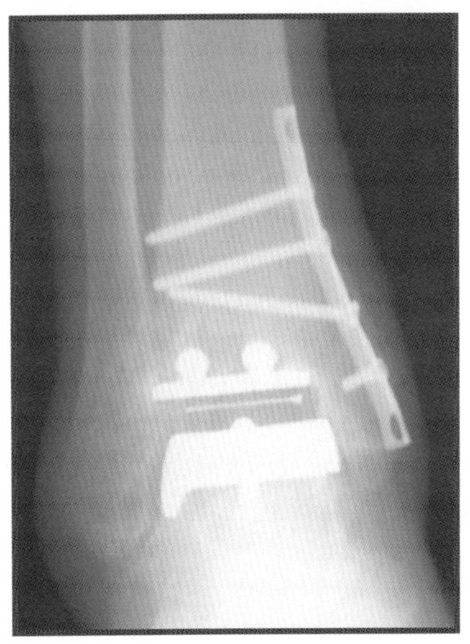

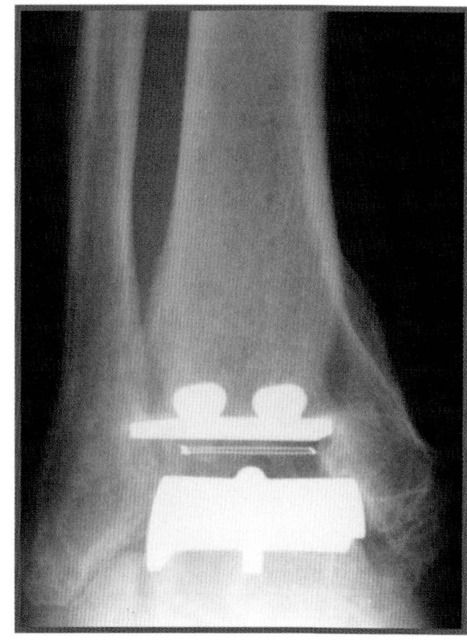

of cases (Lee *et al.*, 2008). In our analysis of the seven studies for this paper, in 1124 TARs, the occurrence of malleolar fracture was reported in 11.2% of the patients (Myerson and Mroczek, 2003; Wood *et al.*, 2008; Haskell and Mann, 2004; Lee *et al.*, 2008; Schuberth *et al.*, 2006; Schutte and Louwerens, 2008; Saltzman *et al.*, 2009). The malleoli are the most common sites of fracture with a reported occurrence of 20% in a study by McGarvey *et al.* (2004). Other studies have described lower rates of fracture in the range of 1–5% (Rippstein *et al.*, 2011; Borenstein *et al.*, 2018). Medial malleolar fractures are more common than lateral malleolar fractures with a respective incidence in 26% vs 10% in one study (Schuberth *et al.*, 2006). When they occur intraoperatively, they can be fixed with cannulated screws or a buttress plate (Figure 3). When they are the result of early weightbearing after surgery in weakened bone, the patient may have to be taken back to surgery for repair (Figures 4 (a)–(c)). Sometimes, they present as a stress fracture that occurs postoperatively which is barely noticed by the patient and will go on to heal spontaneously (Figure 5).

Figure 3. *Intraoperative fracture of the medial malleolus fixed with a buttress plate.*

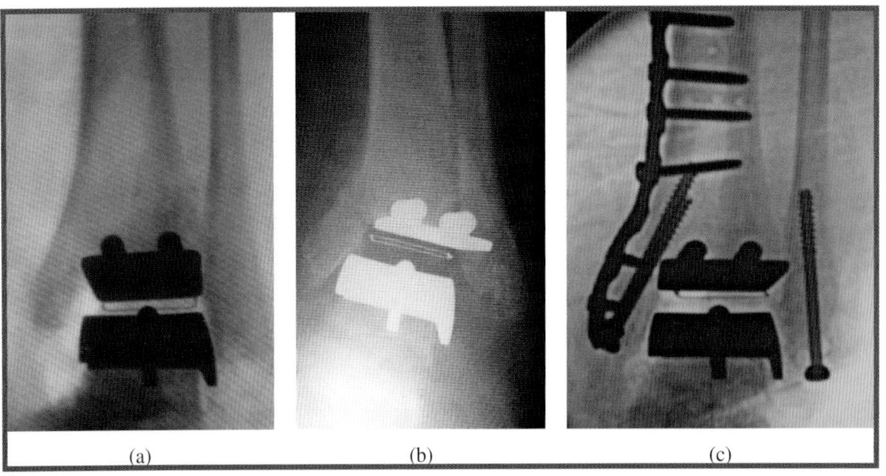

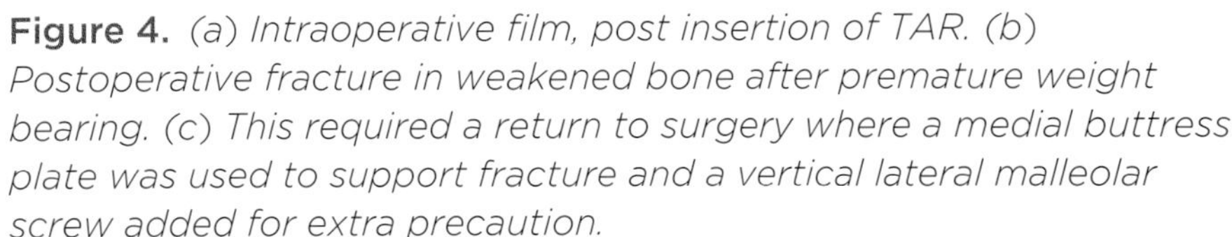

Figure 4. *(a) Intraoperative film, post insertion of TAR. (b) Postoperative fracture in weakened bone after premature weight bearing. (c) This required a return to surgery where a medial buttress plate was used to support fracture and a vertical lateral malleolar screw added for extra precaution.*

Figure 5. *Postoperative stress fracture in the medial malleolus (note callus formation) that went on to heal uneventfully.*

Tibial plafond fractures occur infrequently, with only three cases reported (Schutte and Louwerens, 2008). These fractures can occur when: (1) hardware is removed from the anterior distal tibia (leaving a stress riser) and excessive force is used to insert the prosthesis or (2) an incomplete cut of the posterior cortex of the tibia is made and an osteotome or chisel is used to complete the cut putting pressure on the uncut portion. In general, the incidence of fractures was found to decrease with increasing surgeon experience (Myerson and Mroczek, 2003; Saltzman *et al.*, 2003; Wood *et al.*, 2008; Lee *et al.*, 2008); however, one study by Haskell and Mann (2004) found no difference with increasing experience. In a systematic review carried out by Zaidi *et al.* (2016) of 7942 patients, the incidence of intraoperative medial malleolar fracture was 6% (95%, CI 3.5–9%).

Malleolar fractures are often related to the limited space between the malleoli available for placement of the prosthesis. There is some variability in the shape of the distal tibia and this affects the width of plafond that may be safely resected. Specifically, a distal tibia with a high metaphyseal flare is at greater risk of medial malleolar fracture, because with this morphology, the vertical limb of the tibial resection produces a thin bridge of bone connecting the medial malleolus to the metaphysis. Awareness of such anatomical variations during preoperative planning can help to prevent these fractures.

Another situation with increased risk of medial malleolar fracture is the valgus ankle in which the medial malleolus has been chronically unstressed owing to the deformity and has become osteopenic. In either of these situations, one should have a low threshold to place a prophylactic pin or a cannulated screw to support the bone (Figure 6). Both medial and lateral malleolar fracture can be due to size mismatches between the tibia and the talus as most prosthesis designs require the tibial component to be the same or larger than the talar component. The temptation to test dorsiflexion without the trial components in place should be avoided. As the ankle is dorsiflexed, the wider anterior talus comes into contact with the unprotected malleolus and can cause malleolar fracture. Additionally, it may be preferable to perform Achilles tendon or gastrocnemius releases prior to bone resection, as the ankle must be forcibly

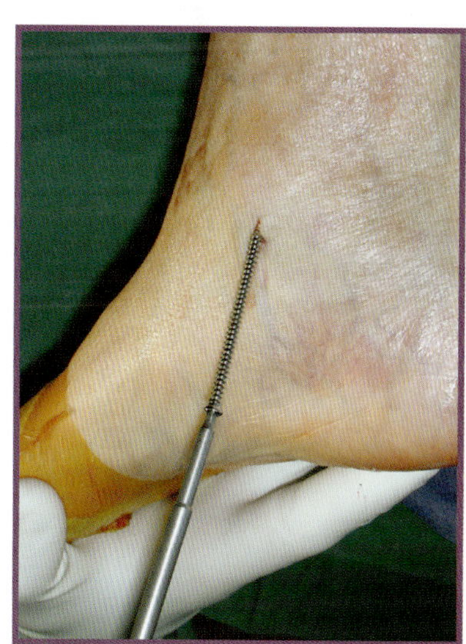

Figure 6. *Intraoperative medial malleolar screw fixation prior to beginning case to reinforce weak medial malleolar bone.*

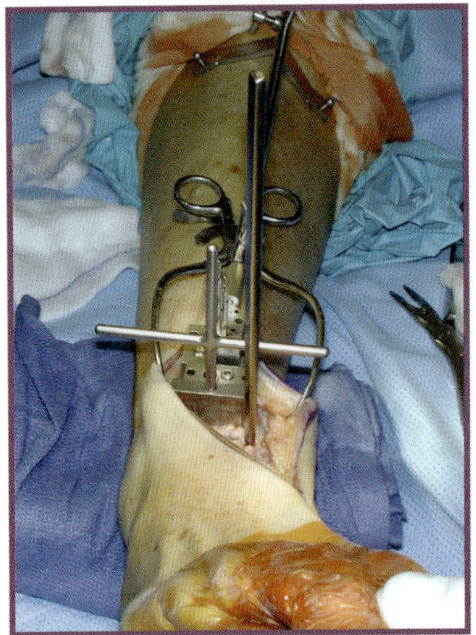

Figure 7. *Alignment of cutting jig parallel with narrow osteotome placed in medial gutter to aid assessment of component axial rotation.*

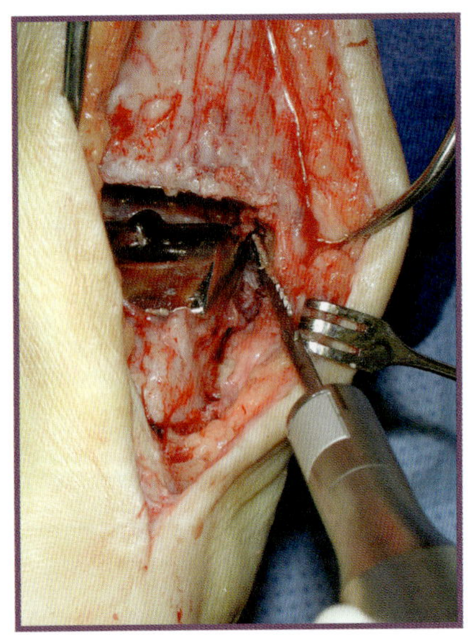

Figure 8. *A fine reciprocating saw used to cut bone in lieu of using osteotomes which can fracture malleoli.*

dorsiflexed during these procedures, putting the malleoli at risk if done after bone resection.

Another cause of malleolar fracture is malrotation of the cutting guide which leads to a resection of a disproportionate posterior portion of the medial or lateral malleolus during the distal tibia cut, thereby weakening it. The fracture usually occurs at times of increased stress on the malleolus such as during component impaction, polyethylene insertion, or forced dorsiflexion (as described above). This problem is best avoided by checking cutting jig alignment with a thin osteotome placed in the medial gutter (Figure 7). Incorrect placement of cutting guides (placed too medially or too proximally) and horizontal overcutting (which creates a cortical stress riser) are also frequent sources of malleolar fracture (Conti and Wong, 2001; Myerson and Mroczek, 2003; Saltzman *et al.*, 2003). Finally, and this cannot be overemphasized, the osteotomes and mallet should be used very sparingly. Small saws are greatly preferred for bone removal because their position can be finely controlled. The senior author uses three saws for TAR surgery; a large 1 cm blade for cutting the distal tibia, a thin oscillating saw for finer transverse cuts, and a fine 3 cm by 0.5 mm reciprocating saw for removal of bone in tight spaces (Figure 8).

Medial malleolar fractures are best fixed with either two parallel screws or a buttress plate (Figure 4). Lateral malleolar fractures sometimes require a one-third tubular plate, but even here cannulated screws put the wound in less jeopardy and with 6 weeks of casting, often heal without a problem. Regardless of the type of fixation, these should be treated with additional time in cast, usually six weeks. The risk of malleolar fractures can be reduced by: (1) preoperative planning, including templating, to ensure appropriate component sizing (for small ankles, a number of orthopedic companies now include talar extra small sizes, e.g. STAR), (2) placement of temporary prophylactic malleolar screws or pins during surgery, (3) careful sizing of the prosthesis during surgery and (4) attention to detail in the determination of the medial — lateral positioning and rotational alignment of the cutting jigs.

Distal tibia fractures may also be caused by excessive tibial resection. The stiffness of the distal tibial trabecular bone decreases rapidly proximal to the subchondral plate (Hvid *et al.*, 1985, Aitken *et al.*, 1985). Over-resection of the distal tibia places the tibial component on weak metaphyseal bone, which is unable to support the load placed across it, leading to fracture. Likewise, placement of an excessively small tibial component, one that lacks cortical support, may lead to similar problems with subsidence or fracture. Tibial over-resection can be prevented by first distracting the joint space prior to pinning the cutting jig and then assessing how far above the apex of the tibial plafond the saw cut will be made. It is also necessary to be aware of weakened anterior tibial bone that may be present with osteoporosis or infarction (Figures 9 (a)–(d)). In these cases, an intramedullary stem on the tibial component may be beneficial. Finally, when making the tibial cut, if there is too much anterior opening, the saw blade will be cutting further above the tibial plafond than desired, which can lead to the fracture of this weaker bone. The senior author (JKD) now cuts all tibiae at 90° in all prostheses to avoid inadvertent excessive anterior slope.

Malleolar Impingement

Malleolar impingement has been reported in the literature with a frequency between 2–6% (Haskell and Mann, 2004; Schuberth *et al.*, 2006; Overley and Beideman, 2015). Impingement is either caused by a size or shape mismatch between the resurfaced talus and the remodelled mortice or by axial malrotation of the components.

Its presentation is usually delayed until the patient has regained some range of motion (ROM). The complaint is usually one of a sharp pain in the region of the anterior portion of the medial malleolus that occurs with dorsiflexion. However, it can also appear laterally, especially if the patient is small (Figure 10). If the symptoms do not abate in a reasonable time period, it may be necessary to debride the gutters or trim the malleolus. This can be accomplished with either an arthroscopic or an open procedure.

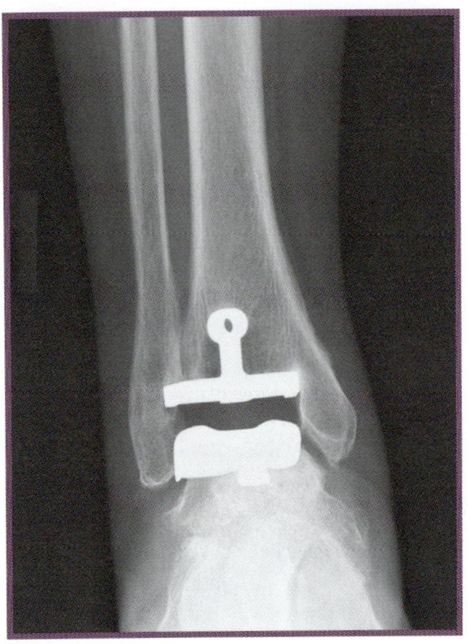

Figure 10. *Patient was very small and even the smallest size in this Salto-Talaris ankle did not allow much space in the lateral gutter. She subsequently underwent arthroscopic lateral gutter resection leading to relief of her symptoms.*

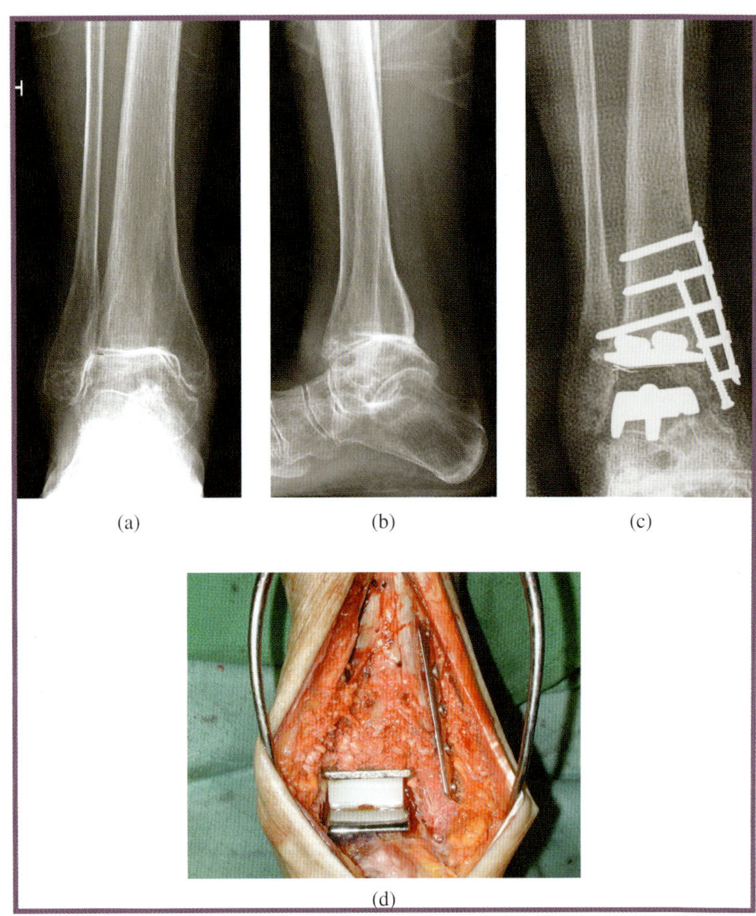

Figure 9. *(a) X-rays from an osteoporotic elderly patient where a delineation between normal and osteopenic bone can be clearly seen on the medial side. (b) A large lip of bone at the anterior tibia was removed, leading to the placement of the prosthesis on the softer metaphyseal bone. (c,d) This resulted in a medial malleolar fracture (despite prophylactic screw) and necessitated a buttress plate for support.*

Impingement can be prevented by careful attention to sizing, medial–lateral positioning, and rotational alignment of the talar component as well as a through intraoperative debridement of the gutters. Sometimes, despite the best sizing, the malleolar component will still abut the malleolus and the bone needs to be trimmed. Sometimes it is the overhang of the prosthesis that will impinge

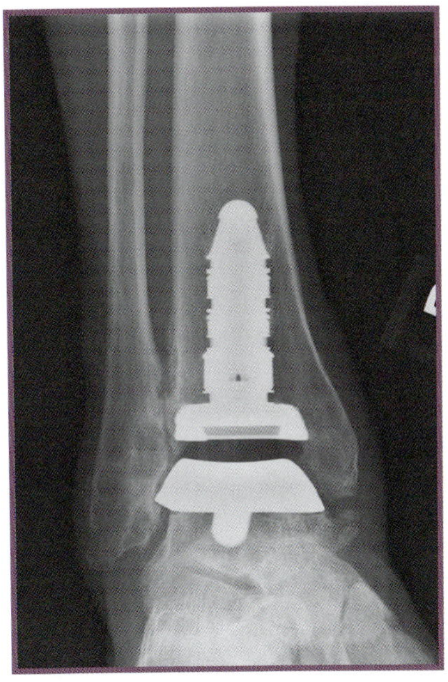

Figure 11. *Here the edge of the talar component is clearly digging into the lateral malleolus.*

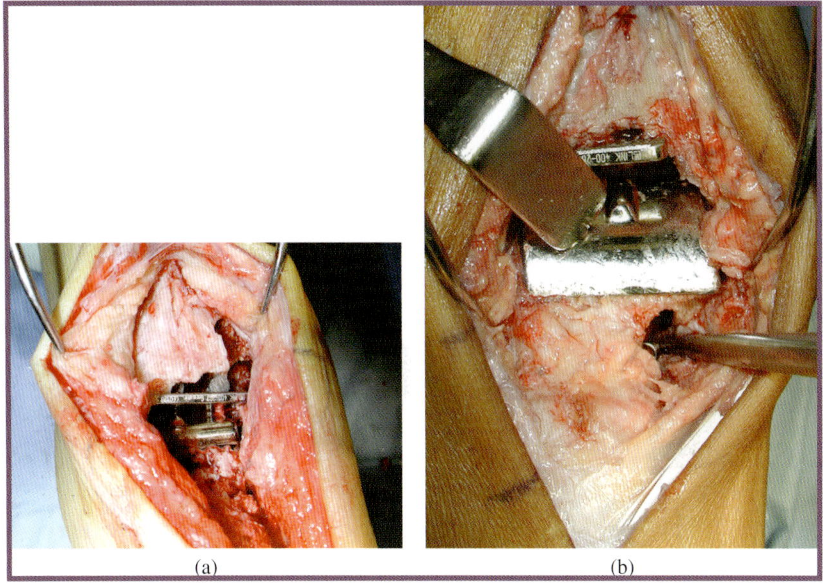

Figure 12. *(a) Osteolysis appearing above the tibial component of a STAR ankle secondary to polyethylene wear without fracture of the polyethylene. (b) Similar cysts were also found below the talar component.*

upon the bone (Figure 11). Taking the time to clean the gutters with a 4 mm wide rongeur will minimize this complication.

Tibial Component Malalignment

Malalignment or malpositioning of the components is the most common problem encountered in ankle replacement. In the six studies reviewed, it occurred in 33% of cases overall, though it ranged widely, from 3% in one study (Haskell and Mann, 2004) to 48% in another (Myerson and Mroczek, 2003). The malaligned or malpositioned prosthesis can lead to decreased ROM, chronic pain (Pyevich *et al.*, 1998), and ankle replacement failure. Failure occurs via a number of progressive problems (Haskell and Mann, 2004), such as excessive polyethylene wear leading to osteolysis (Figures 12 (a) and (b)), component loosening, and polyethylene failure (Figure 13). Malalignment or malpositioning can occur in the frontal, sagittal and coronal planes.

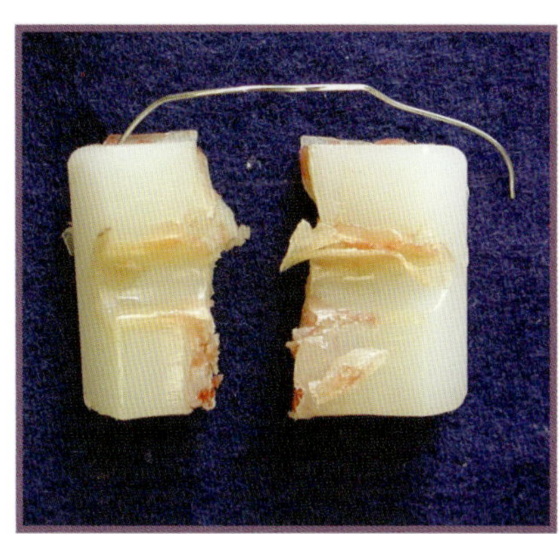

Figure 13. *Fracture of polyethylene component in STAR ankle. Note transverse fracture not in line with the groove.*

Frontal Plane Alignment

Obtaining neutral frontal plane alignment is crucial to the success of the prosthesis. Unfortunately, it is also one of the most difficult things to get right in this procedure. There are a number of preoperative factors that influence the final alignment. The relationship between them is complex and must be thoroughly understood.

Preoperative varus often results from longstanding lateral ligament instability. The incompetent lateral ligaments allow the talus to roll into varus, which then leads to medial chondral overload and subsequent medial sided osteoarthrosis. The degenerative process leads to the formation of osteophytes and contracture of the joint capsule. Thus, the lateral instability may not be initially apparent at the time of surgery. The key to obtaining neutral alignment is soft tissue balancing prior to making the bony cuts. This often requires a complete medial release. The senior author's (JKD) preferred technique is the medial deltoid peel from the tibia (Bonnin *et al.*, 2004). In the procedure, the periosteal tissue and deltoid ligament are sharply incised from the tibia creating a lax sleeve of tissue. The deltoid ligament should not be cut. The technique is analogous to the release of the superficial and sometimes deep medial collateral ligaments performed during arthroplasty of a knee with a varus deformity (Figures 14 (a) and (b)). The author's experience with this technique includes hundreds of cases, with no cases of iatrogenic medial instability. This release of the tethering structures is essential to achieve soft tissue balance.

Preoperative valgus may result from longstanding syndesmotic widening (Figures 15 (a) and (b)) due to unrecognised or untreated syndesmotic injury, or deltoid ligament insufficiency, or fibular malunion (shortened or angulated). It is not known whether restoration of syndesmotic stability is important for stability or wear of the prosthetic ankle.

The key to preventing tibial component malalignment is the use of a full sized image intensifier. The position of the alignment rod in both planes must be carefully scrutinised prior to the placement of

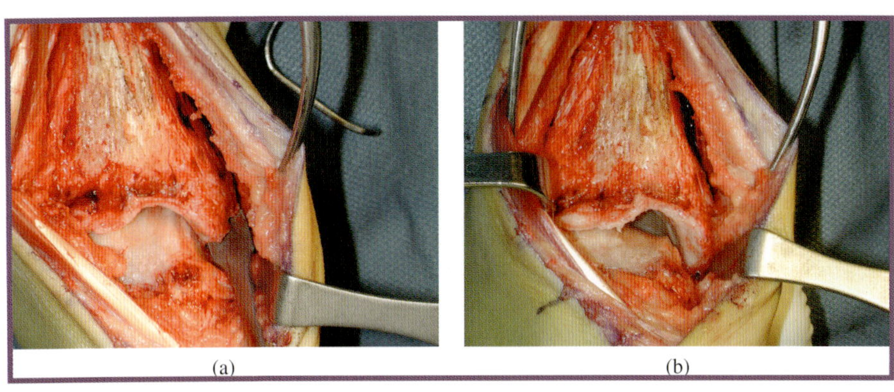

Figure 14. *(a) Varus ankle with invagination of talus into medial tibia. (b) Release of the deltoid ligament from tibia and medial malleolus allows talus to be lifted out of varus.*

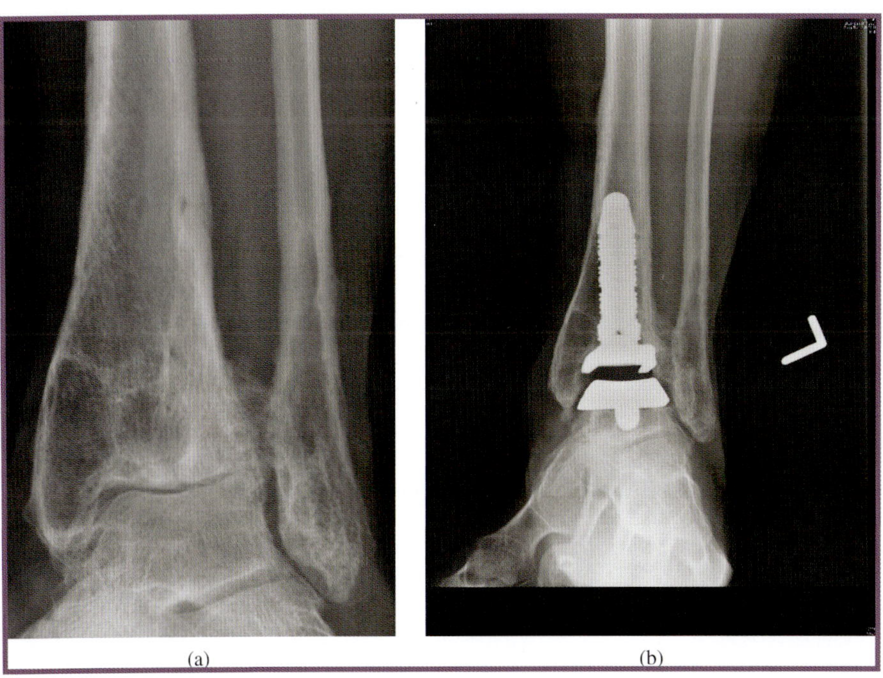

Figure 15. *(a) Preoperative radiograph showing a widened syndesmosis following a Weber C ankle fracture. (b) Postoperative radiograph demonstrates no malalignment.*

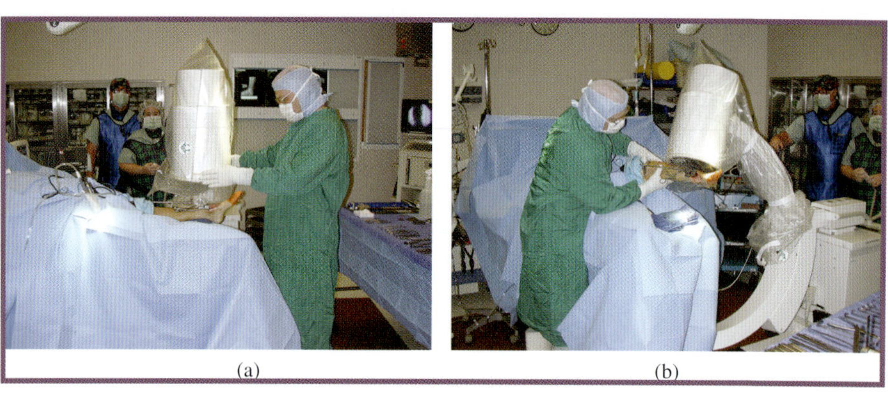

(a)   (b)

Figure 16. *Proper alignment of the cutting jig is established with anteroposterior (a) and lateral (b) fluoroscopic imaging.*

the final fixation pins for the tibial resection guide (Figures 16 (a) and (b)). In contrast, talar component malalignment is prevented by the liberal use of soft tissue balancing. When significant tibial bowing is present, it must be noted preoperatively, as the overall limb alignment is often difficult to assess once the limb is draped. Surgeon experience may play a role in avoiding frontal plane malalignment as an appreciation of the overall tibial axis is gained with experience (Schuberth *et al.*, 2006). However, operating without a large fluoroscope leaves even the most experienced ankle surgeon looking at a very small portion of anatomy to evaluate alignment. Hence, we always use a full sized fluoroscope.

Sagittal Plane Alignment

Sagittal plane alignment is less critical than coronal plane alignment. However, over resection of the anterior tibial cortex places the tibial component on softer bone and can result in component collapse. The senior author recommends a perpendicular cut on the tibia. That way if slight anterior opening occurs, it usually is of no consequence. On the other hand, if one aims for 7° but hits 10°, the talar prosthesis will place increased stress on the anterior tibia, which can then fail. Furthermore, with mobile bearing prostheses,

the insert can move forward when there is too great a slope leading to anteriodorsal polyethylene wear. If one errs by placing a reverse slope on the tibia, the same thing can happen in reverse or the patient may have difficulty getting appropriate dorsiflexion after the surgery. The original tibial resection guide for the STAR ankle utilised a "V"-shaped proximal guide that rested on the proximal tibia. This device did not allow precise control over the flexion extension angle and thus led to a number of coronal plane deformities. The device has since been modified to allow it to be secured to the tibia with a proximal pin placed just below the tibial tubercle. It is the senior author's belief that had the fixed proximal jig been used from the beginning of STAR implantation, many of the coronal plane deformities could have been significantly reduced. This fixed pin is now common practice with many of the jig systems.

Transverse Displacement

Even more unusual, but still possible, is insertion of the tibial component in too lateral or too medial a position. In a large patient, the STAR component, which only comes in 30, 32, 32.5 and 33 mm, may not adequately fill the tibial cut space from side to side (Figure 17). In this situation, it is critical to center the tibial component over the talus and to ensure that there is no instability. Failure to do so will produce a situation in which the polyethylene component can override the metal base plate. The key to preventing this complication is to "measure twice and cut once."

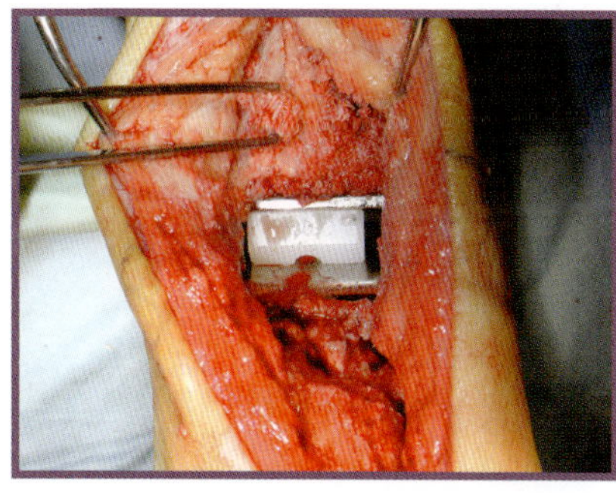

Figure 17. *The cysts in the tibia from Figure 12 have been filled with allograft. However, note the polyethylene still glides over the lateral tibial prosthesis edge because the ankle is so wide.*

Joint Line Malpositioning

The choice of tibial resection level is influenced by a number of factors. Resection of too much distal tibia places the prosthesis on the softer metaphyseal bone, which can lead to tibial component subsidence or tibial fracture. Also, the greater the tibial resection, the narrower the bone bridge connecting the medial malleolus leading to an increased risk of fracture. Moreover, higher resection levels produce a smaller distal tibial surface. This necessitates the use of a

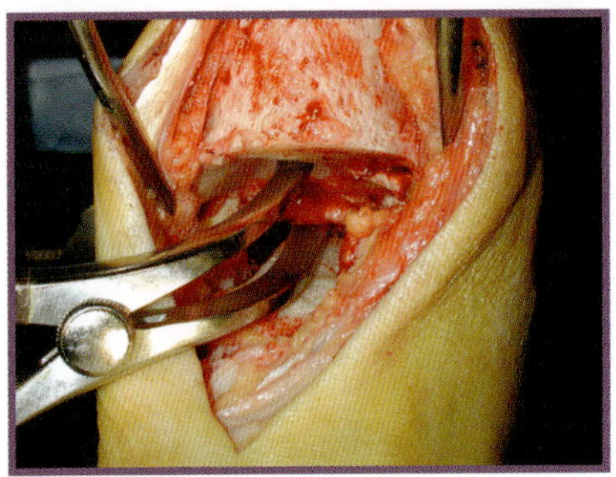

Figure 18. *Smooth lamina spreaders used to open up ankle joint to make visualization better and to ensure a balanced ankle.*

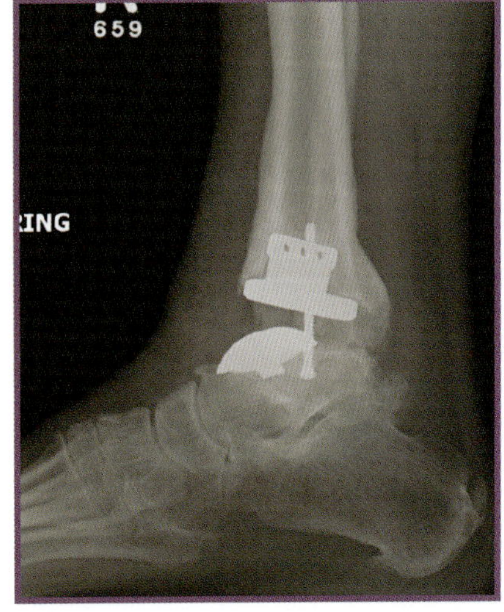

Figure 19. *This patient's foot was brought into too much dorsiflexion when the talus was cut for this Salto Talaris TAR. This places the component anteriorly and in flexion.*

smaller base plate to avoid mediolateral impingement or overhang. On the other hand, under resection leads to either overstuffing the joint (leading to decreased ROM) or over resecting on the talar side (which can lead to talar subsidence). Furthermore, too little resection of bone leaves the cuts in hard sclerotic bone, which may not have the capacity to ingrow onto the prosthesis. Finally, when there has been severe erosion of bone on one side or the other, it is occasionally necessary to resect only to the level of the more deficient side and the full thickness on the other side. Failure to recognise this will result in over resection of the bone. The key to choosing an appropriate joint line is obtaining ligament distraction and balancing prior to pinning the resection jig. This is often accomplished with the use of laminar spreaders (Figure 18) and soft tissue release when necessary.

Talar Component Malpositioning

Similarly, malresection of bone can be accomplished on the talus. Malalignment most often occurs when the talar cut is made with a tibia fixed jig and the foot is not maintained at 90° relative to the tibia. If the foot is plantar flexed, the posterior talus will be cut and the prosthesis will be placed posteriorly and in relative dorsiflexion. If the foot is over dorsiflexed, the anterior portion of the talus will be cut and the resting place for the talus will be anterior and in relative plantar flexion (Figure 19). This relationship is counterintuitive, but understanding this concept will save many ankles from having the talus placed anteriorly, which wears out the polyethylene prematurely from riding on the anterior tibia. Likewise, resecting too much or too little bone on either side of the talus or malpositioning talar fins will lead to incorrect medial–lateral placement of the talar component, which can lead to impingement.

POSTOPERATIVE: EARLY

Deep Vein Thrombosis

Deep vein thrombosis (DVT) has been reported infrequently in association with TAR (Rippstein *et al.*, 2012). Haskell and Mann (2004) reported two cases in their series of 189 patients (Table 2). Knect *et al.* (2004) reported on one case of DVT in their series of 132 patients. In another review of 664 ankle replacements in 637 patients, the DVT rate was 0.45% and the pulmonary embolism (PE) rate 0.15% (Horne *et al.*, 2015). In this group of patients, only those with a prior history of a thromboembolic event or coagulopathy received chemoprophylaxis and there was no significant correlation between risk factors and thromboembolic events. Zaidi *et al.* (2016) recently reported that the incidence of PE within 90 days following primary TAR was 0.51% (95% CI 0.23–1.13) based on over 1000 cases in the UK National Joint Registry. In this study it was found that

Table 2. Early postoperative complications.

Study	Prosthesis	*n*	DVT	Delayed wound healing	Wound dehiscence	Superficial infection	Deep infection	Fracture
Pyevitch (1998)	Agility	86	—	—	—	2	0	—
Myerson (2003)	Agility	50	—	—	2	0	0	—
Haskell (2004)	STAR	189	2	36	—	31	5	4
Henricsson (2007)	mixed	531	—	—	—	—	13	—
Hosman (2007)	Mixed	202	—	—	—	5	1	—
Nelissen (2006)	BP	15	—	—	—	1	—	2
Schuberth (2006)	Agility	50	—	9	1	—	—	—
Lee (2008)	Hintegra	50	—	—	—	6	1	—
Schutte (2008)	STAR	49	—	2	—	—	1	—
Wood (2008)	STAR	143	—	5	5	—	—	10
Saltzman (2009)	STAR	593	—	21	—	—	5	—
Total		1365	2	52	8	45	21	16

Note: % of sample, "—" indicates not reported.

patients with comorbid conditions (Charleston score > 0) were 13 times more likely to develop PE ($p = 0.003$). There were no fatal PE's but the majority of patients received some form of chemical prophylaxis against DVT. Because of reporting methods, however, this study could make no comment on the incidence of DVT.

Despite this very low occurrence rate, the current medicolegal climate necessitates some form of prophylaxis for every patient. At the senior author's institution, every patient receives low dose aspirin and patients at high risk (history of deep venous thrombosis, pulmonary embolism,hypercoagulable state, or oral contraceptive use) receive low molecular weight heparin. The senior author (JKD) also strongly recommends the use of mechanical prophylaxis in all patients. The patient is advised postoperatively to, "Get up once an hour during the day and keep your toes above your nose the rest of the time."

WOUND PROBLEMS

Delayed wound healing, wound dehiscence, superficial and deep infection, are of grave concern around ankle replacements. Indeed, postoperative wound problems are one of the most common complications following TAR, yet many are avoidable. They are due to a number of factors:

(1) The anterior incision splits the anterior tibial angiosome (Attinger *et al.*, 2001) which may lead to devascularisation of one or the other wound edge (Gill, 2004).

(2) The ankle joint and periarticular structures have limited soft tissue covering.

(3) The extensor tendons (particularly the tibialis anterior) have a tendency to bowstring following incision of the extensor retinaculum, which may put pressure on the healing incision from the inside.

Wound problems vary greatly in their severity. They range along a continuum that includes wound erythema, delayed healing with skin necrosis and eschar formation wound dehiscence with exposed tendon (Figure 20), superficial infection, and deep infection. The minor wound complications (erythema, delayed healing, superficial infection) are reported to occur at a rate of 0–19% when using an anterior approach to the ankle (Saltzman *et al.*, 2003; Hintermann and Valderrabano, 2003; Haskell and Mann, 2004; Knecht *et al.*, 2004; Lee *et al.*, 2008; Myerson and Mroczek, 2003; Schuberth *et al.*, 2006; Schutte and Louwerens, 2008; Wood, 2002). Fortunately, major wound complications (deep infection, tissue loss, septic arthritis) are less common, occurring at a reported rate of up to 3% (Saltzman *et al.*, 2003; Haskell and Mann, 2004; Henricson *et al.*, 2007; Hosman *et al.*, 2007; Lee *et al.*, 2008; Myerson and Mroczek, 2003; Pyevich *et al.*, 1998; Schutte and Louwerens, 2008; Valderrabano *et al.*, 2004; Wood, 2002).

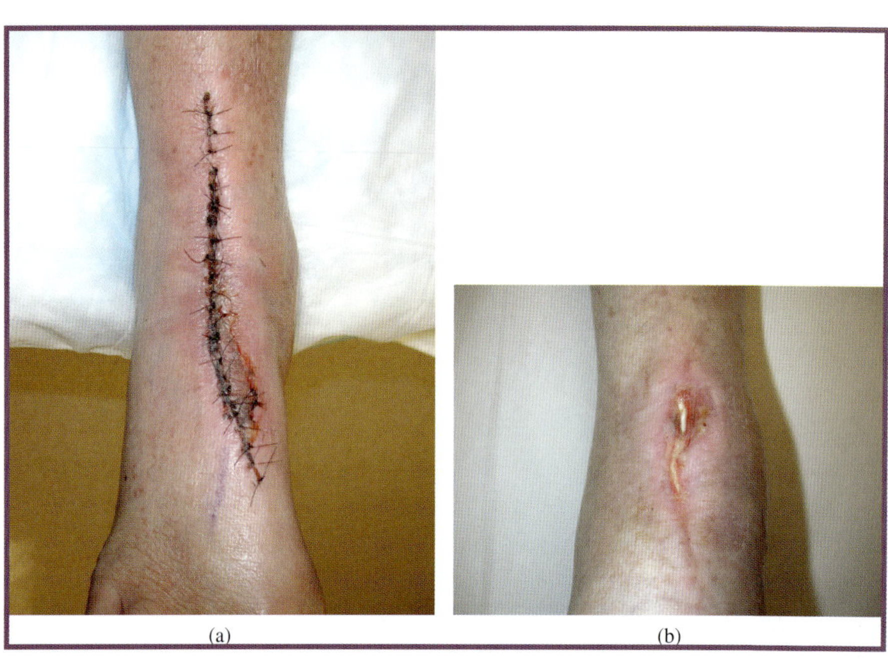

(a)   (b)

Figure 20. *(a) Wound that is mildly erythematous with eschar formation and superficial skin necrosis. (b) Slow wound healing with anterior tibial tendon showing through skin.*

Treatment

Minor wound complications can frequently be treated conservatively with a combination of wound care, immobilisation, and antibiotics. Epidermolysis or wound dehiscence involving up to 1 cm of skin can be treated with immobilisation with or without antibiotics. However, when there is exposed tendon, debridement should be combined with either vacuum-assisted closure (Wound VAC), retinaculum transfer (Figures 21 (a)–(c)), rotation flap coverage (Figures 22 (a) and (b)) or free tissue transfer (Figure 23). Major wound breakdown should be treated like a deep infection.

Deep infections, (those that violate the extensor retinaculum), require early aggressive treatment. Open debridement with appropriate component exchange followed by antibiotics is the treatment

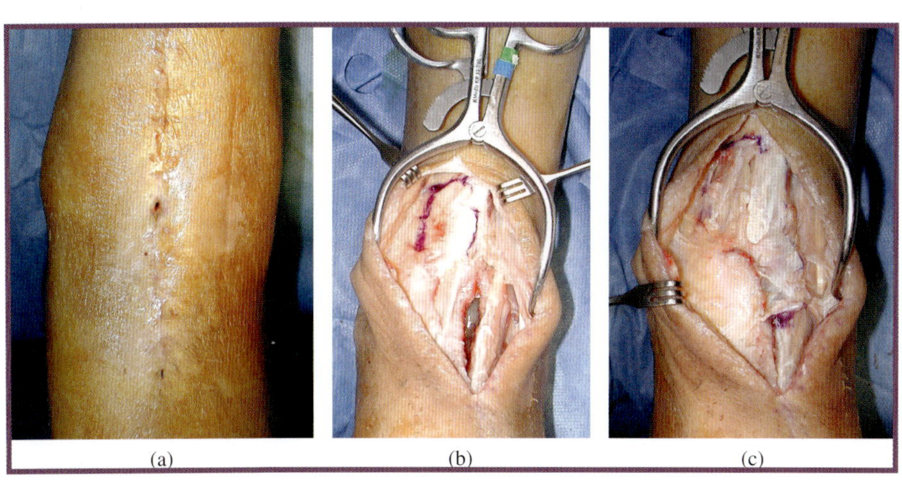

Figure 21. *(a) Patient with a small wound opening anteriorly which was draining purulent material. (b) The infection was found to be limited to the superficial tissues. The retinaculum was outlined above the defect. (c) The infection tract was debrided and irrigated, the retinaculum was turned down to seal the wound, and the skin was closed. Gelpi or other deep retractors may be used to prevent repeatedly retracting the skin edges, thus creating vascular channel blockers which interfere with skin healing.*

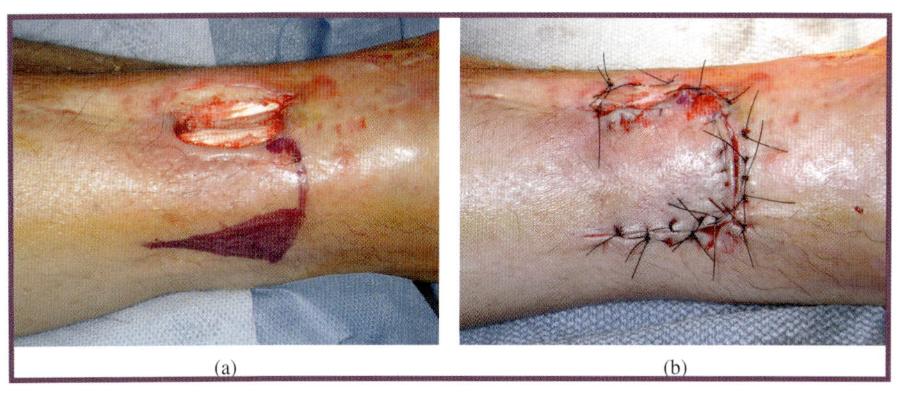

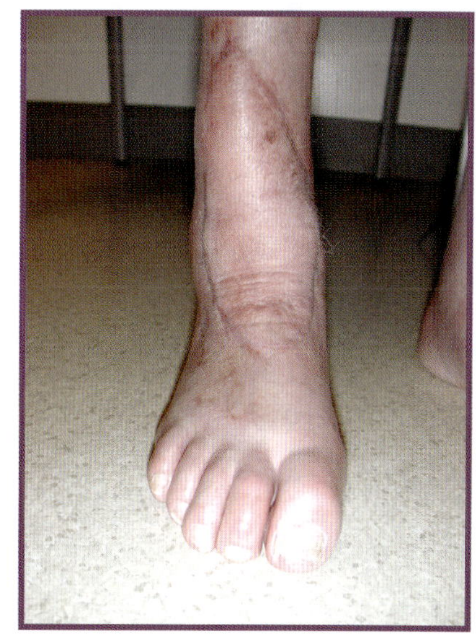

Figure 22. *(a) Wound with extensor tendons showing. Lateral flap outlined with darkened area representing possible are for skin graft. (b) Flap rotated into wound. With lateral freeing up of tissue, the flap was able to be closed laterally.*

Figure 23. *Larger wound necessitated forearm free flap with good result.*

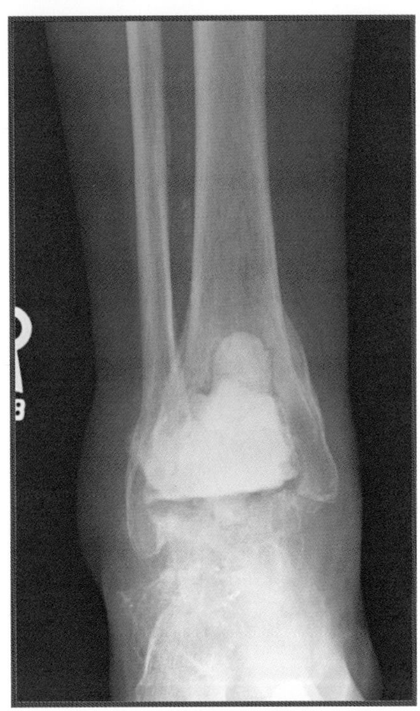

Figure 24. *X-ray of ankle showing removal of the prosthesis and antibiotic spacer in place.*

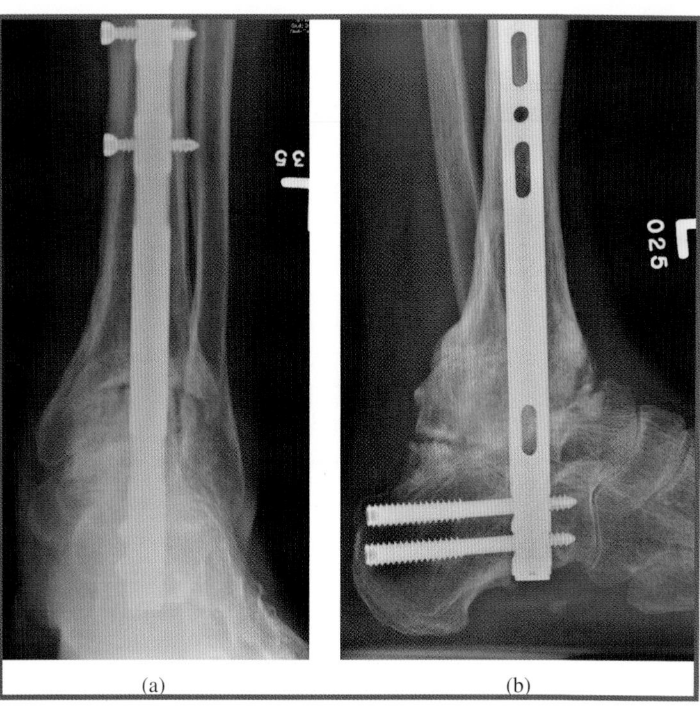

(a)　　　　　　　(b)

Figure 25. *(a) and (b) Post infection removal of implant 1-year postoperative and insertion of tibiotalocalcaneal nail for ankle and subtalar fusion. A femoral head was used to maintain length.*

of choice for a deep infection treated acutely (<6 weeks). More established infections necessitate a more aggressive approach that consists of component removal, placement of an antibiotic spacer block (Figure 24), and 6 weeks of intravenous antibiotics. Often, because the prosthesis is not yet fixed to the bone, it can be easily removed with little loss of bone. Once the infection has been cleared, reimplantation can occur with a larger or different prosthesis. Occasionally, the patient is not a candidate for, or is not willing to, undergo reimplantation in which case tibiotalar or tibiotalocalcaneal arthrodesis may be performed (Figures 25 (a) and (b)).

Some surgeons have even elected to keep the antibiotic spacer as definitive treatment (Myerson *et al.*, 2014).

Prevention

The keys to avoidance of wound problems are optimisation of the healing environment and meticulous handling of the soft tissues. The experience of many surgeons has lead to the adoption of the following set of principles:

(1) Ensure that the patient has an adequate blood supply. If either the dorsalis pedis or posterior tibial pulse cannot be felt, they should be assessed with Doppler ultrasound. If Doppler exam reveals an absent or abnormal pulse, vascular surgery consultation should be obtained.

(2) In rheumatoid patients, withhold disease modifying agents and immunosuppressive medications, if possible, from one to two weeks prior to surgery and until the wound is healed (usually three weeks).

(3) Administer preoperative prophylactic intravenous antibiotics 30 minutes prior to inflation of the tourniquet.

(4) Use a longer incision to avoid unnecessary tension on the wound edges.

(5) Create full thickness flaps without undermining or dissecting layers.

(6) Some authors recommend avoiding self-retaining retractors and only retracting one wound edge at a time in an effort to avoid ischemia, which can lead to wound edge necrosis (Myerson and Mroczek, 2003). In our experience we have found that careful use of Gelpi retractors placed deep (not touching the skin) affords excellent retraction while avoiding placing tension on the wound edges (Figures 21 (b) and (c)).

(7) Meticulous closure of the extensor retinaculum with the foot in dorsiflexion. This often requires an iterative process in which the first few sutures do not fully close the retinaculum, but help to relax the stress in it allowing the subsequent set of sutures to effect the closure.

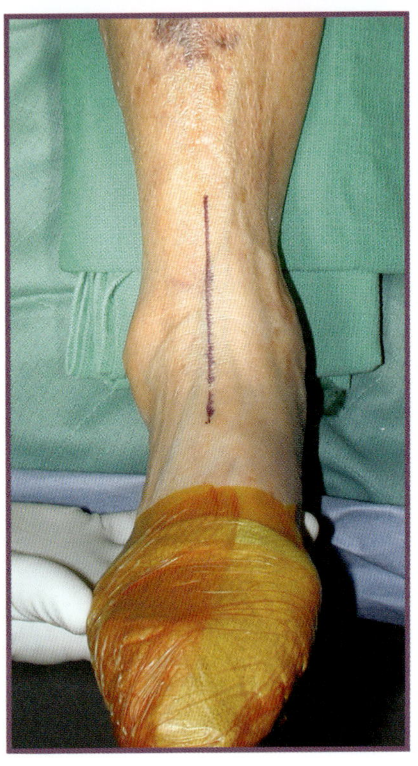

Figure 26. *A straight midline incision is now preferred to allow access to both gutters.*

(8) Use rigid postoperative immobilisation in a cast in dorsiflexion to prevent bowstringing of the extensor tendons. Laying at least three stack of 4 x 8 inch gauze pads over the ankle under the cast can help protect the wound.

(9) Use a postoperative drain, supplemental oxygen and elevation.

The preferred technique of the senior author (JKD) involves a straight 5-inch incision down the middle of the ankle to the midfoot (Figure 26). Previous ankle incisions should be used whenever possible. The skin is then carefully retracted and the retinaculum is opened just lateral to the anterior tibial tendon, avoiding the neurovascular bundle. The deep tissue is then lifted off the anterior tibia and sharply pulled away with a retractor. Immediately, Gelpi retractors are placed deep in the wound to avoid the vascular channel blockage that occurs with repetitive use of skin retractors. At the conclusion of the procedure, the wound is covered with two sets of long sponges placed transversely so that when the ankle is dorsiflexed the dressing does not bunch up but rather each half of the dressing folds at the crack between the dressings. In this manner, the senior author has been able to almost completely avoid soft tissue problems.

SYNDESMOTIC NON-UNION

Only one ankle, the Agility, was designed to rest on the tibia and fibula as a unit. Syndesmotic non-union was reported to occur at a rate of 10–12% (Pyevich *et al.*, 1998, Schuberth *et al.*, 2006). Failure of syndesmotic union often led to component loosening and migration secondary to failure of bony ongrowth onto the prosthesis (Knecht *et al.*, 2004) (Figure 27). Also reported was secondary loosening from collapse of cysts within the bone (Figure 28). This prosthesis is no longer used and thus these complications no longer occur.

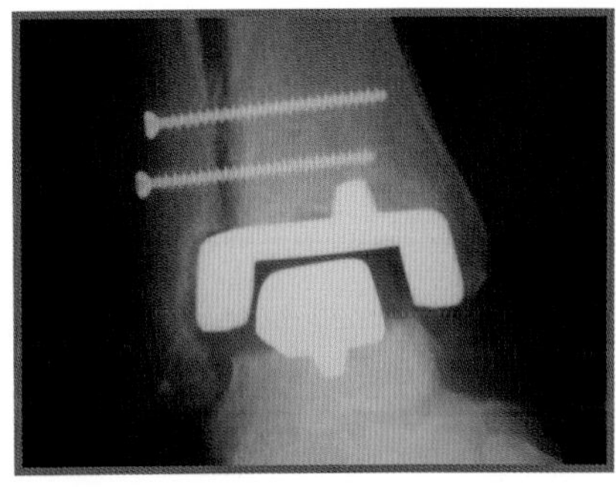

Figure 27. *Agility TAR with syndesmotic non-union leading to loosening of the components.*

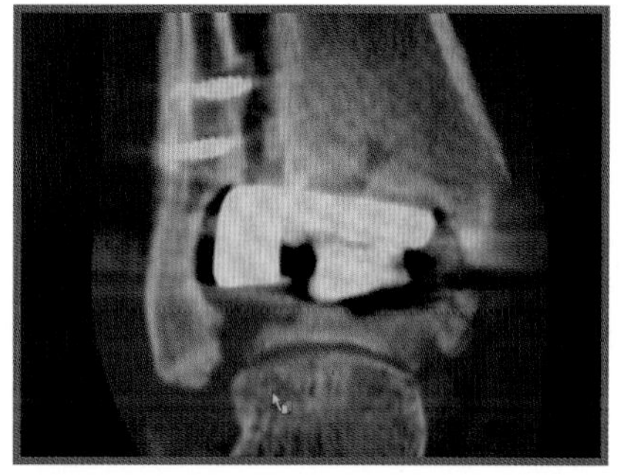

Figure 28. *CT scan showing cystic change around the components of an Agility TAR.*

POSTOPERATIVE: LATE

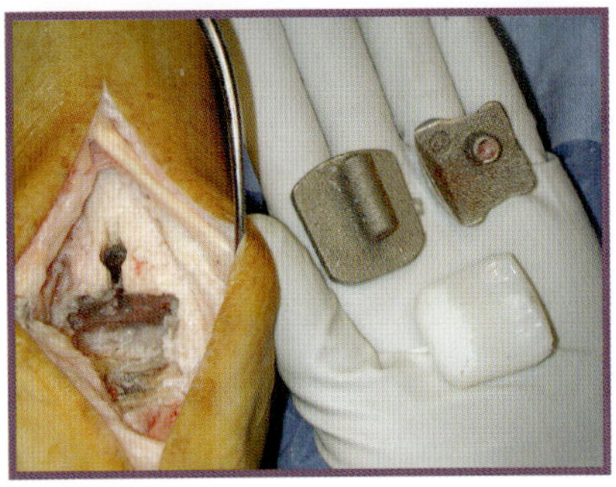

Figure 29. *No ongrowth of bone onto the prosthesis has occurred in this Salto-Talaris ankle seen in Figure 19.*

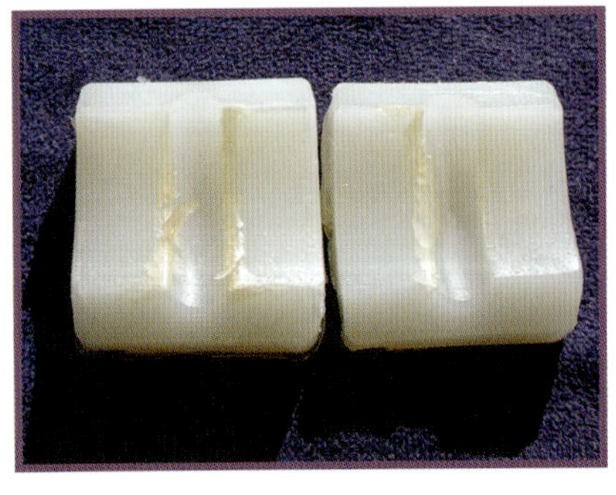

Figure 30. *Bilateral wear of the STAR polyethylene components in this patient featured in Figure 12 led to early osteolysis.*

Osteolysis/Periprosthetic Lucency/Aseptic Loosening

Aseptic loosening ranged from 0% to 6 % in six studies (Fevang *et al.*, 2007, Haskell and Mann, 2004, Henricson *et al.*, 2007, Hosman *et al.*, 2007, Knecht *et al.*, 2004, Lee *et al.*, 2008, Harston *et al.*, 2017), but was reported at 29% (15 of 51 ankles) in one study (Anderson *et al.*, 2003). In that study, seven of the ankles required revision, whereas the remaining eight had radiographic signs of loosening but remained asymptomatic (Pyevich *et al.*, 1998). Aseptic loosening and component migration can result from either failure of bony ongrowth (Figure 29) or periprosthetic osteolysis that occurs in response to polyethylene wear debris (Figure 30).

Failure of bone to ongrow the porous coating of the prosthesis will often manifest as "start-up" pain (pain with the first few steps that then subsides). Stable ongrowth the prosthesis is assessed by for the presence of "spot welds" on radiographs that are indicative of trabecular remodelling at the prosthetic–host interface (Raikin and Myerson, 2006). Ongrowth on the talar side is difficult to assess radiographically in talar components that are concave with sides, thus the interface is shielded from view by the metallic component itself. Thus, CT has been found to be more sensitive than radiographs in detecting the presence and extent of periprosthetic lucency (Hanna *et al.*, 2007).

The total ankle prosthesis produces polyethylene wear debris that is of similar size and particle concentration as that produced by total knee arthroplasty (Kobayashi *et al.*, 2004, Dalat *et al.*, 2013). Malalignment of the prosthesis leads to edge loading which is thought to significantly accelerate the rate of particle production. Even minimal wear of the polyethylene can generate enough particles to create osteolysis (DeOrio and Easley, 2008). The reported incidence of osteolysis is quite variable ranging from 0% to 24% in six studies (Fevang *et al.*, 2007; Nelissen *et al.*, 2006; Schuberth *et al.*, 2006; Schutte and Louwerens, 2008; Valderrabano *et al.*, 2004; Wood *et al.*, 2008). Ballooning osteolysis, without

migration, on the tibial side was reported by Valderrabano *et al.* (2004). These cystic lesions were located at the tibial component-bone interface between fixation bars and occurred in 4.4% of their subjects. This complication occurred only in younger more active patients who had ipsilateral subtalar arthrodesis.

Our understanding of the causes of osteolysis continues to grow and may relate to surgeon factors (such as component malposition) or implant factors. For example, recent studies have shown high rates of osteolysis affecting the Infinity implant of 31% in a series of 64 ankles (Saito *et al.*, 2018) and in another study loosening of the tibial implant leading to high early revision rates within a mean of 13 months following the index procedure (Cody *et al.*, 2018). Other implants such as the AES have been withdrawn from the market due to disproportionately high rates of osteolysis (Koivu *et al.*, 2009; Besse *et al.*, 2010).

Osteolysis is classified as minor if the lytic area extends for less than 1 cm. These lesions should be followed with serial radiographic examination to ensure they are not expanding. On the other hand, lytic areas that are greater than 1 cm in size could represent a significant problem, are almost always the result of polyethylene wear, and require intervention. Treatment consists of addressing both the cysts and the cause of the osteolysis. The cysts should be debrided and bone grafted (Figure 17) and an arthrotomy is often performed to debride synovial and capsular infiltration of polyethylene debris from the joint. This also permits exchange of the polyethylene component. Component alignment and positioning should be assessed and corrected, as malpositioning and malalignment may be the source of the cysts (Figures 31 (a) and (b)). Component fixation should also be assessed as loose components require replacement (DeOrio and Easley, 2008).

Component Subsidence

Talar component subsidence is a recognised issue in ankle arthroplasty. Pyevich *et al.* (1998) reported on talar subsidence

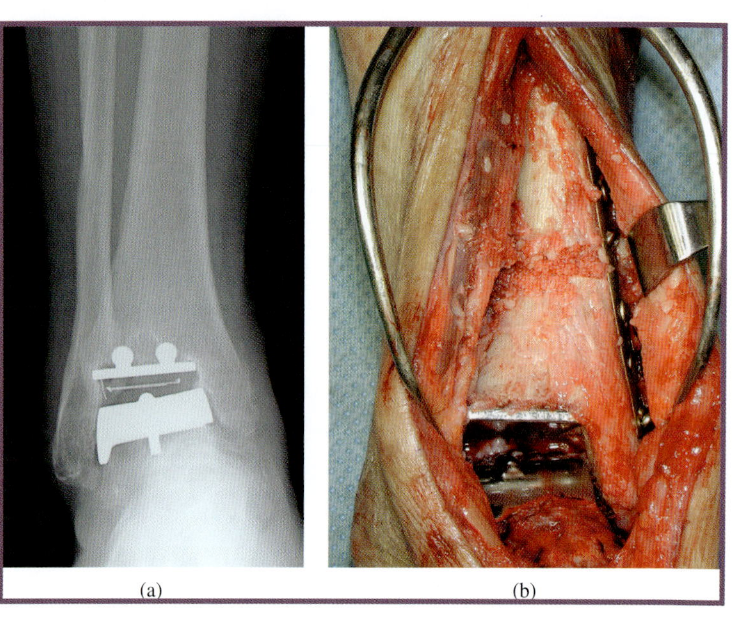

Figure 31. *(a) Preoperative varus deformity in this STAR TAR lead to polyethylene fracture at 3 years after surgery. (b) The varus deformity was corrected with medial opening wedge osteotomy at the time of polyethylene replacement.*

with the Agility prosthesis at rates of 8% (Pyevich *et al.*, 1998) and Schuberth *et al.* (2006) at 10%. The STAR prosthesis has shown rates of subsidence of 1% (Wood *et al.*, 2008) and 0.4% (Fevang *et al.*, 2007). Tibial component subsidence was reported to occur with the Agility ankle at a rate of 14% (Pyevich *et al.*, 1998). Valderrabano (2004) reported a 14% incidence of tibial component tilting in the STAR ankle averaging 6.2° (range 5.1°–9.5°). Whether or not this was secondary to some subsidence is unclear. However, as mentioned previously, the original STAR instrumentation did not include proximal fixation of the jig to the tibia, which resulted in coronal plane malalignment. Recently, Le *et al.*, 2019 suggested that excessive sagittal talar implant inclination angle might be a causative factor. The Canadian group reported that a postoperative talar component inclination angle greater than 22 degrees was associated

with talar component anterior subsidence, defined as a change in that angle of 5 degrees or more between postoperative and last available radiographs (Le *et al.*, 2019).

Component subsidence often occurs in the setting of excessive bony resection as this places the prosthesis on the softer bone that is located proximal or distal to the subchondral plate. It can also occur around cystic areas of ankle replacements (Figure 32). This complication is best avoided by limiting bony resection to the minimum necessary to provide room for the components without overstuffing the joint. Joint distraction with laminar spreaders and ligament balancing with soft tissue releases aid in bone conservation (Schuberth *et al.*, 2006). Talar component subsidence can also occur from avascular necrosis of the talus (DeOrio and Easley, 2008). This occurs most frequently in those prostheses whose instrumentation violates the sinus tarsi, as the blood supply to the body of the talus comes primarily from the artery of the tarsal canal (Tennant *et al.*, 2014). Subtalar arthrodesis, whether performed in a staged or in a concurrent fashion, can also compromise this blood supply leading to avascular necrosis and subsequent talar component subsidence (Figures 33 (a)–(d)).

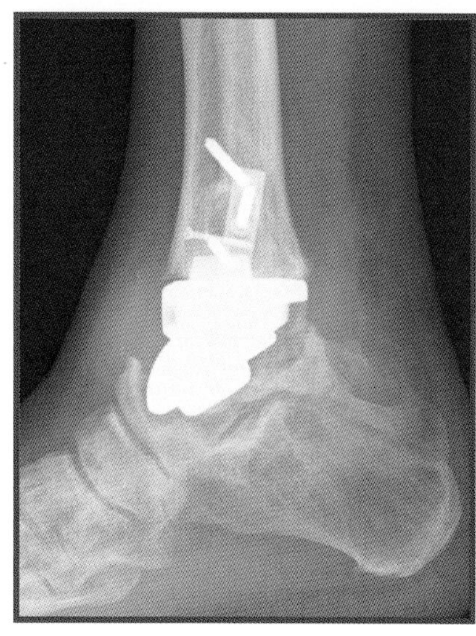

Figure 32. *Collapse of the talar component of an Agility TAR into talar cysts.*

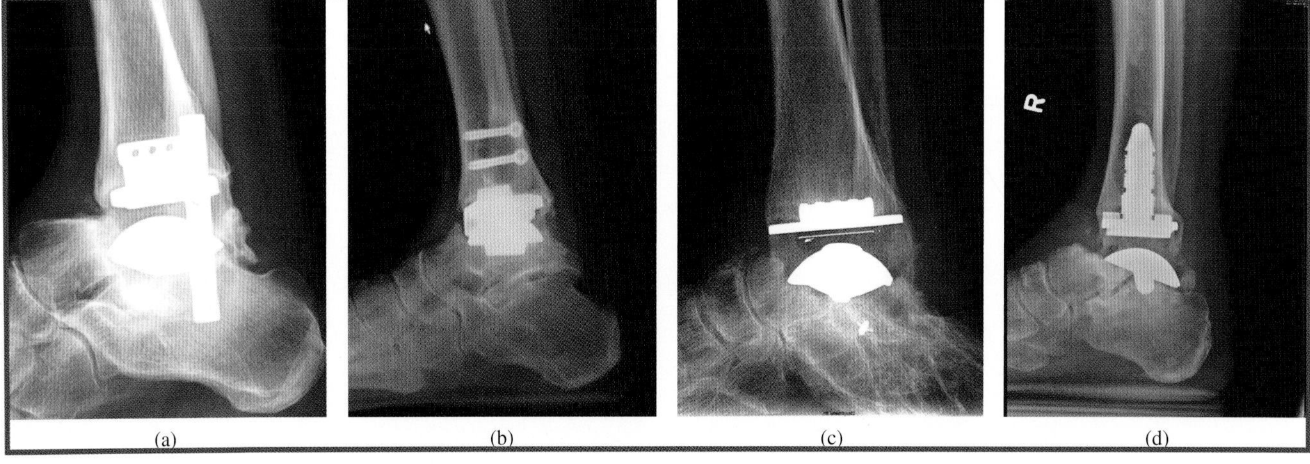

Figure 33. *The talus in various stages of complete collapse with the (a) Salto-Talaris, (b) Agility, (c) STAR with previous subtalar fusion and (d) INBONE TARs.*

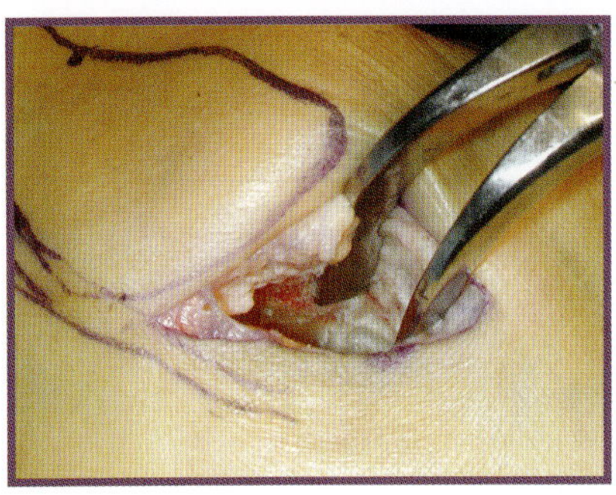

Figure 34. *Only the posterior facet is prepared for arthrodesis when a subtalar arthrodesis is to be performed.*

Limiting subtalar fusions to the posterior facet only, may help prevent this complication (Figure 34).

Polyethylene Fracture

Polyethylene fracture is reported to occur in 0–4% of patients in four studies (Wood *et al.*, 2008, Anderson *et al.*, 2003, Nelissen *et al.*, 2006, Henricson *et al.*, 2007, Rippstein *et al.*, 2012). Most of the reported cases have occurred with the STAR ankle. All these fractures occurred in the coronal plane and not along the longitudinal groove which is oriented in the sagittal plane. This is thought to occur because the curved shape of the talar component places a transverse, longitudinal stress on the polyethylene. As previously mentioned malalignment can hasten polyethylene wear and thus lead to premature fracture of the polyethylene (Figure 13).

Heterotopic Ossification

Heterotopic overgrowth of bone around the medial and lateral margins of the prosthesis can result in painful impingement and loss of ROM (Figures 35 (a)–(c)). The heterotopic bone is most often located posteromedially and is more common in patients with posttraumatic than those with primary osteoarthritis (Valderrabano *et al.*, 2003). It has been reported to occur between 2–63% of ankles (Lee *et al.*, 2008, Valderrabano *et al.*, 2003, Schutte and Louwerens, 2008). It can be prevented by the thorough resection of osteophytes and by the removal of bone fragments and liberal use of irrigation at the time of surgery. The senior author (JKD) cuts out the posterior capsule which often reveals fragments of bone and is thought to be nidus for heterotopic ossification. Postoperatively, symptomatic impingement can be observed or treated with local corticosteroid injection and physical therapy. When conservative treatment fails, open or arthroscopic resection of the bone at the site of impingement is indicated (Raikin and Myerson, 2006).

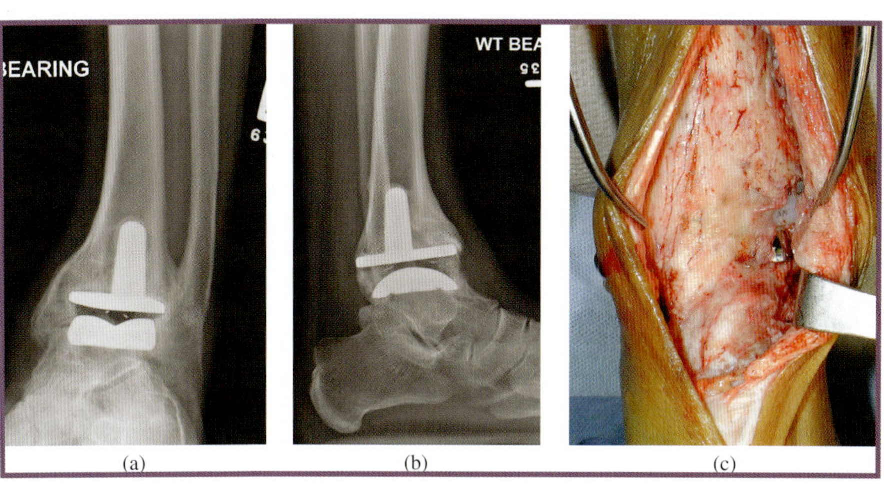

(a)   (b)   (c)

Figure 35. *Radiographs (a) and (b) of a Buechel-Pappas (BP) ankle completely encased in bone. (c) Upon opening this BP ankle for revision, the bone has completely covered the prosthesis.*

Persistent Pain

Pain that persists after TAR is reported to occur at a rate of 0.5–4% in four studies (Wood *et al.*, 2008, Fevang *et al.*, 2007, Henricson *et al.*, 2007, Hosman *et al.*, 2007). The persistence of pain in the ankle must be differentiated from pain in adjacent joints. Adjacent joint pain may be due to arthritis in the talonavicular or subtalar joints. It is often the result of preexisting disease in these joints but only becomes evident following ankle replacement. Ideally, these problems are identified prior to ankle arthroplasty, so that they can be addressed prior to, or at the time of, the replacement. Symptomatic subtalar arthritis should be treated with isolated posterior facet fusion as previously discussed. Bringing the screws from the posterior tuberosity across the posterior facet eliminates the possibility of impairing the blood supply coming through the sinus tarsi. The decision to perform subtalar arthrodesis is more difficult when the patient has only moderate arthrosis and decreased but not absent motion (Figures 36 (a)–(c)).

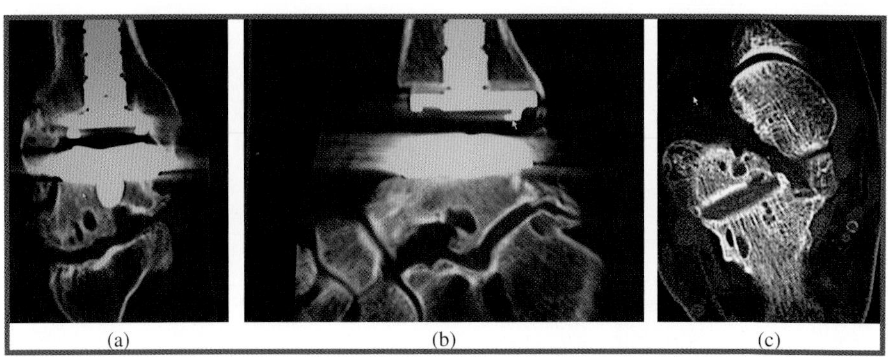

Figure 36. *(a)-(c) Patient underwent INBONE TAR. One year later he complained of pain in the sinus tarsi after doing heavy work. CT scan shows involvement of all areas of the subtalar joint and calcaneal cuboid joint. The patient obtained symptomatic relief for 2 years after a steroid injection into the subtalar joint.*

If a more extensive hindfoot arthrodesis is required, it may be done as a separate procedure preceding the ankle replacement by several months. However, the senior author (JKD) routinely performs double arthrodesis (talonavicular and subtalar joints) in lieu of triple arthrodesis at the time of ankle replacement. The anterior exposure provides easy access to the talonavicular joint and the posterior facet of the subtalar joint is exposed through a small oblique lateral incision which may be done prior to opening the ankle (DeOrio, 2010). Autogenous bone grafting from the ankle and internal fixation of the arthrodeses may be done after the replacement is complete. This is accomplished with two screws coming from the calcaneus into the talus for fixation of the subtalar joint and two or three screws across the talonavicular joint. The calcaneocuboid joint is only addressed in the setting of inflammatory arthropathy or trauma having created both clinical and radiographic arthrosis. A simplified technique is employed, it involves approach to the calcaneocuboid joint through a small lateral incision, preparation of the joint surfaces with an oscillating saw, bone grafting, and fixation with a single screw. Finally, when ankle replacement is performed in patients with a prior triple arthrodesis, the surgeon must take into account the rotational alignment of the forefoot. It may be necessary

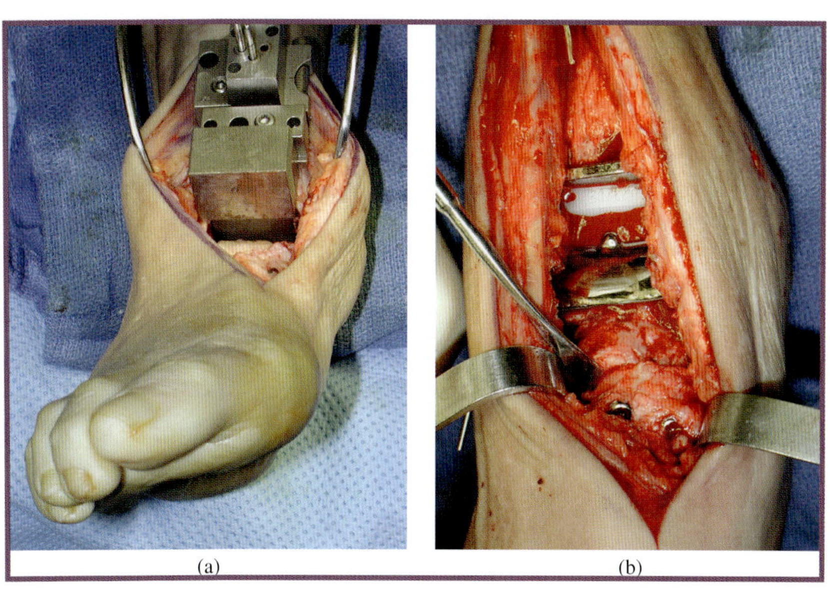

(a)   (b)

Figure 37. *Patient had a prior triple arthrodesis. (a) When the cutting jigs were placed in line with the ankle, her forefoot was in 30° of varus (supination). (b) Therefore she underwent a midfoot (Chopart) osteotomy, derotation and fixation with two large screws.*

to add a midfoot derotation osteotomy to restore a plantigrade foot (Figures 37 (a) and (b)) or to cut the talus slightly asymmetrically to accommodate the hindfoot position (DeOrio, 2013).

Persistent pain, which localises to the ankle joint, has a number of causes. Raikin and Myerson *et al.* (2006) have developed an algorithm to aid in the determination of the source of pain and help guide treatment (Figure 38). They divided the causes based on the timing of the presentation of pain. The early group (less than 3 months) includes wound complications and neuromas. The most common source of persistent pain is failure of the bone to ongrow the prosthesis. This most often occurs when there is inadequate immediate fixation of the prosthesis at the time of surgery. This can be the result of the preoperative loss of bone, avascular bone adjacent to the prosthesis, over resection of bone, or the design of the prosthesis.

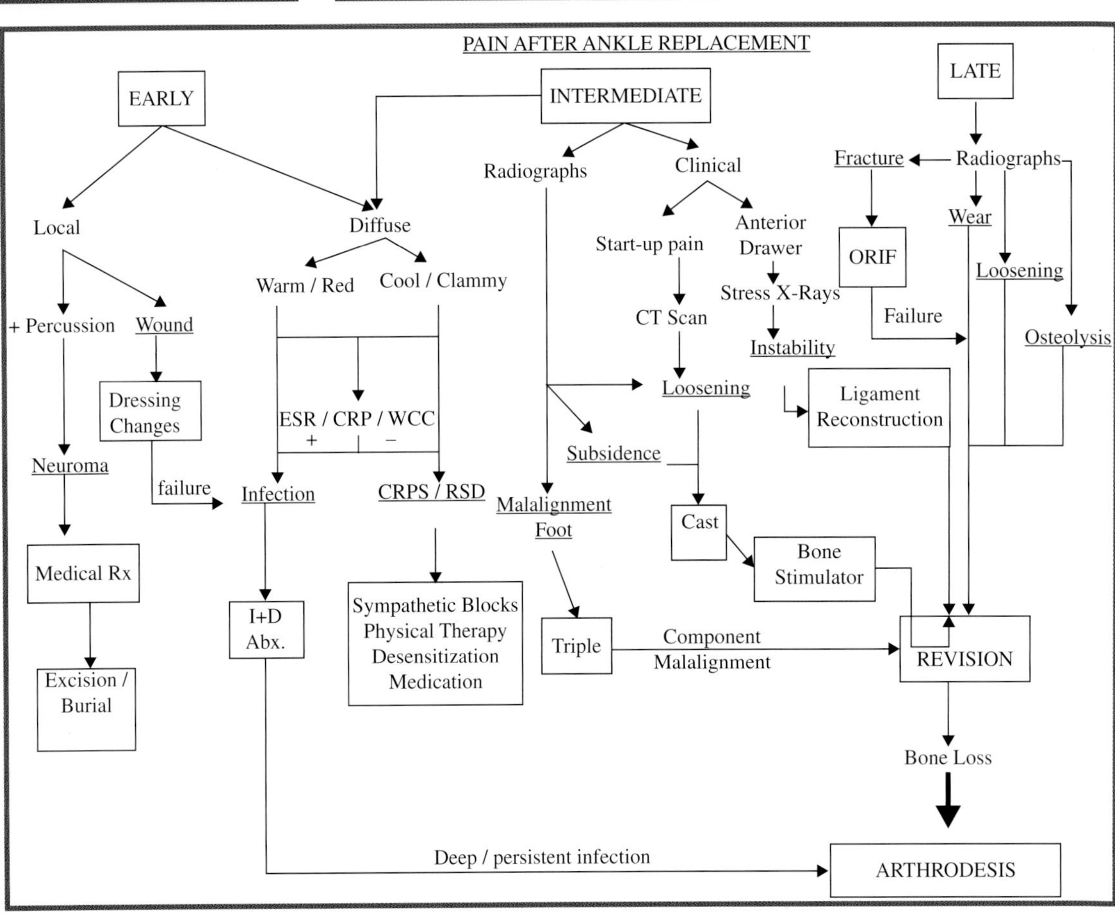

Figure 38. *Algorithm for the diagnosis and management of pain after TAR. Abbreviations: Abx = antibiotics, CRP = C-reactive protein, CRPS = chronic regional pain syndrome, CT = computed tomography, ESR = erythrocyte sedimentation rate, I + D = irrigation and debridement, ORIF = open reduction and internal fixation, RSD = reflex sympathetic dystrophy, Rx = treatment, WCC = white cell count, and XRays = radiographs. (Used with permission from Raikin, S. M., and Myerson, M. S. Figure 3). Since this algorithm was developed, we now also have the option of revision to another ankle replacement as a second stage.*

Pain that appears at an intermediate time after surgery (3–6 months) may be due to a loose prosthesis, chronic regional pain syndrome (CRPS), or infection. CRPS and infection may be difficult to differentiate. History and physical provides some guidance as the complaints in CRPS are often out of proportion

to the physical findings. A limb that is cool, clammy, discoloured, and diffusely painful to touch points toward CRPS. Patients with suspected CRPS should be sent to a pain center for both diagnosis and treatment. Treatment usually consists of nerve blockade, physical therapy for desensitisation and ROM, and often medications which are known to ease neurologic discomfort (e.g. Neurontin (gabapentin) or Lyrica (pregabalin)).

A patient who has fever or chills, an ankle that is warm or erythematous, and has pain with slight movement of the joint should be considered to have an infection until proven otherwise. The suspected infection should be evaluated with a CBC (FBC), ESR, and CRP. When all three of these markers of inflammation are normal, the chance of infection is very low. If any of these markers are abnormal, or if clinical suspicion is high, aspiration of the ankle for cell count with differential and cultures should be performed, and in some circumstances open biopsy is necessary, as a definitive test for infection.

Malalignment, with soft tissue stress, non-union or malunion of a syndesmotic arthrodesis or concurrent osteotomy, and ankle instability are also potential causes of persistent pain presenting in the intermediate period. Ankle instability can be determined with an anterior drawer test and confirmed with stress radiographs.

Persistent pain presenting late (more than 6 months after surgery) should raise the suspicion of component failure, aseptic loosening, malleolar stress fracture, or component subsidence (Fevang *et al.*, 2007, Henricson *et al.*, 2007, Hosman *et al.*, 2007, Wood *et al.*, 2008).

Stiffness

Postoperative stiffness may be due to a multitude of factors. Stamatis and Myerson (2002) divided the factors responsible for stiffness into preoperative, intraoperative, and postoperative factors.

The most important cause of postoperative stiffness is preoperative stiffness. In other words, a contracted joint with a scarred soft tissue envelope will produce a stiff total ankle regardless of the steps that are taken during surgery or after surgery to avoid it. It is important that both the patient and the surgeon recognise this fact and thus have realistic expectations. It is imperative to have an accurate preoperative assessment of ROM and not to be fooled by motion through Chopart's joint. When necessary, plantar flexion dorsiflexion radiographs should be used to isolate tibiotalar motion. Tightness of the gastrocnemius — soleus complex can lead to poor dorsiflexion. Preoperative assessment with the Silfverskiold's test will determine whether gastrocnemius recession or percutaneous triple hemisection is more appropriate. However, even with a negative Silfverskiold's test one study has shown that increased dorsiflexion can be achieved with a gastrocnemius recession alone (DeOrio and Lewis, 2014). Long periods of immobilisation, chronic pain syndromes, inadequate rehabilitation, and the presence of osteophytes are other preoperative factors that can conspire to produce a stiff total ankle (Stamatis and Myerson, 2002).

Intraoperative factors are also important in obtaining the full potential ROM. The extensor tendons of the anterior compartment, particularly the tibialis anterior, are responsible for powering dorsiflexion at the ankle. The extensor retinaculum must be incised to gain access to the ankle. If it is not adequately repaired, the result may be bowstringing of the extensor tendons leading to loss of dorsiflexion power as well as wound healing problems. Axial tension within the joint is a function of the amount of bony resection, soft tissue release, and component thickness. As bone resection and soft tissue release increase, and thinner components are used, the articulation is less stable. Less bony resection and thicker components can lead to joint "overstuffing", which leads to decreased ROM. Stamatis and Myerson (2002) suggested that the deltoid endpoint, the production of firm endpoint within the deltoid when levering the joint with an osteotome, is a useful measure of joint tension. It often arises that the ankle is between sizes in stability. If there is any question about motion, it is better to downsize; so

long as the components still have adequate cortical support. Keep in mind that joint line malpositioning (too proximal or too distal) creates a cam effect, which also limits ROM. Adequate debridement of the anterior and posterior joint spaces as well as the medial and lateral gutters contributes significantly to realising maximal ROM. Furthermore, it is the senior author's opinion that cutting too high an opening angle on the tibia leaves the posterior structures taut further decreasing ROM.

Postoperative factors leading to decreased ROM include prolonged casting in plantar flexion, poorly controlled swelling or pain, and heterotopic bone formation. Dorsiflexion is much more difficult to obtain, and its deficit more noticeable, than plantar flexion. For this reason, as well as to prevent bowstringing of the extensor tendons, the postoperative cast should be applied in slight dorsiflexion. Pain and swelling that occur after the cast has been removed will limit the patient's ability to move their ankle. An intermediate pressure knee high compression hose aids in prevention of excessive swelling, as does elevation once the cast has been removed. Finally heterotopic bone, which forms in the postoperative period, can produce a mechanical block to motion. All bone debris that could act as a nidus for bone formation should be removed at the time of surgery.

Impact of Surgeon Experience

A number of investigators have examined the relationship between complications and surgeon experience (Haskell and Mann, 2004; Lee *et al.*, 2008; Myerson and Mroczek, 2003; Saltzman *et al.*, 2003, 2009, Schuberth *et al.*, 2006; Valderrabano *et al.*, 2004; Wood *et al.*, 2008). Haskell and Mann (2004) compared the rates of perioperative complications encountered during the first 10 to the subsequent 10 cases of STAR TAR performed by 10 surgeons. Patients in the early group had a 3.1 times likelihood of having a perioperative adverse event, and a 3.2 times higher risk of a perioperative wound problem. Similarly, Lee *et al.* (2008) compared the rate of complication in their first 25 to their subsequent 25 Hintegra ankles. They found that overall complication rate decreased by

a factor of three from 60% to 20%, with a four-fold decrease in the number of malleolar fractures. A study by Myerson and Mroczek (2003) compared rates of adverse perioperative events for the first 25 and subsequent 25 cases of Agility TAR by a single surgeon. Perioperative complications (including wound problems, fractures, and tendon or nerve lacerations) decreased from 60% in the initial group to 8% in the subsequent group. The rate of component malposition also decreased by 9%. Another study by Schuberth *et al.* (2006) compared complication rates between their first 25 and subsequent 25 cases of Agility TAR. They found that the rates of intraoperative malleolar fractures, malalignment, syndesmotic nonunion, and need for early component revision decreased between the groups. They found no difference in the rate of wound complications. Wood and Deakin (2003) compared the rates of intraoperative fracture in their first 100 compared to their subsequent 100 cementless, mobile bearing STAR TARs. They found that the incidence fell from 7% in the first 100 ankles, to 2% in the second 100. Saltzman *et al.* (2009) compared adverse events between the pivotal and continued access portions of their study. The pivotal portion of the study contained 158 arthroplasties (16 per surgeon) with variable surgeon experience prior to joining the study group. The continued access portion of the study consisted of the subsequent 435 arthroplasties (43 per surgeon). The incidence of adverse events in the continued access group was found to be significantly less than in the pivotal group. Specifically, a lower incidence of pain, stiffness, edema, and bony changes were found. Nerve injury, fracture, wound problems, and infection was not found to be different between the two groups. In contrast, Spirit *et al.* (2004) found no evidence of a learning-curve effect when the results for the first patients who underwent TAR were compared with the results for later patients. The first 50 patients fared no worse than the next 150 patients in terms of the proportion who had a reoperation and/or failure.

It is also not known whether the type of instruction that the surgeon receives in learning to perform the operation is a factor. Saltzman *et al.* (2003) compared the first 10 TAR performed by three groups

of three surgeons who received different methods of training in the performance of TAR — observation, hands on course, or one-year fellowship. They found that no identified training method had a statistically demonstrable positive impact on preparing surgeons for performing TAR. In terms of hospital/surgeon factors, early revision rates are significantly higher in low volume centres (Zaidi *et al.*, 2016).

CONCLUSION

It is the authors' opinion that ankle replacements will continue to increase in popularity. The frequency of arthrodesis the ankle will in the future continue to decrease. Furthermore, as surgeons gain more experience with the surgical technique, and ankle replacements and the instruments used to put them in become more refined, in all likelihood complications will decrease. However, whether ankle replacement will approach the very low rate of complications for hip and knee remains to be seen.

REFERENCES

Aitken, G. K., Bourne, R. B., Finlay, J. B., Rorabeck, C. H. & Andreae, P. R. 1985. Indentation stiffness of the cancellous bone in the distal human tibia. *Clin Orthop Relat Res*, 264–270.

Anderson, T., Montgomery, F. & Carlsson, A. 2003. Uncemented star total ankle prostheses. three to eight-year follow-up of fifty-one consecutive ankles. *J Bone Joint Surg Am,* 85-A, 1321–1329.

Attinger, C., Cooper, P., Blume, P. & Bulan, E. 2001. The safest surgical incisions and amputations applying the angiosome principles and using the doppler to assess the arterial–arterial connections of the foot and ankle. *Foot Ankle Clin,* 6, 745–799.

Besse, J. L., Colombier, J. A., Asencio, J., Bonnin, M., Gaudot, F., Jarde, O., Judet, T., Maestro, M., Lemrijse, T., Leonardi, C., Toullec, E. & L'afcp 2010. Total ankle arthroplasty in France. *Orthop Traumatol Surg Res*, 96, 291–303.

Bonnin, M., Judet, T., Colombier, J. A., Buscayret, F., Graveleau, N. & Piriou, P. 2004. Midterm results of the salto total ankle prosthesis. *Clin Orthop Relat Res*, 6–18.

Borenstein, T. R., Anand, K., Li, Q., Charlton, T. P., Thordarson, D. B. 2018. A review of perioperative complications of outpatient total ankle arthroplasty. *Foot Ankle Int*, 39(2), 143–148. doi: 10.1177/1071100717738748.

Cody, E. A., Taylor, M. A., Nunley, J. A., II, Parekh, S. G., DeOrio, J. K. 2019. Increased early revision rate with the INFINITY total ankle prosthesis. *Foot Ankle Int*. 40(1), 9–17. doi: 10.1177/1071100718794933. Epub 2018 Sep 3.

Conti, S. F. & Wong, Y. S. 2001. Complications of total ankle replacement. *Clin Orthop Relat Res*, 105–114.

Dalat, F., Barnoud, R., Fessy, M. H., Besse, J. L. & French Association Of Foot Surgery, A. 2013. Histologic study of periprosthetic osteolytic lesions after AES total ankle replacement. A 22 case series. *Orthop Traumatol Surg Res*, 99, S285–S295.

DeOrio, J. K. & Easley, M. E. 2008. Total ankle arthroplasty. *Instr Course Lect*, 57, 383–413.

DeOrio, J. K. 2010. Total ankle replacement with subtalar arthrodesis: Management of combined ankle and subtalar arthritis. *Tech Foot Ankle Surg*, 9, 182–189.

DeOrio, J. K. 2013. Star ankle replacement in ankle arthrosis following triple arthrodesis fused in varus. [Online]. Stryker. Available at: http://www.Star-Ankle.Com/Case-Study/Replacement-Arthrosis-Triple-Arthrodesis-Fused-In-Varus/ [Accessed 2015].

DeOrio, J. K. & Lewis, J. S., Jr. 2014. Silfverskiold's test in total ankle replacement with gastrocnemius recession. *Foot Ankle Int*, 35, 116–122.

Fevang, B. T., Lie, S. A., Havelin, L. I., Brun, J. G., Skredderstuen, A. & Furnes, O. 2007. 257 Ankle arthroplasties performed in norway between 1994 and 2005. *Acta Orthop*, 78, 575–583.

Gill, L. H. 2004. Challenges in total ankle arthroplasty. *Foot Ankle Int*, 25, 195–207.

Hanna, R. S., Haddad, S. L. & Lazarus, M. L. 2007. Evaluation of periprosthetic lucency after total ankle arthroplasty: Helical Ct versus conventional radiography. *Foot Ankle Int*, 28, 921–926.

Harston, A., Lazarides, A. L., Adams, S. B., Jr., DeOrio, J. K., Easley, M. E. & Nunley, J. A., II. 2017. Midterm outcomes of a fixed-bearing total ankle arthroplasty with deformity analysis. *Foot Ankle Int*, 38, 1295–1300.

Haskell, A. & Mann, R. A. 2004. Perioperative complication rate of total ankle replacement is reduced by surgeon experience. *Foot Ankle Int*, 25, 283–289.

Henricson, A., Skoog, A. & Carlsson, A. 2007. The Swedish ankle arthroplasty register: An analysis of 531 arthroplasties between 1993 and 2005. *Acta Orthop*, 78, 569–574.

Hintermann, B. & Valderrabano, V. 2003. Total ankle replacement. *Foot Ankle Clin*, 8, 375–405.

Horne, P. H., Jennings, J. M., DeOrio, J. K., Easley, M. E., Nunley, J. A. & Adams, S. B. 2015. Low incidence of symptomatic thromboembolic events after total ankle arthroplasty without routine use of chemoprophylaxis. *Foot Ankle Int*, 36, 611–616.

Hosman, A. H., Mason, R. B., Hobbs, T. & Rothwell, A. G. 2007. A New Zealand national joint registry review of 202 total ankle replacements followed for up to 6 years. *Acta Orthop*, 78, 584–591.

Hvid, I., Rasmussen, O., Jensen, N. C. & Nielsen, S. 1985. Trabecular bone strength profiles at the ankle joint. *Clin Orthop Relat Res*, 306–312.

Knecht, S. I., Estin, M., Callaghan, J. J., Zimmerman, M. B., Alliman, K. J., Alvine, F. G. & Saltzman, C. L. 2004. The agility total ankle arthroplasty. seven to sixteen-year follow-up. *J of Bone Joint Surg Am*, 86-A, 1161–1171.

Kobayashi, A., Minoda, Y., Kadoya, Y., Ohashi, H., Takaoka, K. & Saltzman, C. L. 2004. Ankle arthroplasties generate wear particles similar to knee arthroplasties. *Clin Orthop Relat Res*, 69–72.

Koivu, H., Kohonen, I., Sipola, E., Alanen, K., Vahlberg, T. & Tiusanen, H. 2009. Severe periprosthetic osteolytic lesions after the ankle evolutive system total ankle replacement. *J Bone Joint Surg Br*, 91, 907–914.

Le, V., Escudero, M., Symes, M., Salat, P., Wing, K., Younger, A., Penner, M. & Veljkovic, A. 2019. Impact of Sagittal Talar inclination on total ankle replacement failure. *Foot Ankle Int*. 26:1071100719847183. doi: 10.1177/1071100719847183.

Lee, K. B., Cho, S. G., Hur, C. I. & Yoon, T. R. 2008. Perioperative complications of hintegra total ankle replacement: Our initial 50 cases. *Foot Ankle Int*, 29, 978–984.

Mcgarvey, W. C., Clanton, T. O. & Lunz, D. 2004. Malleolar fracture after total ankle arthroplasty: A comparison of two designs. *Clin Orthop Relat Res*, 104–110.

Myerson, M. S. & Mroczek, K. 2003. Perioperative complications of total ankle arthroplasty. *Foot Ankle Int*, 24, 17–21.

Myerson, M. S., Shariff, R. & Zonno, A. J. 2014. The management of infection following total ankle replacement: demographics and treatment. *Foot Ankle Int*, 35, 855–862.

Nelissen, R. G., Doets, H. C. & Valstar, E. R. 2006. Early migration of the tibial component of the Buechel–Pappas total ankle prosthesis. *Clin Orthop Relat Res*, 448, 146–151.

Overley, B. D., Jr. & Beideman, T. C. 2015. Painful osteophytes, ectopic bone, and pain in the malleolar gutters following total ankle replacement: management and strategies. *Clin Podiatr Med Surg*, 32, 509–516.

Pyevich, M. T., Saltzman, C. L., Callaghan, J. J. & Alvine, F. G. 1998. Total ankle arthroplasty: A unique design. Two to twelve-year follow-up. *J Bone Joint Surg Am*, 80, 1410–1420.

Raikin, S. M. & Myerson, M. S. 2006. Avoiding and managing complications of the agility total ankle replacement system. *Orthopedics*, 29, 930–938.

Rippstein, P. F., Huber, M., Coetzee, J. C. & Naal, F. D. 2011. Total ankle replacement with use of a new three-component implant. *J Bone Joint Surg Am*, 93, 1426–1435.

Rippstein, P. F., Huber, M. & Naal, F. D. 2012. Management of specific complications related to total ankle arthroplasty. *Foot Ankle Clin*, 17, 707–717.

Saltzman, C. L., Amendola, A., Anderson, R., Coetzee, J. C., Gall, R. J., Haddad, S. L., Herbst, S., Lian, G., Sanders, R. W., Scioli, M. & Younger, A. S. 2003. Surgeon training and complications in total ankle arthroplasty. *Foot Ankle Int*, 24, 514–518.

Saltzman, C. L., Mann, R. A., Ahrens, J. E., Amendola, A., Anderson, R. B., Berlet, G. C., Brodsky, J. W., Chou, L. B., Clanton, T. O., Deland, J. T., DeOrio, J. K., Horton, G. A., Lee, T. H., Mann, J. A., Nunley, J. A., Thordarson, D. B., Walling, A. K., Wapner, K. L. & Coughlin, M. J. 2009.

Prospective controlled trial of star total ankle replacement versus ankle fusion: Initial results. *Foot Ankle Int*, 30, 579–596.

Saito, G. H., Sanders, A. E., de Cesar Netto, C., O'Malley, M. J., Ellis, S. J., Demetracopoulos, C. A. 2018. Short-term complications, reoperations, and radiographic outcomes of a new fixed-bearing total ankle arthroplasty. *Foot Ankle Int*, 39(7), 787–794. doi: 10.1177/1071100718764107. Epub 2018 Mar 28.

Schuberth, J. M., Patel, S. & Zarutsky, E. 2006. Perioperative complications of the agility total ankle replacement in 50 initial, consecutive cases. *J Foot Ankle Surg*, 45, 139–146.

Schutte, B. G. & Louwerens, J. W. 2008. Short-term results of our first 49 Scandanavian total ankle replacements (Star). *Foot Ankle Int*, 29, 124–127.

Spirt, A. A., Assal, M. & Hansen, S. T., Jr. 2004. Complications and failure after total ankle arthroplasty. *J Bone Joint Surg Am* 86-A, 1172–1178.

Stamatis, E. D. & Myerson, M. S. 2002. How to avoid specific complications of total ankle replacement. *Foot Ankle Clin*, 7, 765–789.

Tennant, J. N., Rungprai, C., Pizzimenti, M. A., Goetz, J., Phisitkul, P., Femino, J. & Amendola, A. 2014. Risks to the blood supply of the talus with four methods of total ankle arthroplasty: A cadaveric injection study. *J Bone Joint Surg Am*, 96, 395–402.

Valderrabano, V., Hintermann, B., Nigg, B. M., Stefanyshyn, D. & Stergiou, P. 2003. Kinematic changes after fusion and total replacement of the ankle: Part 1: Range of motion. *Foot Ankle Int*, 24, 881–887.

Valderrabano, V., Hintermann, B. & Dick, W. 2004. Scandinavian total ankle replacement: A 3.7-year average followup of 65 patients. *Clin Orthop Relat Res*, 47–56.

Wood, P. L. 2002. Experience With the star ankle arthroplasty at Wrightington hospital, UK. *Foot Ankle Clin*, 7, 755–764, vii.

Wood, P. L. & Deakin, S. 2003. Total ankle replacement. The results in 200 ankles. *J Bone Joint Surg Br*, 85, 334–341.

Wood, P. L., Prem, H. & Sutton, C. 2008. Total ankle replacement: Medium-term results in 200 Scandinavian total ankle replacements. *J Bone Joint Surg Br*, 90, 605–609.

Zaidi, R., MacGregor, A., Cro, S., Goldberg, A. J. 2016. Pulmonary embolism and mortality following total ankle replacement: A data linkage study using the NJR data set. *BMJ Open* 6:e011947. doi:10.1136/bmjopen-2016-011947.

Zaidi, R., Macgregor, A. J., Goldberg, A. 2016. Quality measures for total ankle replacement, 30-day readmission and reoperation rates within 1 year of surgery: A data linkage study using the NJR data set. *BMJ Open*, 6(5), e011332. doi: 10.1136/bmjopen-2016-011332.

TOTAL ANKLE REPLACEMENT IN DEFORMITY

J. C. Coetzee and P. Rippstein

Summary

Varus, valgus, or complex deformities add a major challenge to the total ankle replacement (TAR). It is important to deal with any such deformity either before, or at the time of the TAR.

A simple analogy is to compare the ankle joint to the tyres on a car. If the wheel balance is off, the tyres will wear out quickly. Even if the tyres are replaced, the new ones will also wear out quickly if the balance is not restored. The same goes for the ankle. If there is uneven wear in the ankle due to ligamentous instability or axial malalignment, replacing the joint without correcting the abnormalities will lead to early failure.

INTRODUCTION

As the surgeon becomes experienced in total ankle replacement (TAR), there is a tendency to attempt more than the straight forward ankle deformity. Significant varus or valgus can be especially challenging. One should be cognizant of all the pitfalls and know how to deal with the difficult ankle, and there should also be a clear understanding that the greater the varus or valgus, the harder the procedure, and the less predictable the outcome of ankle replacement.

Varus or valgus due to pure bone erosion at the level of the ankle seldom poses an extra-ordinary challenge, and can usually be corrected with the standard bone cuts. The majority of varus or valgus ankles will, however, have an element of ligamentous imbalance. If the imbalance is not corrected at the time of surgery, the lifespan of the implant will be compromised. One of the challenges in the future will not be whether an ankle replacement is a viable option, but whether an ankle replacement is the correct option in a specific situation.

The causes and treatment options for varus and valgus ankles are presented in Tables 1 and 2.

Table 1. Cause and treatment options for varus ankles.

Varus ankle	
Cause	**Treatment**
Bone erosion — usually post-traumatic.	Tibial bone cut might correct the alignment.
Bone erosion and lateral ligament laxity.	Tibial bone cut helps, but ligament balancing also needed.
Lateral ligament laxity and hindfoot deformity.	Ligament balancing and hindfoot and/or forefoot correction.

Table 2. Cause and treatment for valgus ankles.

Valgus ankle	
Cause	**Treatment**
Bone erosion — usually post-traumatic.	Tibial bone cut might correct the alignment.
Bone erosion and lateral ligament instability.	Tibial bone cut helps, but ligament balancing also needed.
Posterior tibial tendon dysfunction (PTTD) with deltoid rupture.	Very difficult and complex to repair. Include deltoid and extensive foot reconstruction. Might not be suitable for TAR.

LEG ALIGNMENT

Malalignment at the ankle can be caused, or accentuated, by malalignment of the entire extremity. Some deformities are simple to recognise, for example extreme genu varum or valgum, and it is obvious that it should be corrected. Subtle genu varum or valgum deformities will also influence the ankle replacement. The authors believe that the tibial alignment should follow the mechanical axis of the leg, which does not always correspond to the anatomical axis. It is recommended to take full-length standing X-rays of both lower extremities as part of the preoperative work-up (Figure 1).

Any deformity in the leg will negatively affect the ankle by tilting the ankle joint which can lead to shear stresses within articular cartilage, as well as changes in contact pressures.

These deformities need to be corrected prior to addressing the ankle by replacement. It is not only mandatory to reduce the contact pressure on the replaced ankle, but there is also evidence that one might actually delay the need for a replacement by correcting the alignment and reducing the pressure (Pagenstert *et al.*, 2007; Stamatis *et al.*, 2003).

Contact surface area can decrease by up to 40% with angular malalignment, creating increased contact pressures in residual surface contact. Contact pressures are maximised as the level of the deformity gets closer to the ankle joint. Tarr *et al.* (1985) found that distal tibial deformities created the highest contact pressures, with sagittal plane deformities having the greatest effect. A 15° anterior bow caused a 40% increase in contact pressure, while posterior bowing of 15° caused a 42% increase.

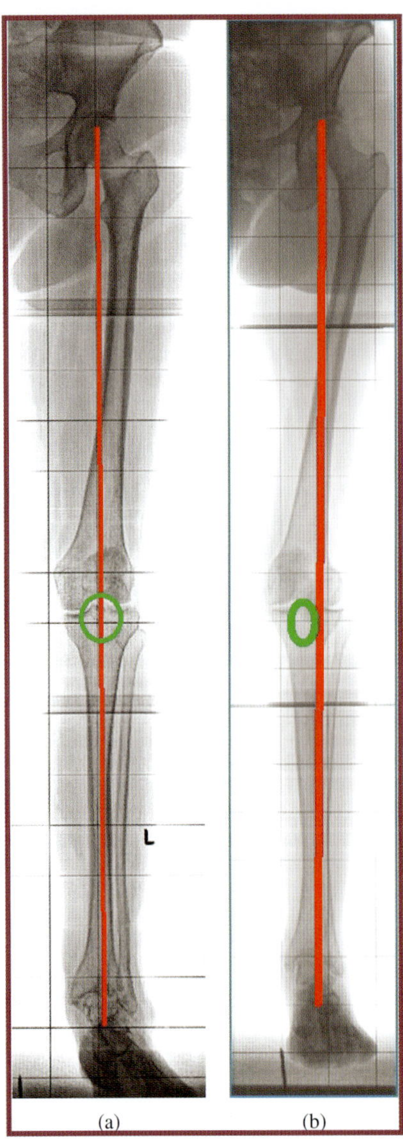

Figure 1. *Long leg standing X-rays should be standard preoperative protocol for total ankle replacement planning. The ideal ankle should be perpendicular to the mechanical axis. If there is a varus or valgus malalignment of the leg, the mechanical and tibial axis might not be the same. This will change to the position of the external tibial rod placement in preparation for the tibial bone cut. (a) The mechanical axis goes through the center of the tibial tuberosity. The alignment guide (if used) can therefore be placed center over the tibial tuberosity. (b) A valgus knee due to lateral compartment DJD is shown here. The mechanical axis runs through the lateral compartment. The tibial alignment guide (if used) should be lateral to the center of the proximal tibia. If the implantation is being performed using Patient Specific Instrumentation (PSI) this planning takes place preoperatively based on 3 dimensional scanning.*

FOOT ALIGNMENT

A stable plantigrade foot is essential for a successful ankle replacement. Specific attention should be given to the muscle balance of the foot. In valgus deformities it is common to have a chronic posterior tibial tendon dysfunction with secondary foot deformities. In varus ankles the peroneal tendons might be compromised. Certain trends are common — a cavo-varus foot with varus ankle deformities, and a plano-valgus foot in valgus ankles. Failure to address these issues will compromise the long-term result of the ankle replacement.

The preoperative X-rays should include long leg alignment films and weight bearing foot X-rays. The lateral ankle view should include the entire foot.

VARUS ANKLES

As mentioned above one should look at the entire leg when determining all the factors contributing to the deformity. There might be a supramalleolar deformity, in addition to a hindfoot varus that needs to be corrected. Once all the extra-articular deformities are noted, one can concentrate on the ankle joint itself. Not all varus ankles are created equal. The varus deformity could be due to bone erosion alone, a combination of bone erosion and lateral instability, or due to primarily ligamentous instability (Figures 2–4).

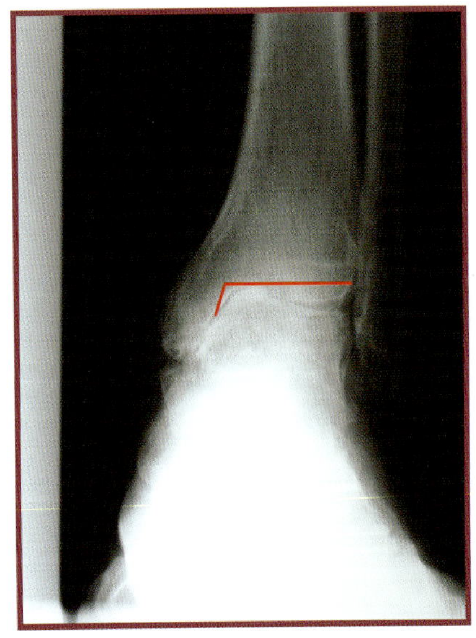

Figure 2. *Most of the varus in this ankle is due to true posttraumatic bone erosion. The patient sustained a severe pilon fracture 10 years ago, and presented with a stiff painful ankle. Clinical examination showed no varus/valgus instability and limited plantar flexion and dorsiflexion with the usual dense scar tissue from multiple surgeries. This is classified as a stage 1 varus ankle and is easily corrected with the normal tibial bone cut required for a TAR.*

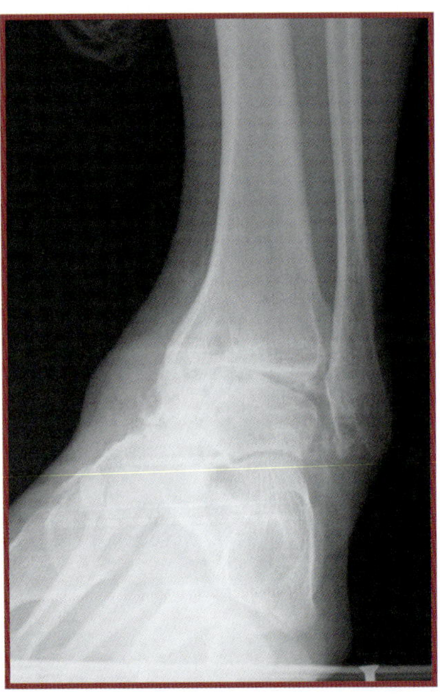

Figure 3. *In this example, there is medial tibial erosion, but also obvious lateral ankle instability. This ankle, we classify as a stage 2 varus ankle, will need more than a simple correction of the bone alignment. A lateral ligament reconstruction will be critical to the success of the ankle replacement.*

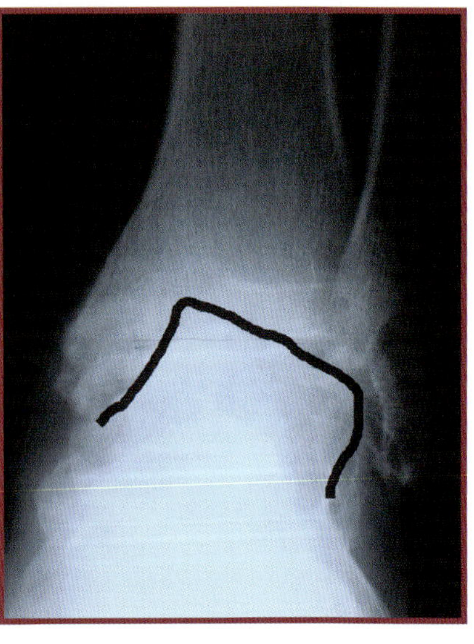

Figure 4. *Severe collapse of the ankle into varus with secondary subtalar joint changes. This ankle, which we classify as stage 3 varus, is a very difficult ankle to reconstruct, even with adding a lateral ligament reconstruction and may require the subtalar joint to be addressed.*

Table 3 describes the various types of varus deformity which in the authors opinion show a progressively more complex problem that is more difficult to manage. In this chapter we describe how to manage the various stages.

Table 3. Classification of varus deformity at the ankle.

Stage 1
- Varus due to medial bone erosion or tibial plafond malunion.
- No or minimal lateral instability.
  - Usually posttraumatic after ankle or tibial plafond fractures.
- No ectopic bone medial or lateral.
- No widening of the lateral joint line.
- No subluxation of the subtalar joint.

Stage 2
- Medial bone erosion and lateral ligament instability/ insufficiency.
  - Could be postfracture, but majority due to chronic lateral instability.
  - Could be completely, or partially passively corrected.
- Widening of the lateral joint line.
- Ectopic bone mainly lateral along the talus, preventing reduction of the talus in the mortise.
- No subluxation of the subtalar joint.

Stage 3
- Fixed deformity with severe medial malleolar and plafond bone erosion and complete lateral ligament instability.
- Not passively correctable.
- Widening of the lateral joint line.
- Subtalar joint subluxed with fixed hindfoot varus or valgus.

MANAGEMENT OF VARUS DEFORMITIES

Most varus deformities can be corrected if a stepwise diligent approach is used, and one does not stop until the ligament balance is equal and the bone alignment corrected.

Deformity correction should be performed from proximal to distal. Significant knee malalignment is dealt with a knee replacement or appropriate distal femur or proximal tibia osteotomy. As a general rule, deformity of more than 10° should probably be addressed and is usually performed as a separate staged procedure.

Tibial shaft alignment/angulation issues of more than 10° are usually posttraumatic and should also be addressed prior to the ankle replacement.

Subtle alignment issues above the ankle joint might not need surgical correction, but care should be taken to take them into account when placing the external tibial cutting guide. In the end, the distal tibial cut should be perpendicular to the mechanical axis of the leg and parallel to the floor (Figure 5).

The surgical approach to the ankle is the same for varus or valgus deformities. The standard midline anterior incision in the interval between extensor hallucis longus and tibialis anterior is used to expose the ankle.

The additional surgical procedures to correct the alignment at the ankle depend on the severity and mechanism of the varus deformity.

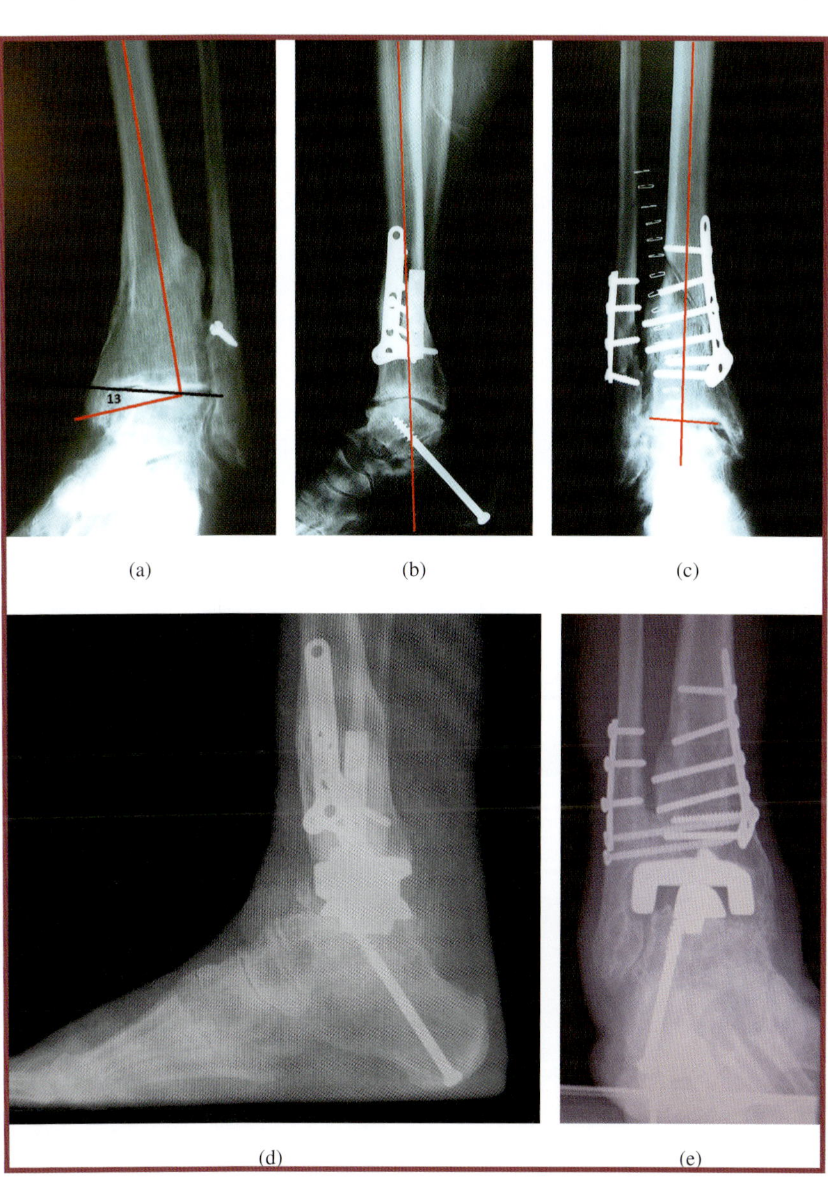

Figure 5. *(a) An AP view showing a 13° varus through the ankle joint after a previous tibial/fibula fracture malunion. Note, there was also a 30 degree recurvatum of the tibia on the lateral radiograph. (b,c) A biplane corrective osteotomy was done to realign the mechanical axis of the tibia. The patient did fine for about 1 year, before a TAR was done as a second stage. (d,e) 8 years after the corrective osteotomy of the tibia, 7 years after the ankle replacement. Alignment is excellent and there is minimal signs of subsidence and no clinical problems.*

STAGE 1 VARUS

This usually presents with posttraumatic bone erosion or, more commonly, tibial plafond malunion with little if any ligamentous laxity. The majority of these will be relatively simple where the tibial bone cut will resolve the varus bone erosion. The initial distal tibia bone cut should be perpendicular to the long axis of the tibia/mechanical axis of the leg — and not parallel to the joint line. The external cutting guide should be placed with care, and fluoroscopy should be used to ensure the alignment of the cutting block prior to making the first cut. The tibial cut should be at least at the level of the most proximal part of the erosion. This usually means that very little bone is removed from the medial tibial plafond, while more bone is removed from the lateral side of the tibia. There should be adequate tensioning on the ligaments to ensure stability of the ankle. This might be more predictable with an ankle replacement system that has several options in polyethylene insert thickness (Figure 6).

It is important to test the varus valgus stability of the ankle once the trial components are in place. If there is a significant discrepancy in medial/lateral stability, it has to be corrected. The options will be discussed below.

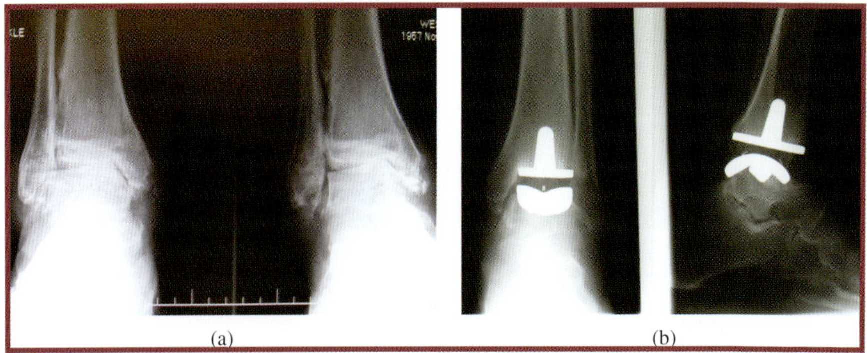

Figure 6. *(a) and (b) Preoperative X-rays show mild bony erosion on the AP and mortise views. On the postoperative X-rays it is obvious that the deformity was completely corrected with an appropriate distal tibial bone cut and tensioning of the ligaments with the correct thickness polyethylene spacer.*

STAGE 2 VARUS

A combination of factors contributes to the difficulty obtaining reduction and correction with varus ankle deformities. On the lateral side there is invariably heterotopic bone built-up in the gutter, involving the lateral side of the talus and the medial side of the distal fibula.

The medial malleolus is often eroded, resulting in shortening or contracture of the deltoid ligament, medial capsule and tibialis posterior tendon sheath. Without addressing both gutters it will be impossible to rotate the talus back into the mortise.

The lateral gutter debridement is fairly uniform among surgeons. An osteotome or chisel is used to aggressively remove the osteophytes from the lateral talus and medial fibula. There should be no bone block to reduction/rotation of the talus. If it is still not possible to rotate the talus back in place, one can assume the medial structures are tight.

There are different methods of releasing the medial structures. Some surgeons prefer to release the deep deltoid from the talus by sliding an osteotome or knife down the medial border of the talus until the entire deep portion is released. Great care should be used not to damage the neurovascular structures on the medial side. This approach works well if the ligament imbalance was not overly severe (see Table 4).

Table 4. Methods of balancing the medial side of the joint in a varus ankle.

Mild medial contracture	Slide osteotome down the medial talus to release the deep deltoid of the talus.
Severe medial contracture	Release all or nearly all of the superficial and deep deltoid by dissecting a periosteal/ligament flap of the medial malleolus, starting anterior, working posterior. Might also include the tibial posterior tendon sheath.
Mild or severe contracture	Distal sliding osteotomy of the medial malleolus.

Others advocate releasing the deltoid of the medial malleolus in one large, complete ligament/periosteal flap. The advantage is that one can do a complete or near complete release of the deltoid to balance severe discrepancies between medial and lateral stability. The medial flap usually scars down fairly quickly, and iatrogenic valgus instability has not proven to be an issue.

An alternative to a deltoid release is to perform a medial malleolar distal sliding osteotomy. With an ankle replacement where the medial malleolus is not compromised, the procedure is fairly simple. Distal displacement of the medial malleolus creates a functional lengthening of the deltoid ligament complex without destabilising the medial structures. Advocates of this procedure feel that as a rule internal fixation is not necessary, and the period of immobilisation after the replacement should be enough to allow the osteotomy to heal. There is however a real concern that the osteotomy will weaken the medial malleolus, and lead to non- or delayed union, which in turn will delay the start of range and motion and rehabilitation. It is technically easy, but the complications might outweigh the potential benefits.

Once the ankle joint is mobile and passively correctable to neutral in the ankle mortise, the hindfoot alignment is evaluated. If there is a tendency to a varus deformity below the ankle, a lateralising or lateral closing wedge calcaneal osteotomy should be done to correct the mechanical axis. This is done through a 5 cm incision along the lateral border of the calcaneus. The sural nerve and peroneal tendons are protected (usually anterior to the incision). A small retractor is placed halfway between the Achilles insertion and subtalar joint and wrapped around the superior border of the calcaneus. A second retractor is placed plantarly around the calcaneus. If there is a true calcaneus varus a lateral closing wedge osteotomy is done and immobilised with a staple and/or screw. If the plan is to move the mechanical axis more laterally to protect the lateral ligament repair, a lateralising calcaneal osteotomy is done. The maximum the calcaneus can translate safely is about 10 mm. The lateralising osteotomy is immobilised with a screw (Figure 7).

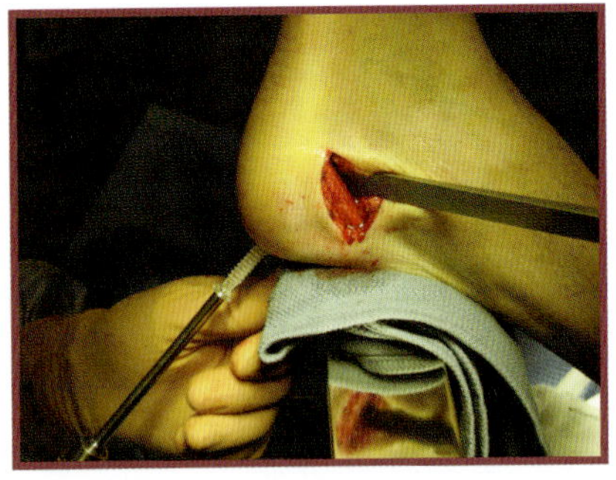

Figure 7. *Significant lateral translation of the plantar aspect of the calcaneus to change the mechanical axis of the hindfoot to correct a varus thrust.*

With the components in place the ankle is tested for stability and ligament balance. In about 50% of cases the ankle will be adequately balanced at this point, especially if an aggressive medial release was done. Tensioning is done by adding polyethylene thickness. It is also important to remember to start by taking very little bone from the tibia in a very lax ankle.

However, if there is more than 3 mm difference in laxity there should be a low threshold to add a lateral ligament reconstruction to ensure long-term stability (see Table 5). In some cases there is little, if any true ligamentous tissue left on the lateral side after chronic instability.

A Brostrom lateral ligament repair is still the mainstay procedure, but there are cases where the lateral tissue is thin and attenuated due to long-standing instability. If there is a good tissue, a Brostrom should suffice. If not, an augmentation should be added.

My (CC) preferred augmentation method in TAR is a very simple, reliable, non-anatomic repair using part of the peroneus brevis tendon. This technique is used in older, low demand patients, or if there is insufficient tendon length to bring it down to the talar neck. A separate lateral incision is used to expose the lateral side of the ankle and peroneal tendons. Through this incision the lateral gutter debridement is done or completed. Once the final ankle replacement components are in place, a Brostrom type lateral repair is done (Figure 8).

Table 5. Options for lateral ankle ligament reconstruction.
• Conventional Brostrom repair if there is adequate tissue.
• Non-anatomic repair using peroneus brevis.
• Use of a split peroneus brevis tendon in a anatomic reconstruction If the peroneal tendon is healthy and in good condition.
• Anatomic allograft reconstruction.   o If the peroneus is compromised or if it is the surgeons choice to use allograft.

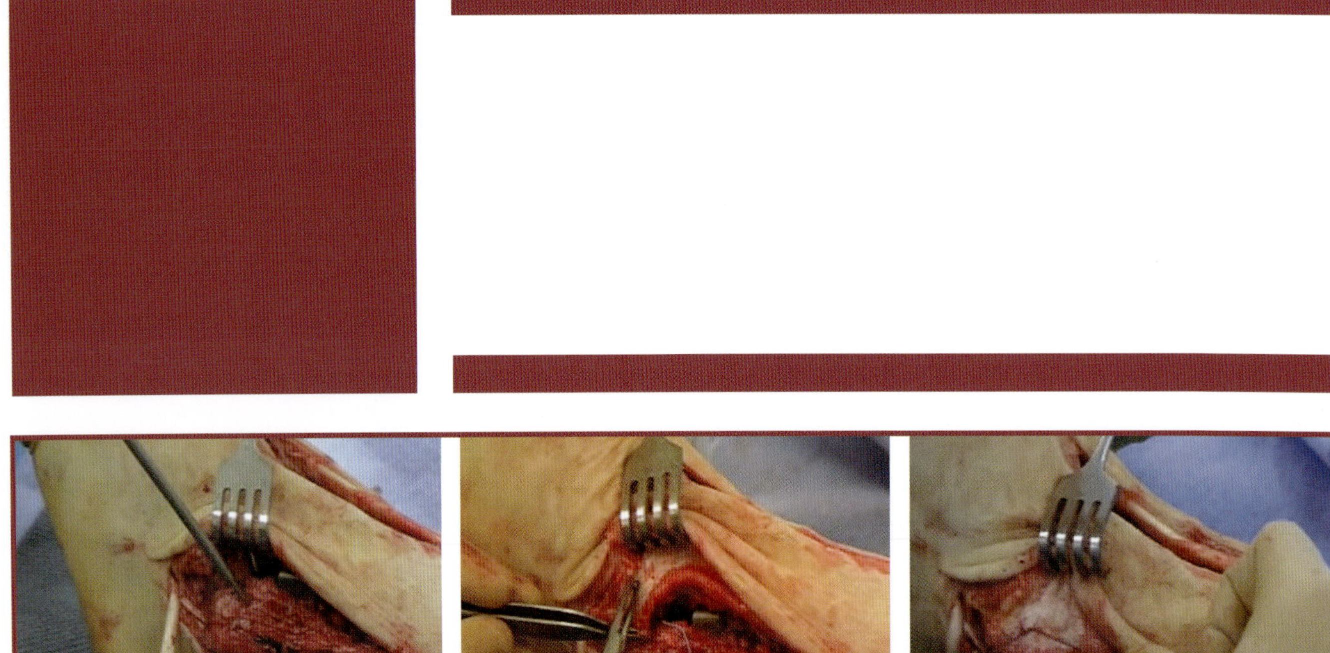

(a)   (b)   (c)

Figure 8. *(a)–(c) With the initial dissection, the soft tissue flap is left intact on the talus and calcaneus. This allows for a Brostrom type lateral ligament repair. The soft tissue flap is advanced in a single layer and anchored into the fibula with bone anchors.*

As a rule, one half of the peroneus brevis tendon is harvested. If the tendon has signs of pathology or a tear, the entire tendon is used with the assumption that a diseased tendon would not work as a motor, but could be used for a static repair. The distal attachment is kept intact, and the tendon is harvested as far proximal as possible. The peroneus brevis is then routed over the Brostrom repair over the lateral side of the ankle to the anterolateral tibia. Under adequate tension it is secured with a staple onto the tibia. This is done under enough tension to prevent the joint from tilting into varus, but one should not pull the joint into valgus either. This is a non-anatomic repair and will limit inversion, but not necessarily anterior drawer stability. The Brostrom repair appears to add enough anterior translational stability in addition to the inherent anterior stability of the joint replacement components.

Other options are more conventional repairs. A split peroneus brevis, other autologous or allograft tendon could be used as a near anatomic repair of the calcaneofibular ligament. The distal attachment in the 5th metatarsal is kept intact, while half of the tendon is harvested as far proximal as possible. The tendon is then routed through a drill hole in the fibula and anchored under adequate tension with the ankle in neutral varus/valgus alignment and at 90°. The stump of the tendon could also be anchored to the talar neck under tension.

Another option is to do a true anatomic repair. I (CC) usually use a semitendinosus allograft. The reasoning is two-fold. The peroneus brevis is a natural everter of the foot. By using it to do a lateral ligament repair, you "sacrifice" a secondary stabiliser of the ankle. Even the best peroneal autograft has limited length. With an allograft there is no limit in how the tendon is routed or fixed (Figure 9).

A drill hole is made from the "footprint" of the calcaneal attachment of the calcaneofibular ligament on the lateral side of the calcaneus in a plantar medial direction. The allograft tendon is then routed from lateral to plantar medial into the calcaneus. A drill hole is then made at the tip of the fibula to exit anterior on the fibula — roughly where the CFL and ATFL attachments would have been. The tendon is routed through this drill hole and pulled down to the talar neck. A drill hole is made through the talar neck from the footprint of the talar attachment of the ATFL through the talus to the medial side. With the ankle in neutral in all planes the tendon is tensioned by pulling medial on both the talar and calcaneal sutures attached to the tendon and tenodesis screws inserted on the lateral side of the talus and calcaneus. This method allows for long bone tunnels through the talus and calcaneus, easy tensioning and fixation, and therefore reliable reconstruction (Figure 10).

At this point the foot is re-evaluated and associated deformities corrected. Once the ankle ligaments are stable, the foot alignment should be assessed. If there is forefoot driven hindfoot varus (plantarflexed first ray) a dorsal closing wedge osteotomy should be done of the 1st metatarsal. If it is felt that some of the varus is due to an over pull of the peroneus longus, the longus should be lengthened or preferably tenodesed to the brevis to act as an everter instead of a 1st ray plantar flexor.

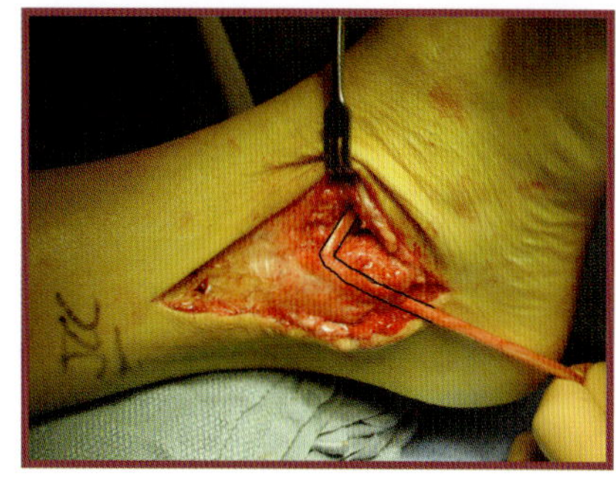

Figure 9. *With an allograft, or free tendon graft, there is enough length to do an anatomic reconstruction of the lateral ligament complex.*

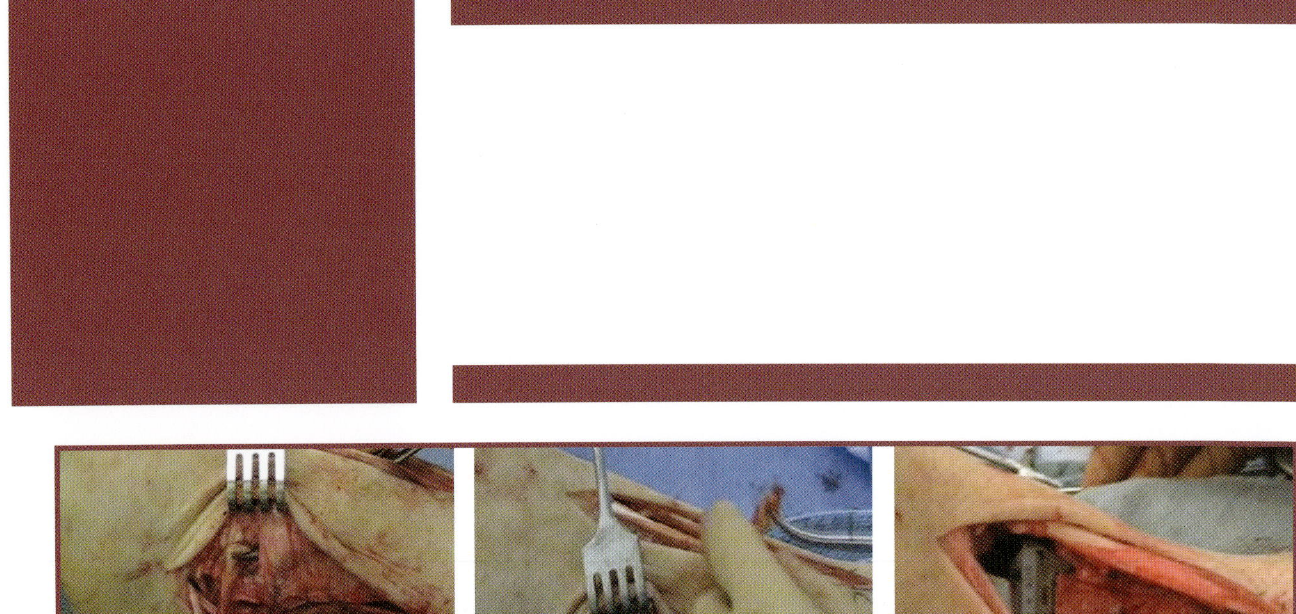

Figure 10. *(a)–(c) Half of the peroneus brevis is rerouted over the Brostrom ligament repair, anterior over the lateral side of the ankle joint and fibula. It is then anchored to the tibia under adequate tension to provide a very strong check reign to inversion.*

It is very seldom that a subtalar or talo-navicular fusion is done at the same time, unless if it is done secondary to a chronic tibialis posterior tendon dysfunction. We have moved away from fusing these two joints at the time of the TAR, even if they appear to be arthritic on X-rays. The fact that the ankle moves better after the replacement, appears to protect the surrounding joints and one might be able to avoid or delay fusions. Fusing the talo-navicular or subtalar joint at the time of the TAR also poses a theoretical higher risk of creating a serious vascular insult to the talus.

STAGE 3 VARUS

There is definitely a school of thought that these severe, complex varus or valgus deformities are better treated with a fusion instead of a replacement (Smith and Wood, 2007). In contrast, more recent work from the Canadian Group suggests that more complex patients (COFAS 3&4) may do better from an ankle replacement than a fusion (Penner, 2018).

The basic approach is the same as for a Stage 2, but the subtalar and midfoot instability should also be addressed. These patients will need either a subtalar or a triple arthrodesis to correct and stabilise their hindfoot prior to the ankle replacement and lateral ligament repair.

They are at best unpredictable and should not be attempted until the surgeon is completely comfortable with straightforward cases. It might be best to do this as a two stage procedure. The first stage will be a correction of the foot deformity and ligament imbalance. It usually includes a subtalar or triple arthrodesis, forefoot surgery as needed, and a lateral ligament reconstruction. Once this is healed the ankle replacement is done.

If there is significant bone erosion it might force the issue to do it all as a one stage procedure. This is a major undertaking and should be very well planned.

VALGUS DEFORMITIES

Not all valgus deformities on X-ray are due to medial ligament compromise. In fact, a large percentage of mild to moderate valgus deformity on weightbearing imaging studies are a result of chronic lateral instability. This will become apparent during the replacement, and should then be dealt with as discussed above (Figure 11).

A clinical indication that the valgus is due to a lateral instability is a normal foot.

The other end of the spectrum are the true, and often severe, valgus deformities, almost always secondary to chronic failure of the medial structures and PTTD. In these situations over time the

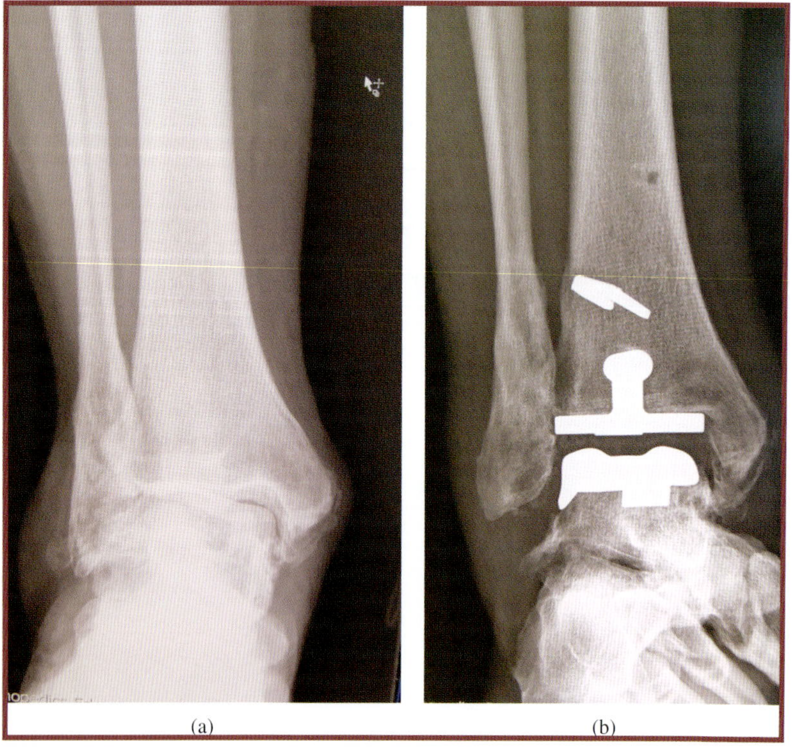

(a)   (b)

Figure 11. *(a) This is an example of an ankle that was in a little valgus on X-ray, but proofed to be a lateral ligament instability during surgery. (b) A lateral ligament reconstruction was done anchoring the peroneus brevis into the tibia with a staple.*

Table 6. Causes and treatment for valgus deformity in the ankle.	
Posttraumatic lateral bone erosion or collapse (similar to stage 1 varus).	Usually correctable with standard tibial bone cut.
Uneven wear due to lateral ligament instability, especially if syndesmotic instability. (Yes, it can cause a valgus collapse; not always varus!).	Manage like a stage 2 varus ankle, but a deltoid release is seldom indicated. Lateral reconstruction should be done.
Chronic tibialis posterior tendon dysfunction with secondary deltoid failure and forefoot changes.	Very difficult to salvage. A deltoid reconstruction is needed as well as an extensive mid and forefoot reconstruction. Best option might be an ankle fusion.

progressive valgus force results in deltoid ligament dysfunction and incompetence. In end stage cases there will be severe dorso-lateral peri-talar subluxation and a fixed valgus of the talus in the mortise.

Additionally there could be compensatory forefoot deformities including forefoot supination due to medial column instability. As mentioned, the severe foot deformities might be the clue that this is a deltoid instability valgus, and not a lateral ligament issue (Table 6).

The general approach is similar to that of a varus ankle. With a valgus ankle there might be medial gutter bone overgrowth that should be removed. A limited lateral release should be done to allow the talus to reduce in the mortise.

A valgus deformity can be more difficult to correct than a varus deformity. There is no local structure (peroneus brevis on the lateral side) to reliably replace the deltoid ligament with. A primary deltoid repair is never strong enough. If there is a decent tibialis posterior tendon left it could be used as a ligament substitution. It can be left attached distally and under tension anchored into the medial malleolus or distal tibia. This is a non-anatomical repair and has proven to be unreliable at best.

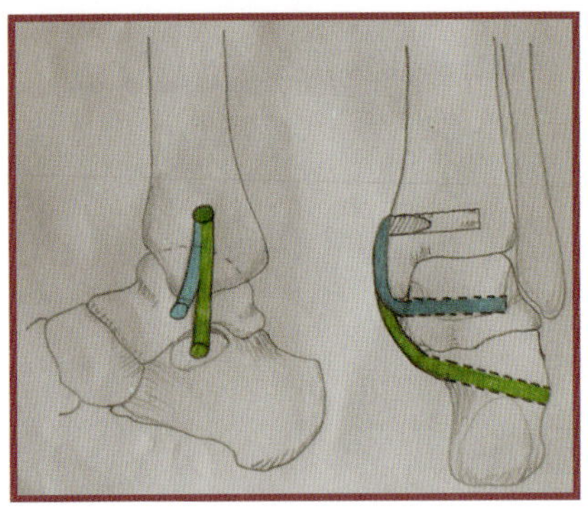

Figure 12. *Illustration of the medial allograft technique where two ends of tendon allografts are inserted into the body of the talus and sustentaculum of the calcaneum and then appropriately tensioned and fixed to the medial tibia with a biotenodesis screw.*

Myerson advocated an allograft technique where he creates a deep and superficial deltoid. It is anchored into the distal tibia and two grooves are created to attach one arm in the talus and one in the calcaneus (Gibson and Prieskorn, 2007) (Figure 12).

It is advisable to correct the foot deformities prior to the ankle replacement (Gauvain *et al.*, 2017). In mild to moderate deformities, this could include a medialising calcaneal osteotomy, PTT repair and augmentation with flexor Digitorum longus (FDL) tendon, gastrocnemius slide and medial ray stabilisation if indicated.

In longstanding PTTD, the foot deformity should be addressed either before or as part of the TAR. If there is minimal erosion or collapse of the ankle joint, it might be more predictable to correct the foot and stabilise the deltoid as a first stage, and then do the ankle replacement later. This could include a talo-navicular, subtalar, or triple arthrodesis to correct and stabilise the hindfoot. With the hindfoot reduced under the ankle the forefoot will almost inevitably be in forefoot supination. This is corrected with a plantar flexion fusion through the naviculo-cuneiform or cuneiform-1st metatarsal joint. With the foot stabilised the deltoid is tested. If there is an obvious instability, the deltoid ligament should be repaired/reconstructed. The patient should be immobilised for at least 6 weeks to allow soft tissue and bony healing. We believe one should re-examine the ankle at 3 to 6 months before going ahead with an ankle replacement. If the ankle appears to be stable an ankle replacement could be attempted. If the deltoid reconstruction failed even with the foot reconstruction an ankle replacement is not indicated, and fusion should be considered (Figure 13).

In some cases, there will be significant lateral erosion of the talus or tibia secondary to the longstanding valgus force on the ankle. In these cases reconstruction of the foot without correcting the ankle joint at the same time will lead to certain failure of the deltoid repair. The ankle replacement and foot reconstruction should therefore be done as a single procedure. This is a major endeavour, and the failure rate is fairly high. The cost benefit ratio should be carefully weighed. It might be best to fuse these ankles (Figure 14).

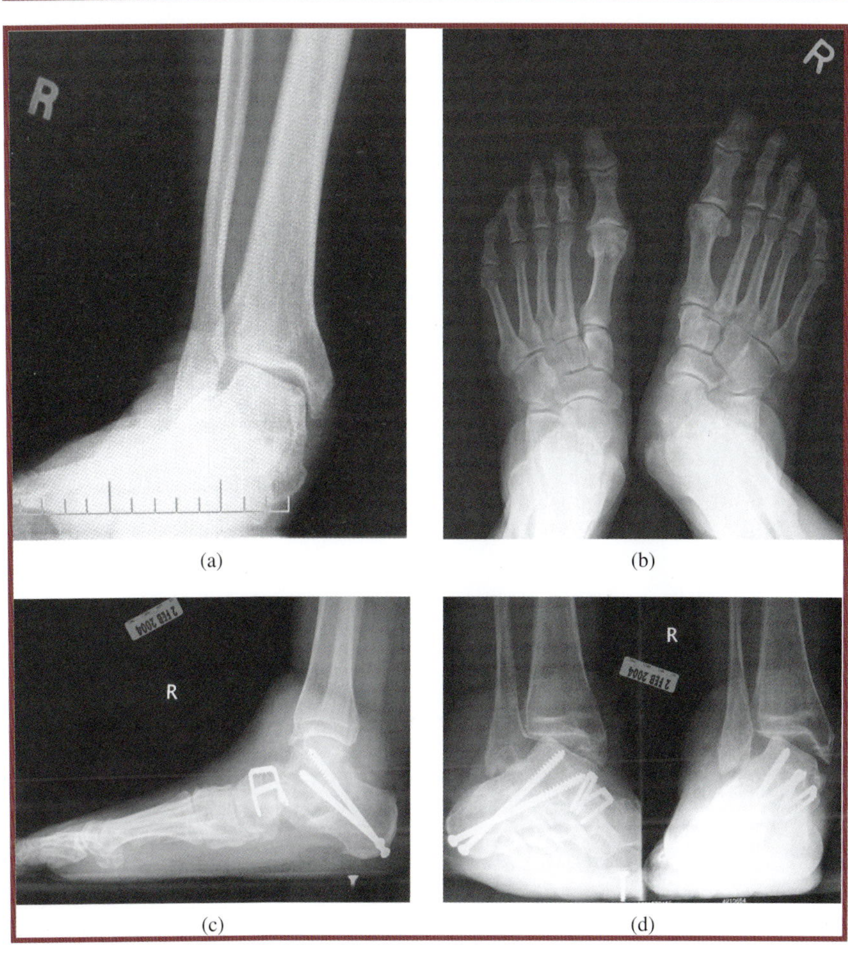

Figure 13. *(a)-(d) This patient presented with a grade 3 PTTD and chronic deltoid instability. The ankle joint was not eroded. The decision was made to do a triple arthrodesis and deltoid repair as a first stage — or even definitive treatment. Even with this aggressive approach the patient return 3 months later with even a more severe deformity. The only salvage at this point is an ankle fusion.*

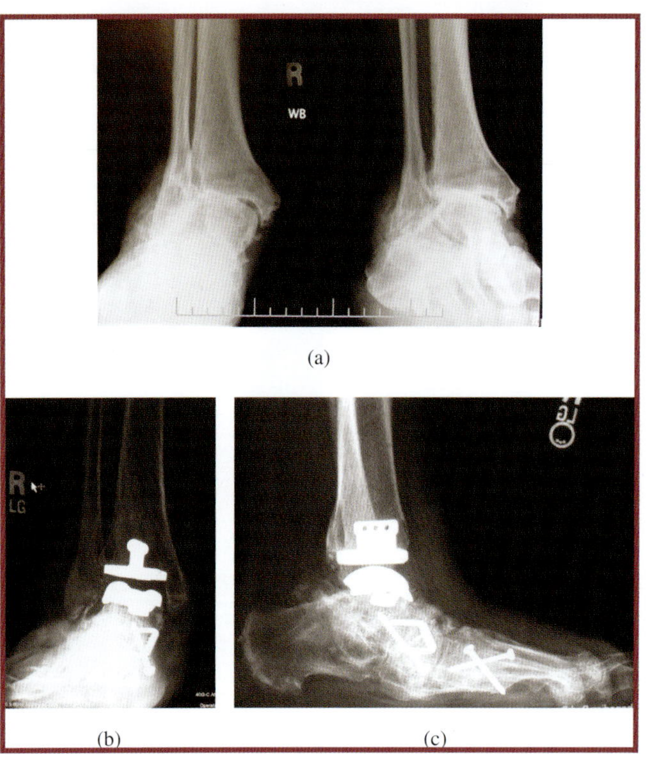

Figure 14. *(a, b) This patient presented with a longstanding tibialis posterior tendon dysfunction, Grade 4, with severe erosion of the ankle resulting in a fixed deformity. If a TAR is considered one has to correct the foot and ankle in a single setting. This is always a major endeavour and the failure rate might be unacceptably high. (c) A lateral view 6 months after a simultaneous TAR, deltoid reconstruction, subtalar, and talonavicular fusion as well as a 1st tarso-metatarsal fusion to correct a forefoot supination deformity. All the fusions healed and the alignment is reasonable. Figure 14(b) however show the ankle already collapsing back into valgus, with failure almost inevitable.*

CONCLUSIONS

It is likely that one will encounter a large percentage of patients with complex deformities around the ankle. Alignment issues are fairly simple to address and there is universal acceptance that it should be done, either prior to, or at the time of the replacement.

Varus or valgus deformities at the ankle create some controversy, especially when it comes to whatever method is best or most reliable. There is no controversy however, for the need to have perfect balance between the medial and lateral stability of the ankle.

In the end the surgeon should experiment and determine which method, or combination of techniques yields the most reproducible result in their hands.

There is agreement that most varus deformities are amenable to reconstruction.

Severe valgus, especially with deltoid insufficiency, has the highest failure rate, and should be attempted with great caution. In most hands the best treatment for those will still be a fusion.

Even though it might technically be possible to do, the complication rate, especially early failure rates can be unacceptably high.

REFERENCES

Gauvain, T. T., Hames, M. A. & Mcgarvey, W. C. 2017. Malalignment correction of the lower limb before, during, and after total ankle arthroplasty. *Foot Ankle Clin*, 22, 311–339.

Gibson, V. & Prieskorn, D. 2007. The valgus ankle. *Foot Ankle Clin*, 12, 15–27.

Pagenstert, G. I., Hintermann, B., Barg, A., Leumann, A. & Valderrabano, V. 2007. Realignment surgery as alternative treatment of varus and valgus ankle osteoarthritis. *Clin Orthop Relat Res*, 462, 156–168.

Penner, M. J., Wing, K., Glazebrook, M. & Daniels, T. 2018. The effect of deformity and hindfoot arthritis on midterm outcomes of ankle replacement and fusion: A prospective COFAS multi-centre study of 890 patients. *Foot Ankle Orthop*, 3, S107–S108. https://doi.org/10.1177/2473011418S00098.

Smith, R. & Wood, P. L. 2007. Arthrodesis of the ankle in the presence of a large deformity in the coronal plane. *J Bone Joint Surg Br*, 89, 615–619.

Stamatis, E. D., Cooper, P. S. & Myerson, M. S. 2003. Supramalleolar osteotomy for the treatment of distal tibial angular deformities and arthritis of the ankle joint. *Foot Ankle Int*, 24, 754–764.

Tarr, R. R., Resnick, C. T., Wagner, K. S. & Sarmiento, A. 1985. Changes in tibiotalar joint contact areas following experimentally induced tibial angular deformities. *Clin Orthop Relat Res*, 199, 72–80.

ANKLE REPLACEMENT IN COMORBIDITY

K. Georg and N. Espinosa

Summary

The indications for total ankle replacement (TAR) has extended greatly from simple isolated ankle joint degeneration into cases with complex foot deformity or instability. In addition, TAR has been increasingly employed in patients with significant comorbidities such as diabetes, inflammatory arthritis, or neurological disease. This chapter outlines the specific surgical and perioperative considerations that need to be addressed when managing patients with significant associated comorbidities.

INTRODUCTION

Over the last 40 years the design, instrumentation, and surgical technique of total ankle replacement (TAR) have considerably improved. Despite the fact that mid- to long-term outcomes are not comparable to those in hip or knee arthroplasty, TAR certainly has become a viable alternative to ankle fusion. In addition, a growing knowledge of TAR biomechanics and additive surgical procedures (e.g. osteotomies, ligament reconstructions, etc.) provide a new base to extend the indications from simple degenerative joint disease into those cases with simultaneous complex foot deformity or instability.

Besides this, TAR is considered in patients with comorbidity such as diabetes, inflammatory arthritis, or neurological disease. This chapter aims to give an overview over considerations that have to be made in these patient groups and reports on outcomes published in the literature.

The following points speak in favour of TAR when treating secondary and end-stage ankle arthritis:

- Joint replacement preserves motion and a more normal gait pattern consequently decreasing stress on the midfoot and subtalar joints lowering the risk of subsequent joint degeneration.
- Patients suffering from ankle joint degeneration due to systemic disease often present with bilateral pathology. While ankle arthrodesis may give good mid- to long-term functional results if performed unilaterally, this may be less so if performed bilaterally.

- Postoperative mobilisation after TAR can be allowed full weight-bearing and protected in a walker if no additional corrective osteotomies, joint fusions, or ligament reconstructions are performed. Therefore, muscle wastage is lower than if a non-weight-bearing regimen is required after ankle fusion. Furthermore, patients with systemic disease often suffer from additional upper limb problems, impeding mobilisation on crutches, thus making them wheel-chair bound after surgery if weight-bearing is not allowed. Therefore, the postoperative rehabilitation is likely to be faster and better tolerated in these patients who frequently present with poor muscle function.
- Patients with systemic disease frequently have an adapted lifestyle with decreased physical demands. Theoretically, this may lead to longer implant survival.

RHEUMATOID ARTHRITIS AND OTHER INFLAMMATORY DISEASE

About 10–50% of patients with rheumatoid arthritis suffer from hindfoot involvement often combined with a planovalgus deformity (Schill and Wetzel, 2011; Rippstein and Naal, 2011). In contrast, varus deformity develops 3 times less frequently (Wood *et al.*, 2007).

When considering TAR in a rheumatoid patient, any hindfoot deformity must be addressed in order to balance the hindfoot and to achieve good short- to long-term clinical outcomes (Saltzman, 2000). Small hindfoot deformities (usually less than 10° of tilt) may be corrected using the cutting jig while preparing the tibial and talar surfaces (Barg *et al.*, 2012) (Figure 1). In contrast, when there is a hindfoot valgus of more than 10°, additional interventions have to be considered depending on severity and location of deformity.

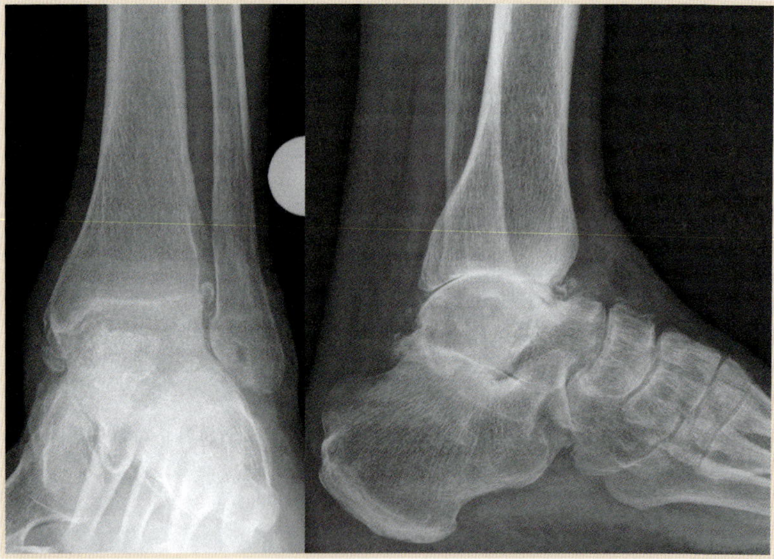

Figure 1. *Anteroposterior and mediolateral X-rays of a 49-year-old patient with severe ankle joint degeneration due to rheumatoid arthritis. Typically, generalised joint space narrowing and subchondral sclerosis is found. Osteophyte formation is minor. Absence of a severe deformity makes this patient an ideal candidate for joint replacement; however, subtalar fusion may additionally be required for symptomatic osteoarthritis.*

Procedures may include supramalleolar osteotomy, lengthening/ rotational osteotomy of the distal fibula, corrective calcaneal osteotomy (sliding osteotomies, lateral column lengthenings, etc.), medial ligament reconstruction, or corrective fusions (Barg *et al.*, 2012).

Besides deformity aspects and concomitant adjacent joint arthritis, concerns in rheumatoid patients include bone fragility and an elevated risk of infection (Besse *et al.*, 2010).

Investigating risk factors for incision-healing complications after total ankle arthroplasty Raikin *et al.* (2010) showed that underlying inflammatory arthritis increased the risk for major wound complications requiring reoperation by an odds ratio of 14. Several studies have shown that the continuation of immunosuppressive medications with steroids, methotrexate, or even tumour-necrosis factor-alpha does not increase the risk of perioperative infection (Bibbo and Goldberg, 2004; Jain *et al.*, 2002). It is therefore been suggested to continue disease suppressive treatment in these patients during the perioperative period (Sean *et al.*, 2012; Hayashi *et al.*, 2012; Wood *et al.*, 2007).

Another concern when implanting a TAR in patients suffering from inflammatory joint disease is the poor bone stock due to prolonged steroid administration. Bone quality plays an important role for stable fixation; however, the limits of permissible bone-density are not known (Bibbo, 2013). Studies have found that the bone quality in rheumatoid patients is sufficient for stable fixation of arthroplasty implants, and sufficient to allow protected full weight-bearing during the postoperative rehabilitation (Rippstein and Naal, 2011). Any identified bone cyst may be filled with allo- or autograft (Bibbo, 2013).

Another possible complication due to poor bone stock is the increased risk of medial malleolar fracture. In our practice, and if there is a possible risk of intraoperative fracture of the medial malleolus, we perform prophylactic percutaneous screw fixation before starting joint preparation for the prosthesis whilst care is

taken to avoid medial notching during tibial preparation
(San Giovanni *et al.*, 2006).

There remains a paucity of long-term results available in the literature
regarding TAR implantations in patients with rheumatoid arthritis.
However, mid-term results are promising with survival rates of
80–95% and revisions rates of 5–20% reported (Hirao *et al.*, 2017;
Kraal *et al.*, 2013; Schill and Wetzel, 2011). Registry data showed
5-year survival rates in patients with rheumatoid arthritis not
statistically significantly different from non-rheumatoid patients
(Henricson *et al.*, 2007). A summary of published series on ankle
replacement in patients with inflammatory arthritis is given in Table 1.

Table 1. Published series on ankle replacement in patients with inflammatory arthritis.

Publication	Number of ankles/patients (patients)* Implant**	Follow-up	Clinical and radiological outcome***	Complications/revisions
Bonnin *et al.* (2011)	23/? (87) Salto	Mean 8.9 years	Mean AOFAS score improved from 22 to 76.3 (±14.8) (not statistically significant different to score reached by osteoarthritis group)	3 revisions in rheumatoid group: • 1 deep infection • 1 polyethylene fracture • 1 tibial cyst
Doets (2006)	93/76 (93) BP	Mean 8 years	Satisfaction rate 84% (good to excellent) Mean AOFAS Score 77 (73–81) Mean KAS 76 (72–97) Survival rate at 8 years 84%	Early complications: • 20 malleolar fractures • 11 distal tibial fractures • 8 impaired wound healing • 3 infection Revision rate 16.1%: • 6 aseptic loosening • 2 deep infection • 6 axial deformity • 1 impaired wound healing

Table 1   (*Continued*)

Publication	Number of ankles/patients (patients)* Implant**	Follow-up	Clinical and radiological outcome***	Complications/revisions
Kofoed (1995)	13/11 (25) STAR	Mean 9.5 years	Mean KAS 92 (no statistically significant difference between the osteoarthritis and rheumatoid arthritis group for the first 10 years)	Revision rate 2.7% (overall): • 1 deep infection No malleolar fracture
Jensen and Linde (2009)	33/26 (26) TPR	Max 23 years	Survival rate at 5 years 91% Survival rate at 10 years 85%	
Nishikawa *et al.* (2004)	27/21 (21) TNK	Mean 6 years (1–14)	Mean AOFAS score 66 (32–90) Survival rate at 14 years 77% Rad. 48% tibial component sintering, 33% talar sintering	• 10 aseptic loosening (3 revised) • 1 impaired wound healing • 1 malleolar fracture
Schill and Wetzel (2011)	38/38 (38) STAR	10–15 years	Satisfaction rate 77% good-excellent Rad. 13% talar component sintering	Revisions for: • 5 impaired wound healing • 2 severely impaired wound healing requiring surgical flap • 4 conversions to arthrodesis • 6 exchange of inlay • 2 exchange talar component
	43/100 (?) TARIC	Min 2 years	Mean AOFAS score improved from 41 to 76	2 revisions
San Giovanni *et al.* (2006)	31/31 (23) BP	Mean 8 years (5.0–12.2)	Mean AOFAS score 81 (40–92) Satisfaction rate 89% Rad. 82% implants stable	Revision Rate 6.4% Intraoperative malleolar fractures 32% Postoperative complication rate 29%: • 4 wound dehiscence • 4 stress fractures • 1 medial malleolar non-union

(*Continued*)

Table 1   (*Continued*)

Publication	Number of ankles/patients (patients)* Implant**	Follow-up	Clinical and radiological outcome***	Complications/revisions
Su (2004)	27 Second gen.	Mean 6.4 years	Mean AOFAS score 81 Rad. 88.5% implants stable	Rad 11.5% tibial lytic zones
Van der Heide *et al.* (2009)	58/54 (54) BP/STAR	Mean 2.7 years (1–9)	Mean KAS 73 (21–92) Survival rate 92%	Revision rate (removal) 9.6%: • 4 deep infection • 1 aseptic loosening Complications: • 13 malleolar fracture • 1 post. Tibial plafond fracture
Wood (2007)	211/201 (201) STAR/BP	—	Survival rate at 8 years 88%, improved to 97% for those with well-preserved preoperative hindfoot alignment Survival rate at 10 years 83%	9% malleolar fracture 15% impaired wound healing (reduced to 3% with surgeons' increased experience)

Notes:
*Number of ankles/patients with inflammatory arthritis included/Total number of patients included in the study.
**BP: Buechel-Pappas (Endotec); Salto (Tornier); STAR: Scandinavian TAR (Small Bone Innovations); TARIC (Implantcast);
TNK: Takakura-Nara-Kyocera (Kyocera); TPR: Thompson-Parkridge-Richards.
***AOFAS: American Foot and Ankle Society Hindfoot-Score (max 100 points); KAS: Kofoed Ankle Score (max 100 points).

TAR is a valuable option when treating rheumatoid patients. Mid-term results compare favourably to patients with primary or post-traumatic osteoarthritis. Even though wound healing problems and malleolar fractures are a concern in rheumatoid patients, perioperative complication rates are acceptable. In some series, in spite of the potentially increased risk, significantly lower complication rates in rheumatoid patients have been found (3%) when compared with patients suffering from either primary or posttraumatic osteoarthritis (10%) (Rippstein and Naal, 2011; Rippstein *et al.*, 2011).

The use of cement in ankle arthroplasty is controversial. In a recent series of ankle replacements in Japanese rheumatoid patients who underwent a cemented mobile bearing implant, although the mid-term patient-reported outcomes and implant retention rate were satisfactory, the radiographic findings were less so, with migration of the tibial component and subsidence of the talar component found in 21.1% and 28.9% ankles, respectively (Yano *et al.*, 2019).

GOUTY ARTHRITIS

With a prevalence of up to 3%, gout is a very common inflammatory arthritic condition (Harris *et al.*, 1995). In 44–67% of patients, gout attacks the first metatarsophalangeal joint; however, up to 26% of patients reported the first occurrence at the ankle joint (Chen *et al.*, 2003; Roddy *et al.*, 2007). Despite this, severe ankle osteoarthritis secondary to gout is rare (Saltzman *et al.*, 2005). Recurrent gouty attacks, synovitis, and implant failure have been shown after total hip or knee replacement and may also be a concern for total ankle replacement (Barg *et al.*, 2011a; Blyth and Pai, 1999; Freehill *et al.*, 2010; Ortman and Pack, 1987).

The only study reviewing results after TAR in gouty arthritis has been published by Barg *et al.* (2011c). The study included a group of 16 patients with a mean preoperative duration of gout of 7.8 years (range 2.3–26.7 years) in whom 19 ankle joint replacements were performed. No intra- or perioperative complications occurred.

Revisions were necessary in one patient with bilateral aseptic implant loosening 4.7 years after primary joint replacement and in one patient, a medial sliding osteotomy had to be performed due progressive valgus deformity. At a mean follow-up of 5.1 years (2.1–9.1 years), average VAS pain scores had significantly decreased from 7.5 (5 to 10) to 1.2 (0 to 3), AOFAS hindfoot scores had significantly increased from on average 38 (15 to 77) to 75 (64 to 92) points and all categories of the SF-36 score were significantly improved. No patient recalled recurrent gouty attacks and all but one patient were satisfied with the result of the procedure. These results are comparable to other series dealing with TAR in terms of rate of complications, revisions, and functional improvement. Thus, with the limitations of the sparse knowledge we have so far, there is no contraindication to TAR in patients with gouty arthritis. However, an interdisciplinary approach must always be considered when treating these patients.

HAEMOPHILIA

When treating haemophiliac patients, providing them with adequate substitution of factors is absolutely important in order to avoid orthopaedic interventions. Prophylactic supplementation that starts in early childhood has been shown to be beneficial and cost-effective and may prevent or halt destructive processes within the target joints (ankle, elbow, knee, and shoulder) (Berdel *et al.*, 2010). However to date, there remain many patients who receive insufficient factor replacement and improper physical therapy. In combination with poor patient education, these factors are responsible for recurrent intra-articular bleeds and consecutive synovitis — both of which lead to haemophilic arthropathy (Serban *et al.*, 2008). The pathophysiology of chondral damage is a consequence of chronic inflammation and the direct toxic effects of blood (Pasta *et al.*, 2008). Cyst formation is common and secondary to multiple bleeds, and can be extensive.

Due to recurrent bleeds into the growth plate, deformities may develop (usually valgus deformities) leading to malalignment with altered force transmissions across the hindfoot and local overloads enhancing the detrimental effect of joint destruction (Pasta *et al.*, 2008).

Over time and with ongoing ankle arthropathy, anterior distal tibia osteophyte formation results in reduced dorsi-flexion of the ankle joint leading to a fixed equinus deformity.

Sequentially, the midfoot joints become overloaded and deteriorate (Berdel *et al.*, 2009).

Talar flattening may occur, resulting in a planovalgus deformity (Pasta *et al.*, 2008) (Figure 2).

It is therefore important to appreciate the pathomechanisms and possible spectrum of foot deformity aspects that can be encountered whilst planning surgery on haemophilic patients.

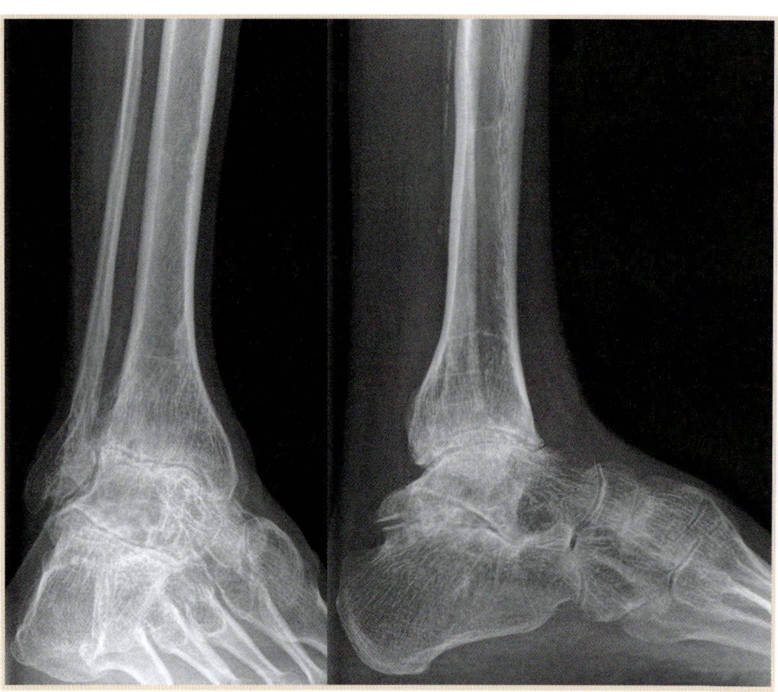

Figure 2. *Anteroposterior and mediolateral X-rays of a 55-year-old patient suffering from advanced haemophiliac arthropathy. Joint line valgus malalignment likely due to growth disturbance following bleedings into the epiphyseal plate is present. Anterior osteophyte formation limits ankle dorsal extension. Beginning talar flattening can be observed.*

In the very early stage of disease and when only chronic synovitis but no severe ankle arthropathy is present, arthroscopic synovectomy and debridement can be considered and may be of value (Rodriguez-Merchan EC, 2017).

In case of concurrent deformity, corrective osteotomies are effective to balance the hindfoot, and in the presence of equinus deformity an Achilles tendon lengthening procedure (open) represents a powerful option.

However, in case of end-stage ankle arthritis, either ankle fusion or TAR should be taken into consideration (Serban *et al.*, 2008).

As the disease commonly shows bilateral affliction, preservation of residual joint motion to maintain a more normal gait pattern and to protect adjacent joints from secondary degeneration appears to be a reasonable approach. TAR therefore represents a viable option.

When performing TAR on patients with haemophilia, there are specific concerns. Wound healing problems due to recurrent bleeding are critical. The soft-tissue coverage around the ankle is less when compared with the hip or knee and therefore even a small hematoma and persistent bleeding in the postoperative period may cause impaired wound healing. Meticulous intraoperative haemostasis and proper perioperative application and control of factor substitution are therefore mandatory. Another issue is the insufficient talar bone stock due to flattening of the talus, which makes proper placement of the talar component more difficult. Under some specific circumstances, this problem may be overcome using a bone block augmentation on top of the talus, to implant the talar component (Scholz and Scholz, 2008), but extreme caution must be used, as it is possible that the flattening is secondary to avascular necrosis.

With regard to the data obtained from the literature, some studies on hip and knee arthroplasty in patients with haemophilia report higher rates of aseptic loosening and deep infection (Bossard *et al.*, 2008; Preis *et al.*, 2017). In contrast, there are only a limited number of studies on the outcome of ankle arthroplasty in haemophilic patients. However, as summarised in Table 2, these report acceptable mid-term outcomes with low complication rates. In experienced hands, ankle arthroplasty can therefore be seen as a valuable alternative to ankle fusion, but peri- and postoperative management of the patients has to be organised in close collaboration with an experienced haematologist (Preis *et al.*, 2017).

Table 2. Summary of case series reporting on ankle replacement in patients with haemophilia.

Publication	Number of ankles/ patients Implant*	Follow-up	Clinical and radiological outcome**	Complications/revisions
Eckers *et al.* (2017)	12	Mean 9.6 years (3.3–17.8)	Estimated implant survival was 94% at 5, 85% at 10 and 70% at 15 years, respectively. Pain score 2/10 (range, 0–6) on the VAS. Range of motion (ROM) had increased significantly. The AOFAS hindfoot score averaged 81 points (range, 73–90). All radiographs revealed component loosening or periprosthetic radiolucency.	Three cases required revision surgery.
Preis *et al.* (2017)	14	Mean 5.8 years (2.0–9.2)	VAS significantly decreased from 8.5 +/– 0.9 (range = 0.8–10) to 1.3 +/– 1.6 (range = 0–6). Significant functional improvement including ROM and American Orthopaedic Foot and Ankle Society (AOFAS) hindfoot score was observed.	One patient sustained an intraoperative medial malleolar fracture. In two patients, delayed wound healing was observed. In one patient, open arthrolysis was performed due to painful arthrofibrosis.
Barg *et al.* (2010)	10/8 Hintegra	Mean 5.6 years (2.7–7.6)	AOFAS score improved from mean 38 (8–57) to 81 (69–95). VAS pain score decreased from 7.1 (4–9) to 0.8 (0–3). ROM increased from on average 18.3° (0–34°) to 27.3° (15–35°). Rad. 100% of components stable.	No intra- or perioperative complications. 1x Revision: • 1x arthrolysis and Achilles tendon lengthening due arthrofibrosis.
Van der Heide *et al.* (2006)	5/3 (3) BP	Median 4.3 years (1–8.7)	AOFAS score improved from 35–40 to 87–90. Rad 100% of components stable.	None

Notes:
*BP: Buechel–Pappas (Endotec); Hintegra (Integra LifeScience).
**AOFAS: American Foot and Ankle Society Hindfoot-Score (max 100 points); VAS pain score: Visual analogue pain score (max 10 points); ROM: ROM.

HEREDITARY HAEMOCHROMATOSIS

Hereditary hemochromatosis is an autosomal recessively inherited disease leading to iron overload due to increased intestinal absorption. The most commonly underlying mutation is estimated to be found homozygous in 1 of 200 individuals (Carlsson, 2009). The classic clinical triad of hemochromatosis is a darkened skin, diabetes, and cirrhosis (bronze diabetes). However, it occurs in end-stage disease and is rarely seen in orthopaedic practice where most patients present with fatigue and non-specific arthritis — often the first manifestation of disease. Besides the metacarpophalangeal joints several authors consider the ankle as a target joint in patients suffering from hemachromatosis. In most patients, onset of ankle pain starts before the age of 45 years. An increased sensitivity to cartilage damage or reduced reparative capacity has been postulated (Carlsson, 2009). Phlebotomy to decrease iron load does not substantially relieve joint pain, unlike its effects on other symptoms of the disease. The radiographic pattern of ankle osteoarthritis has been reported to be predominantly anterolateral joint space narrowing, bony eburnation, osteophyte formation, and cysts in the distal tibia or talus in the anterior aspect of the joint (Figure 3) (Carlsson, 2009).

In the absence of other systemic diseases or history of trauma in patients below 55–60 years of age with longstanding ankle pain, laboratory testing (including iron levels, iron-binding capacity, and serum ferritin levels) may be determined and genetic testing be performed if iron-saturation levels are above 50% or elevated ferritin levels are found (Carlsson, 2009).

When preparing the patient for surgery it is important to take into consideration any cardiomyopathy or impaired liver function that could potentially lead to coagulopathy.

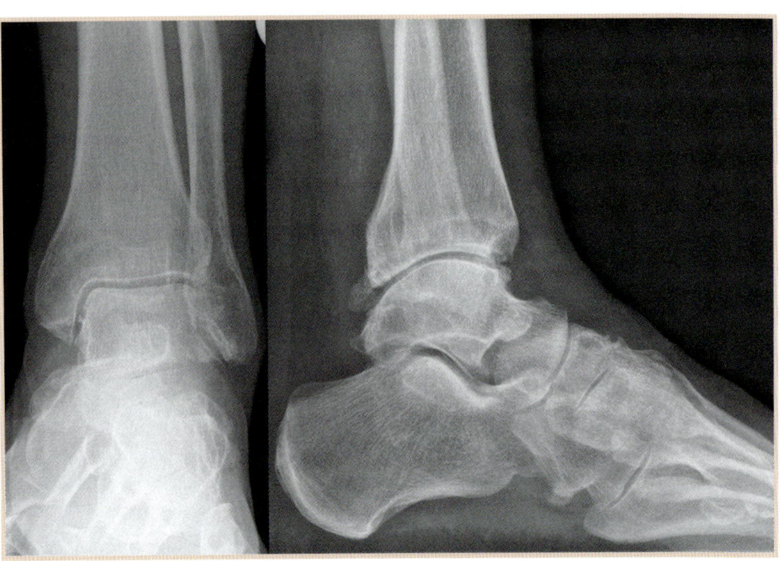

Figure 3. *Anteroposterior and mediolateral X-rays of a 62-year-old patient with intermittent ankle pain due secondary arthritis in hemochromatosis. Joint space width is still largely preserved. Beginning anterolateral especially talar-sided osteophyte and cyst formation may be noted.*

Not much has been published regarding the treatment of patients suffering from hemochromatosis. Table 3 summarises the most important studies. So far, the largest series of TAR in haemochromatosis patients was published by Barg *et al.* in 2011. All 16 patients (five with bilateral ankle replacement) had substantial pain relief at an average follow-up of 5.3 years with a rate of revision similar to that reported in other series not exclusively treating hemochromatosis patients (Barg *et al.*, 2011a).

Table 3. Case series of TAR with hemochromatosis patients included (published after 1999).

Publication	Number of ankles/ patients* implant**	Follow-up	Clinical and radiological outcome***	Complications/revisions
Barg *et al.* (2011a)	16/21 (16) Hintegra	Mean 5.3 years (range 3.1–8.6)	Pain VAS decreased from average 6.7 to 1.9. AOFAS Score increased from average 46 to 84. SF-36 improved for all categories. Rad. no implant loosening.	No wound healing problems. Intraoperative complications: • 1x A.dorsalis pedis artery laceration at concomitant tarsometatarsal arthrodesis. 4x Reoperations: • 1x debridement of a tibial cyst. • 1x subfibular debridement and lateral ligament reconstruction. • 2x arthrolysis with Achilles tendon lengthening.
Carlsson (2009)	7/10 (7)	—	No information on outcome or complications given.	
Davies and Saxby (2006)	4/5 (4) STAR	3–4 years	Outcome: Reported by all patients as favourable.	Intraoperative complication: • 1x medial malleolar fracture.
Fevang *et al.* (2007)	4/4 (257)	—	Norwegian Arthroplasty Registry. No details on the subgroup of patients with haemochromatosis given.	
Hintermann (1999)	2/2 (50) STAR	Min. 1 year	No details on patients with hemochromatosis given, higher satisfaction and AOFAS-pain scores for patients with systemic disease or primary osteoarthritis as compared to patients with posttraumatic osteoarthritis.	
Hosman *et al.* (2007)	2/2 (202)	—	New Zealand National Joint Registry. No details on the subgroup of patients with haemachromatosis given.	

Notes:
*Number of patients/ankles with hemochromatosis, in brackets: total number of ankle replacements included in the case series with or without hemochromatosis.
**Hintegra (Integra); STAR: Scandinavian TAR (small bone innovations).
***AOFAS: American Foot and Ankle Society Hindfoot-Score (max 100 points); VAS pain score: Visual analogue pain score (max 10 points); ROM: range of motion.

DIABETES

As for total hip or knee replacement diabetes is not an absolute contraindication to ankle replacement surgery (Bibbo, 2013). However, the patient must be compliant and well-treated with diabetic therapy and the surgeon must rule out significant secondary complications such as vascular disease, neuropathy (including Charcot arthropathy), and impaired immunosystem function (Wukich *et al.*, 2010). Wukich *et al.* showed in series of over 1000 patients who underwent any type of orthopaedic foot and ankle surgery an up to five-fold increased risk of postoperative infection in diabetic patients (13.2% vs 2.8% in non-diabetic patients (Wukich *et al.*, 2010) and 9.5% vs 3.5%, respectively (Wukich *et al.*, 2011)). Patients with well-adjusted and uncomplicated diabetes do not reveal any increased risk of infection (Wukich *et al.*, 2010).

The presence of peripheral neuropathy seems to be a major risk factor regarding the development of infection (Armstrong *et al.*, 2006; Costigan *et al.*, 2007; Wukich *et al.*, 2010). During clinical examination, it is mandatory to verify any loss of peripheral sensibility, diminished Achilles tendon reflexes and sense of vibration. In addition — and where needed — a neurophysiological examination may be advised before indicating joint replacement surgery.

Particular attention to vascular status must be paid if patients concomitantly have a history of nicotine abuse. The anterior ankle skin coverage is always thin and vulnerable. In the company of peripheral arterial occlusive disease, the risk of impaired wound healing is increased. Thus, proper handling of soft tissues is essential to avoid that complication. Sometimes preoperative angiography is needed to estimate the risk. When impaired perfusion is confirmed, TAR is contraindicated.

Surgical site infection puts the patient at risk for periprosthetic joint infection. For total hip and knee replacements in diabetic patients, several studies have shown an increased risk for periprosthetic infection within the first year postoperative (Iorio *et al.*, 2012; Jamsen *et al.*, 2010, 2012; Peersman *et al.*, 2001). Pedersen *et al.* (2010) have shown an increased risk for total hip replacement revision due to deep infection in a mid- to long-term follow-up with a relative risk of 1.43. In a study by Malinzak *et al.* (2009), diabetic patients were three times as likely to develop periprosthetic joint infection as non-diabetics at a minimum 2-year follow-up. Choi *et al.* (2014) showed that patients in a diabetic group had significantly higher failure rates of primary TAR than in the non-diabetic group. The uncontrolled diabetic subgroup had a significantly poorer outcome than the non-diabetic group and a higher rate of delayed wound healing. The incidence of early-onset osteolysis was higher in the diabetic group than in the non-diabetic group. These results suggest that diabetes mellitus, especially with poor glycaemic control, negatively affects the short- to mid-term outcome after TAR. In a retrospective study of 813 primary TARs with 50 diabetic patients, TAR was found to provide pain relief and improve function in patients with diabetes and ankle arthritis. While patients with diabetes were heavier and had worse ASA preoperative grades, they did not have a significantly different complication or infection rate to the non-diabetic population (Gross *et al.*, 2015).

In conclusion, TAR in our opinion is not an absolute contraindication in diabetic patients; however, sequels of diabetes should be ruled out preoperatively and diabetic control should be optimised. Patients qualifying for joint replacement should be informed of their increased risk of deep infection not only perioperatively, but also in a mid- to long-term view.

NEUROLOGICAL DISORDERS

Neuromuscular disorders are often considered a contraindication to TAR as muscle function is needed for proper balancing. Progressive loss of muscle strength or contraction may corrupt a primarily well-functioning prosthesis. However, one must be aware of the natural history of a neuromuscular disease and patients with a stationary functional deficit for example due to cardiovascular stroke or peroneal palsy may nevertheless be treated with ankle replacement if accompanied with selected tendon transfers (as shown by Bibbo (2013) and Bibbo *et al.* (2011)).

Morgan *et al.* reported on a case in which a TAR was performed in a patient with polio with satisfactory muscle function who had a subjectively excellent outcome at 2.5 years postoperatively (Morgan *et al.*, 2012). Beside these case reports, we are not aware of publications reporting on the outcome of TAR in patients with neuromuscular disorders and we believe ankle replacement in this group of patients can only be indicated in a few carefully selected cases.

GENERALISED HYPERMOBILITY

Ligamentotaxis is of great importance for ankle arthroplasty to ensure adequate tension at and around the tibiotalar joint. Lack of ligamentous restraint with recurrent subluxations places the joint at risk for continuous edge loading with early failure or even dislocation.

TAR has been suggested to be absolutely contraindicated in generalised widespread hyperlaxity (Besse *et al.*, 2010), but each patient must be considered on their merits.

OBESITY

The proportion of overweight patients continually increases in industrialised nations and obesity has been recognised as a risk factor for a poor outcome in hip and knee arthroplasty (Bourne *et al.*, 2007).

For ankle arthroplasty, continuously increased load may also lead to an early implant failure. However, Baker *et al.* (2009) reviewed the data on 36 such patients after ankle replacement and after a follow-up of mean 5 years no association with reduced outcome or need for secondary surgery was found. Gross *et al.* (2016) also found no difference in complication, infection, or failure rates in obese patients, but did find lower FAOS pain and SF-36 scores at mean 44.7-month follow-up.

A larger case series of overweight patients with a BMI > 30 kg/m^2 was published by Barg *et al.* (2011b). They evaluated 123 TARs in 118 patients over a follow-up period of 2 to 10 (mean 5.7) years. The total AOFAS scores improved in these patients from 35 (range 8–78) points to 75 (51–95) points; intraoperative complications occurred in 7.3% and 18.7% underwent some type of secondary surgery. Implant revision or conversion to arthrodesis, due to aseptic loosening, had to be performed in six patients resulting in a 6-year survival rate of 93%. Of note, they recorded a rate of deep venous thrombosis over twice as high compared to the rate observed in all patients who underwent TAR (9.8% vs 3.9%).

Schipper *et al.* (2016) showed that there was a significantly reduced 5-year survival in patients with a BMI of > 30 and more than 5-years follow-up (mean 7.7 years). In a review of the literature, 17.8% of patients with a BMI > 30 and >12-months follow-up developed a complication requiring a revision surgical procedure. The most commonly reported surgeries were revision of the metallic components and ankle gutter debridement (Sansosti *et al.*, 2017).

While necessity of general antithrombotic prophylaxis in hindfoot surgery is still under debate, it should therefore be considered in these patients.

Overall, there is not enough clear evidence to class obesity as a contraindication to TAR.

REFERENCES

Armstrong, D. G., Lavery, L. A., Frykberg, R. G., Wu, S. C. & Boulton, A. J. 2006. Validation of a diabetic foot surgery classification. *Int Wound J*, 3, 240–246.

Baker, J. F., Perera, A., Lui, D. F. & Stephens, M. M. 2009. The effect of body mass index on outcomes after total ankle replacement. *Ir Med J*, 102, 188–190.

Barg, A., Elsner, A., Hefti, D. & Hintermann, B. 2010. Haemophilic arthropathy of the ankle treated by total ankle replacement: A case series. *Haemophilia*, 16, 647–655.

Barg, A., Elsner, A., Hefti, D. & Hintermann, B. 2011a. Total ankle arthroplasty in patients with hereditary hemochromatosis. *Clin Orthop Relat Res*, 469, 1427–1435.

Barg, A., Knupp, M., Anderson, A. E. & Hintermann, B. 2011b. Total ankle replacement in obese patients: Component stability, weight change, and functional outcome in 118 consecutive patients. *Foot Ankle Int*, 32, 925–932.

Barg, A., Knupp, M., Kapron, A. L. & Hintermann, B. 2011c. Total ankle replacement in patients with gouty arthritis. *J Bone Joint Surg Am*, 93, 357–366.

Barg, A., Pagenstert, G. I., Leumann, A. G., Muller, A. M., Henninger, H. B. & Valderrabano, V. 2012. Treatment of the arthritic valgus ankle. *Foot Ankle Clin*, 17, 647–663.

Berdel, P., Schott, D., Pagenstert, G., Pennekamp, P., Oldenburg, J., Wirtz, D. C., Seuser, A. & Gravius, S. 2009. Upper ankle joint prostheses in haemophilia patients. *Hamostaseologie*, 29(Suppl 1), S65–S68.

Berdel, P., Pagenstert, G., Randau, T., Schott, D., Taubner, A., Oldenburg, J., Seuser, A., Wirtz, D. C. & Gravius, S. 2010. Algorithm for the treatment of the haemophilic arthropathia of the upper ankle joint. *Hamostaseologie*, 30(Suppl 1), S93–S96.

Besse, J. L., Colombier, J. A., Asencio, J., Bonnin, M., Gaudot, F., Jarde, O., Judet, T., Maestro, M., Lemrijse, T., Leonardi, C., Toullec, E. & L'afcp 2010. Total ankle arthroplasty in France. *Orthop Traumatol Surg Res*, 96, 291–303.

Bibbo, C. & Goldberg, J. W. 2004. Infectious and healing complications after elective orthopaedic foot and ankle surgery during tumor necrosis factor-alpha inhibition therapy. *Foot Ankle Int*, 25, 331–335.

Bibbo, C., Baronofsky, H. J. & Jaffe, L. 2011. Combined total ankle replacement and modified bridle tendon transfer for end-stage ankle joint arthrosis with paralytic dropfoot: Report of an unusual case. *J Foot Ankle Surg*, 50, 453–457.

Bibbo, C. 2013. Controversies in total ankle replacement. *Clin Podiatr Med Surg*, 30, 21–34.

Blyth, P. & Pai, V. S. 1999. Recurrence of gout after total knee arthroplasty. *J Arthroplasty*, 14, 380–382.

Bonnin, M., Gaudot, F., Laurent, J. R., Ellis, S., Colombier, J. A. & Judet, T. 2011. The salto total ankle arthroplasty: Survivorship and analysis of failures at 7 to 11 years. *Clin Orthop Relat Res*, 469, 225–236.

Bossard, D., Carrillon, Y., Stieltjes, N., Larbre, J. P., Laurian, Y., Molina, V. & Dirat, G. 2008. Management of haemophilic arthropathy. *Haemophilia*, 14(Suppl 4), 11–19.

Bourne, R., Mukhi, S., Zhu, N., Keresteci, M. & Marin, M. 2007. Role of obesity on the risk for total hip or knee arthroplasty. *Clin Orthop Relat Res*, 465, 185–188.

Carlsson, A. 2009. Hereditary hemochromatosis: A neglected diagnosis in orthopedics: a series of 7 patients with ankle arthritis, and a review of the literature. *Acta Orthop*, 80, 371–374.

Chen, S. Y., Chen, C. L., Shen, M. L. & Kamatani, N. 2003. Trends in the manifestations of gout in Taiwan. *Rheumatology (Oxford)*, 42, 1529–1533.

Choi, Wj, L. J., Lee M., Park Jh, Lee, Jw. 2014. The impact of diabetes on the short- to mid-term outcome of total ankle replacement. *Bone Joint J*, 96-B, 1674–1680.

Costigan, W., Thordarson, D. B. & Debnath, U. K. 2007. Operative management of ankle fractures in patients with diabetes mellitus. *Foot Ankle Int*, 28, 32–37.

Davies, M. B. & Saxby, T. 2006. Ankle arthropathy of hemochromatosis: a case series and review of the literature. *Foot Ankle Int*, 27, 902–906.

Doets, H. C., Brand, R. & Nelissen, R. G. 2006. Total ankle arthroplasty in inflammatory joint disease with use of two mobile-bearing designs. *J Bone Joint Surg Am*, 88, 1272–1284.

Eckers, F., Bauer, D. E., Hingsammer, A., Sutter, R., Brand, B., Viehofer, A. & Wirth, S. H. 2017. Mid- to long-term results of total ankle replacement in patients with haemophilic arthropathy: A 10-year follow-up. *Haemophilia*, 24(2), 307–315.

Fevang, B. T., Lie, S. A., Havelin, L. I., Brun, J. G., Skredderstuen, A. & Furnes, O. 2007. 257 Ankle arthroplasties performed in Norway between 1994 and 2005. *Acta Orthop*, 78, 575–583.

Freehill, M. T., Mccarthy, E. F. & Khanuja, H. S. 2010. Total knee arthroplasty failure and gouty arthropathy. *J Arthroplasty*, 25, 658 E7–E10.

Gross, G. C., Green, C. L., Deorio, J. K., Easley, M., Adams, S., Nunley, J. A., II. 2015. Impact of diabetes on outcome of total ankle replacement. *Foot & Ankle Int*, 36, 1144–1149.

Gross, C. E., Lampley, A., Green, C. L., DeOrio, J. K., Easley, M., Adams, S. & Nunley, J. A., II. 2016. The effect of obesity on functional outcomes and complications in total ankle arthroplasty. *Foot & Ankle Int*, 37, 137–141.

Harris, C. M., Lloyd, D. C. & Lewis, J. 1995. The prevalence and prophylaxis of gout in England. *J Clin Epidemiol*, 48, 1153–1158.

Hayashi, M., Kojima, T., Funahashi, K., Kato, D., Matsubara, H., Shioura, T., Kanayama, Y., Hirano, Y. & Ishiguro, N. 2012. Effect of total arthroplasty combined with anti-tumor necrosis factor agents in attenuating systemic disease activity in patients with rheumatoid arthritis. *Mod Rheumatol*, 22, 363–369.

Henricson, A., Skoog, A. & Carlsson, A. 2007. The Swedish ankle arthroplasty register: an analysis of 531 arthroplasties between 1993 and 2005. *Acta Orthop*, 78, 569–574.

Hintermann, B. 1999. Short- and mid-term results with the Star total ankle prosthesis. *Orthopade*, 28, 792–803.

Hirao, M., Hashimoto, J., Tsuboi, H., Ebina, K., Nampei, A., Noguchi, K., Tsuji, S., Nishimoto, N. & Yoshikawa H. 2017. Total ankle arthroplasty for rheumatoid arthritis in Japanese patients: A retrospective study of intermediate to long-term follow-up. *JB JS Open Access*, 2(4), e0033. doi: 10.2106/JBJS.OA.17.00033.

Hosman, A. H., Mason, R. B., Hobbs, T. & Rothwell, A. G. 2007. A New Zealand National Joint Registry review of 202 total ankle replacements followed for up to 6 years. *Acta Orthop*, 78, 584–591.

Iorio, R., Williams, K. M., Marcantonio, A. J., Specht, L. M., Tilzey, J. F. & Healy, W. L. 2012. Diabetes mellitus, hemoglobin A1c, and the incidence of total joint arthroplasty infection. *J Arthroplasty*, 27, 726–729 E1.

Jain, A., Witbreuk, M., Ball, C. & Nanchahal, J. 2002. Influence of steroids and methotrexate on wound complications after elective rheumatoid hand and wrist surgery. *J Hand Surg Am*, 27, 449–455.

Jamsen, E., Nevalainen, P., Kalliovalkama, J. & Moilanen, T. 2010. Preoperative hyperglycemia predicts infected total knee replacement. *Eur J Intern Med*, 21, 196–201.

Jamsen, E., Nevalainen, P., Eskelinen, A., Huotari, K., Kalliovalkama, J. & Moilanen, T. 2012. Obesity, diabetes, and preoperative hyperglycemia as predictors of periprosthetic joint infection: A single-center analysis of 7181 primary hip and knee replacements for osteoarthritis. *J Bone Joint Surg Am*, 94, E101.

Jensen, N. C. & Linde, F. 2009. Long-term follow-up on 33 TPR ankle joint replacements in 26 patients with rheumatoid arthritis. *Foot Ankle Surg*, 15, 123–126.

Kofoed, H. 1995. Cylindrical cemented ankle arthroplasty: A prospective series with long-term follow-up. *Foot Ankle Int*, 16, 474–479.

Malinzak, R. A., Ritter, M. A., Berend, M. E., Meding, J. B., Olberding, E. M. & Davis, K. E. 2009. Morbidly obese, diabetic, younger, and unilateral joint arthroplasty patients have elevated total joint arthroplasty infection rates. *J Arthroplasty*, 24, 84–88.

Morgan, S. S., Brook, B. & Harris, N. J. 2012. Is there a role for total ankle replacement in polio patients? A case report and review of the literature. *Foot Ankle Surg*, 18, 74–76.

Nishikawa, M., Tomita, T., Fujii, M., Watanabe, T., Hashimoto, J., Sugamoto, K., Ochi, T. & Yoshikawa, H. 2004. Total ankle replacement in rheumatoid arthritis. *Int Orthop*, 28, 123–126.

Ortman, B. L. & Pack, L. L. 1987. Aseptic Loosening of a total hip prosthesis secondary to Tophaceous gout. A case report. *J Bone Joint Surg Am*, 69, 1096–1099.

Pasta, G., Forsyth, A., Merchan, C. R., Mortazavi, S. M., Silva, M., Mulder, K., Mancuso, E., Perfetto, O., Heim, M., Caviglia, H. & Solimeno, L. 2008. Orthopaedic management of haemophilia arthropathy of the ankle. *Haemophilia*, 14(Suppl 3), 170–176.

Pedersen, A. B., Mehnert, F., Johnsen, S. P. & Sorensen, H. T. 2010. Risk of revision of a total hip replacement in patients with diabetes mellitus: A population-based follow up study. *J Bone Joint Surg Br*, 92, 929–934.

Peersman, G., Laskin, R., Davis, J. & Peterson, M. 2001. Infection in total knee replacement: A retrospective review of 6489 total knee replacements. *Clin Orthop Relat Res*, 15–23.

Preis, M., Bailey, T., Jacxsens, M. & Barg, A. 2017. Total ankle replacement in patients with haemophilic arthropathy: Primary arthroplasty and conversion of painful ankle arthrodesis to arthroplasty. *Haemophilia*, 23, E301–E309.

Raikin, S. M., Kane, J. & Ciminiello, M. E. 2010. Risk factors for incision-healing complications following total ankle arthroplasty. *J Bone Joint Surg Am*, 92, 2150–2155.

Rippstein, P. F., Huber, M., Coetzee, J. C. & Naal, F. D. 2011. Total ankle replacement with use of a new three-component implant. *J Bone Joint Surg Am*, 93, 1426–1435.

Rippstein, P. F. & Naal, F. D. 2011. Total ankle replacement in rheumatoid arthritis. *Orthopade*, 40, 984–986, 988–990.

Roddy, E., Zhang, W. & Doherty, M. 2007. Are joints affected by gout also affected by osteoarthritis? *Ann Rheum Dis*, 66, 1374–1377.

Rodriguez-Merchan, E. C. 2017. Management of hemophilic arthropathy of the ankle. *Cardiovasc Hematol Disord Drug Targets*, 17, 111–118.

Saltzman, C. L. 2000. Perspective on total ankle replacement. *Foot Ankle Clin*, 5, 761–775.

Saltzman, C. L., Salamon, M. L., Blanchard, G. M., Huff, T., Hayes, A., Buckwalter, J. A. & Amendola, A. 2005. Epidemiology of ankle arthritis: Report of a consecutive series of 639 patients from a tertiary orthopaedic center. *Iowa Orthop J*, 25, 44–46.

San Giovanni, T. P., Keblish, D. J., Thomas, W. H. & Wilson, M. G. 2006. Eight-year results of a minimally constrained total ankle arthroplasty. *Foot Ankle Int*, 27, 418–426.

Sansosti, L. E., Van, J. C. & Meyr, A. J. 2017. Effect of obesity on total ankle arthroplasty: A systematic review of postoperative complications requiring surgical revision. *J Foot Ankle Surg*, 57(2), 353–356.

Schill, S. & Wetzel, R. 2011. Total ankle arthroplasty for rheumatoid arthritis]. *Z Rheumatol*, 70(5), 417–422.

Schipper, O. N., Denduluri, S. K., Zhou, Y. & Haddad, S. L. 2016. Effect of obesity on total ankle arthroplasty outcomes. *Foot & Ankle Int*, 37, 1–7.

Scholz, R. & Scholz, U. 2008. The total ankle replacement for severe arthropathy in haemophilia. *Hamostaseologie*, 28(Suppl 1), S40–S44.

Sean, N. Y., Xavier, C. & Assal, M. 2012. Total ankle replacement for rheumatoid arthritis of the ankle. *Foot Ankle Clin*, 17, 555–564.

Serban, M., Mihailov, M. D., Poenaru, D., Pop, L., Branea, I., Bataneant, M., Lacatusu, A., Barna, L., Tepeneu, N. & Schramm, W. 2008. Orthopedic approach of haemophiliacs. A single center experience in Romania. *Hamostaseologie*, 28(Suppl 1), S52–S54.

Su, E. P., Kahn, B. & Figgie, M. P. 2004. Total ankle replacement in patients with rheumatoid arthritis. *Clin Orthop Relat Res*, 32–38.

Van Der Heide, H. J., Novakova, I. & De Waal Malefijt, M. C. 2006. The feasibility of total ankle prosthesis for severe arthropathy in haemophilia and prothrombin deficiency. *Haemophilia*, 12, 679–682.

Van Der Heide, H. J., Schutte, B., Louwerens, J. W., Van Den Hoogen, F. H. & Malefijt, M. C. 2009. Total ankle prostheses in rheumatoid arthropathy: Outcome in 52 patients followed for 1–9 years. *Acta Orthop*, 80, 440–444.

Wood, P. L., Crawford, L. A., Suneja, R. & Kenyon, A. 2007. Total ankle replacement for rheumatoid ankle arthritis. *Foot Ankle Clin*, 12, 497–508, vii.

Wukich, D. K., Lowery, N. J., Mcmillen, R. L. & Frykberg, R. G. 2010. Postoperative infection rates in foot and ankle surgery: A comparison of patients with and without diabetes mellitus. *J Bone Joint Surg Am*, 92, 287–295.

Wukich, D. K., Mcmillen, R. L., Lowery, N. J. & Frykberg, R. G. 2011. Surgical site infections after foot and ankle surgery: A comparison of patients with and Without diabetes. *Diabetes Care*, 34, 2211–2213.

Yano, K., Ikari, K. & Okazaki, K. 2019. Radiographic outcomes of mobile-bearing total ankle arthroplasty for patients with rheumatoid arthritis. *Foot Ankle Int*, 40(9), 1037–1042. doi: 10.1177/1071100719851469. Epub 2019 May 31.

MANAGING THE FAILED ANKLE REPLACEMENT

T. M. Clough and M. T. Karski

Summary

The outcome of ankle joint replacement, has greatly improved since the 1980s and the argument put forward by Hamblen (1985) that the ankle joint cannot be replaced is no longer valid. Registries exist for total ankle replacement (TAR) in the UK, Sweden, Norway, Finland, and New Zealand (Fevang *et al.*, 2007; Henricson *et al.*, 2007; Hosman *et al.*, 2007; Skytta *et al.*, 2010; Tomlinson and Harrison, 2012). Results are not as good as those for hip and knee arthroplasty, but continue to improve (Haddad *et al.*, 2007). The Scandinavian Total Ankle Replacement (STAR) prosthesis has one of the longest track records. A 10-year survival of the STAR prosthesis was reported to be 80% (Wood *et al.*, 2008b). A 15 year survival for the STAR prosthesis on a cohort of 200 patients has recently been reviewed to be 76% (Clough *et al.*, 2019). Two studies have demonstrated 91% survival for the STAR TAR at 19 years (Frigg *et al.*, 2017), and 73% survival at 15 years (Palanca *et al.*, 2018). Other implant designs to report long-term results have reported approximately similar survival rates (Buechel Sr *et al.*, 2004; Knecht *et al.*, 2004). Buechal *et al.* (2004) reported on his prosthesis, with a 92% 10-year survival for the BP TAR.

TAR is being increasingly performed for the patient with ankle arthrosis both in the UK and world-wide. This does lead to increasing numbers of failures presenting, usually to specialist centres. We report on our algorithm for the management of these difficult and challenging cases.

MECHANISMS OF TAR FAILURE

It is essential when considering treatment and management options for the failed TAR, to fully understand the mechanisms of failure, as this will dictate treatment options. Mechanisms of failure can be condensed into the following subgroups, though two or more mechanisms may co-exist in the same patient.

(1)   Aseptic loosening.
(2)   Component malposition.
(3)   Recurrent edge loading.
(4)   Malleolar fracture.
(5)   Infection.
(6)   Chronic pain (in the absence of radiographically significant abnormalities).

Aseptic Loosening

Aseptic loosening is thought to be due to osteolysis from macrophage activation, secondary to polyethylene wear debris. This failure mechanism was the rationale for the adoption of the mobile bearing principle. Theoretically this reduces wear debris by having high congruency between the components, thereby reducing edge loading. Because the polyethylene bearing is mobile on the flat metal implant surface, this then creates low-contact stresses when compared to a fixed bearing device with high congruency, thus reducing shear stresses at the bone–implant interface. Although these theoretical advantages; therefore, exist with this design concept, and have been used clinically for many years in total knee replacement (TKR) surgery, the long-term clinical results in TKR have not shown any improved outcome or survival when compared to fixed bearing TKR designs (Zeng *et al.*, 2013). The incidence of aseptic loosening does vary dramatically with ankle implant design.

The AES implant has been reported to have prohibitively high-aseptic loosening rates (Koivu *et al.*, 2009; Kotnis *et al.*, 2006; Besse *et al.*, 2010, Di Iorio *et al.*, 2017; Koivu *et al.*, 2017) and has now been withdrawn from the market. Significant osteolysis can result in catastrophic failure as demonstrated in Figure 1.

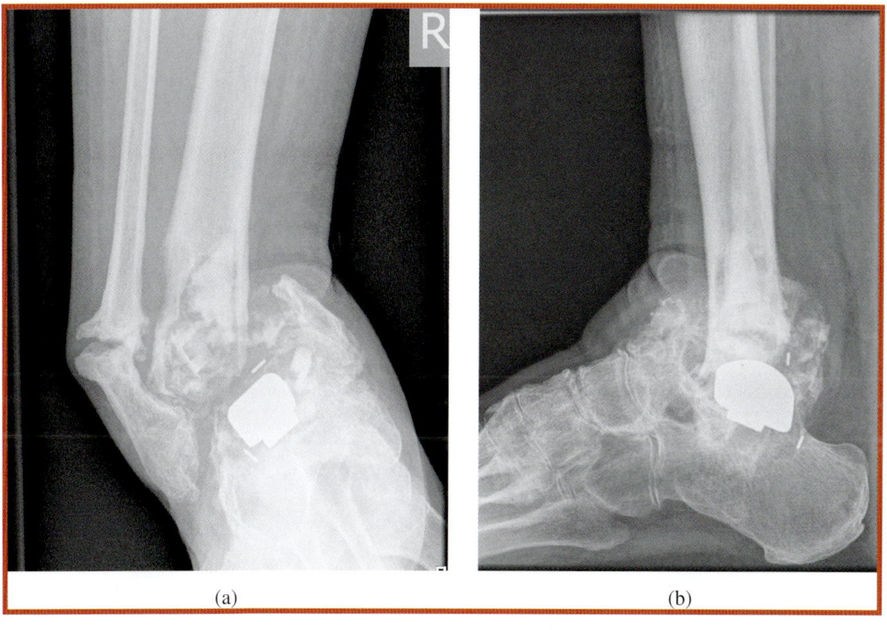

(a) (b)

Figure 1. *(a) and (b) Shows catastrophic failure with hindfoot malposition resultant from collapse following gross osteolysis and destruction, secondary to wear debris, in a first generation ankle replacement (thought to be the "Liverpool" ankle replacement where the tibial component was all polyethylene).*

Component Malposition

Component malposition usually relates to technical error at the time of implantation and is easily defined radiologically. With increasing familiarity of both the surgical approach and technique, as well as new developments of implantation such as intraoperative fluoroscopy and patient specific instrumentation, this complication should be minimised (Figure 2(a) and (b)).

Recurrent Edge Loading

The ideal surgical candidate for TAR has a neutrally aligned degenerate ankle. Caution should be exercised in recommending TAR in patients where the heel is in significant varus or valgus malalignment, as early failure has been shown to be more frequent in these subgroups (Haskell and Mann, 2004; Henricson *et al.*, 2007; Wood and Deakin, 2003). The cautious surgeon will not undertake

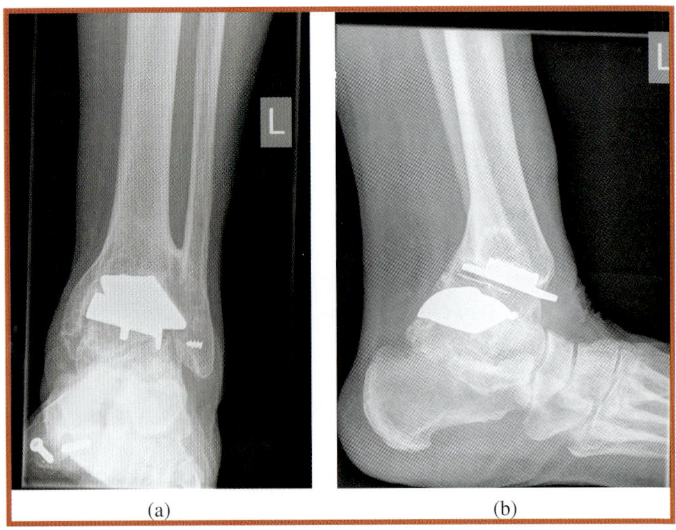

Figure 2. *(a) and (b) Postoperative X-ray with significant component malposition.*

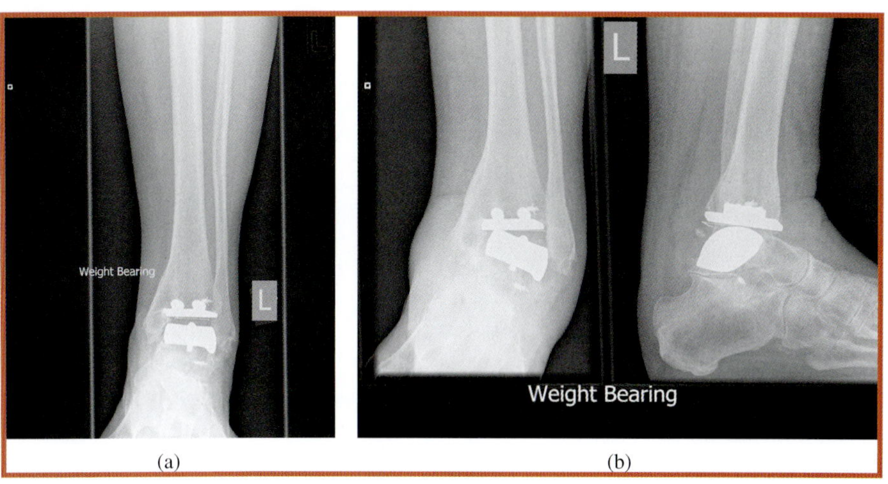

(a)   (b)

Figure 3. *TAR performed in a patient with ankle arthrosis and a degree of lateral ligament concomitant instability. (a) The patient had a lateral ligament reconstruction at the time of the original TAR surgery, and (b) about 3 years later, the ankle developed recurrent hindfoot drift, instability and edge loading.*

replacement when the deformity is greater than 15° (Wood *et al.*, 2008a) (Figure 3). Additional procedures such as corrective os calcis osteotomy, lateral ligament reconstruction, fibular shortening osteotomy, deltoid ligament release, and tibialis posterior tendon lengthening have all been described and used to correct the hindfoot deformity at the time of TAR in an attempt to get the hindfoot axis to neutral (Hobson *et al.*, 2009; Gauvain *et al.*, 2017). Despite these efforts, and even if all goes well in the early period, recurrent drift and edge loading are still not uncommon.

Malleolar Fracture

The overall incidence of malleolar fracture with TAR has been reported to vary from 3% to 20% (Clough *et al.*, 2018; McGarvey *et al.*, 2014). Other studies have described lower rates of fracture in the region of 1–5% (Rippstein *et al.*, 2011; Borenstein *et al.*, 2017). Malleolar fracture can happen either early or late. Early fracture

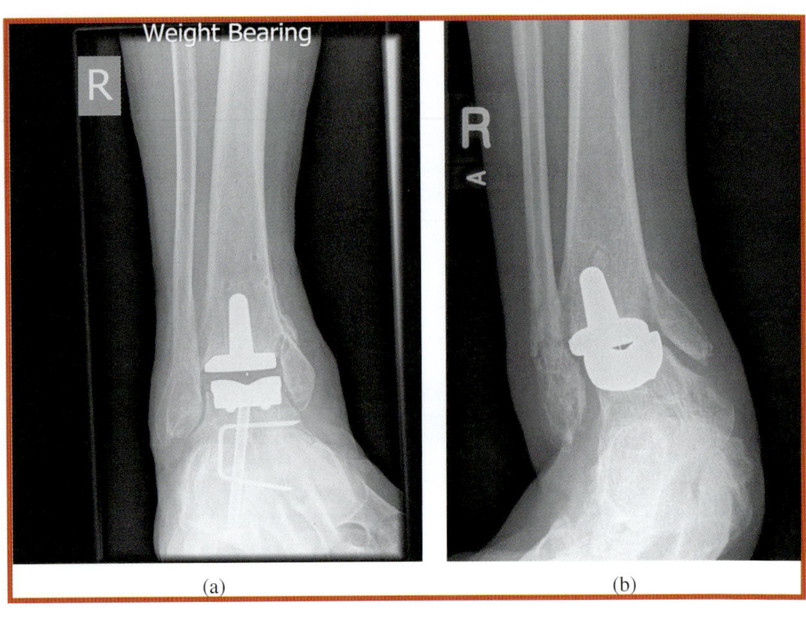

Figure 4. *(a) Medial malleolar fracture. (b) Combined medial and lateral malleolar fracture.*

(intraoperative or perioperative) rates can vary both with surgical experience and also with osteoporotic or soft rheumatoid bone. Late malleolar fracture is often secondary to recurrent hindfoot drift/deformity into either varus or valgus, and is essentially a stress fracture, though can be an acute injury (Figure 4).

Infection

As with any arthroplasty, deep infection in a TAR is a tragic and disappointing complication. The incidence of failure from deep infection is reported to vary from 1% to 4% (Buechel Sr *et al.*, 2004; Wood *et al.*, 2010). A systematic review has reported the rate of superficial infection as 2.4% and deep infection as 1.1%, although these figures are clearly subject to reporting bias (Zaidi *et al.*, 2013).

Safe Failure

Having examined the patient and identified the predominant mechanisms of failure, the authors believe that the treatment strategy for revision should address that failure mechanism. Clearly for some people, two or more failure mechanisms may co-exist, and if so, all these need to be addressed. For some, it is interesting to note that whilst the prosthesis may have radiologically failed; clinically, the patient can survive with minimal symptoms. Cooke reported this as "safe failure" (Cooke, 2007). This is usually due to the implant essentially becoming non-functional. This can happen for example with component subsidence in a neutrally aligned heel, whereby loading will then shift off the component and onto the

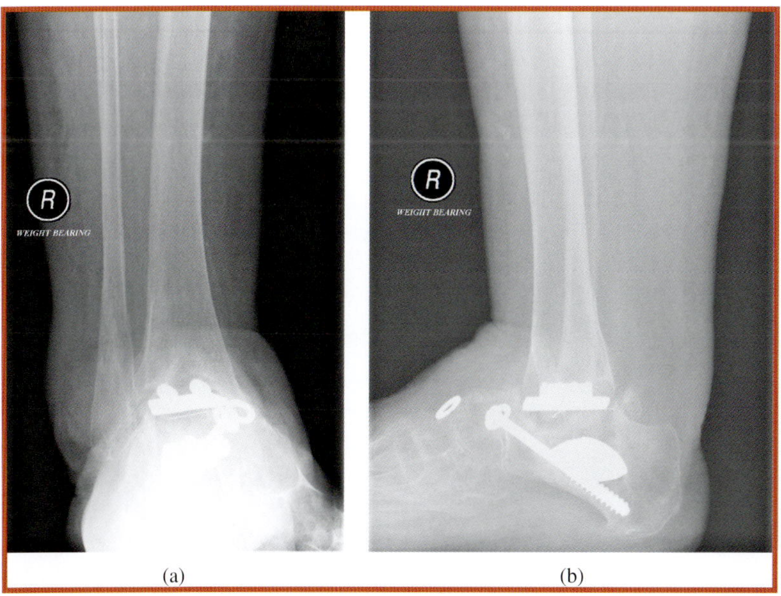

Figure 5. *(a) AP and (b) Lateral X-rays of Safe Failure. The STAR talar implant has subsided into a new stable position and the patient's symptoms settled.*

contact area between both the medial and lateral malleoli and the talus. Careful monitoring is required in these patients with regular clinical and radiological review, certainly initially, but it is the authors experience that once "safe failure" occurs, then it rarely progresses onto actual clinical failure (Figure 5).

Chronic Pain — Radiologically Normal

In some circumstances the radiographs look entirely normal but the patient still has pain (Figure 6). This is a more challenging problem and it is important to look for causes outside of the joint for example in the soft tissues or in the adjacent joints.

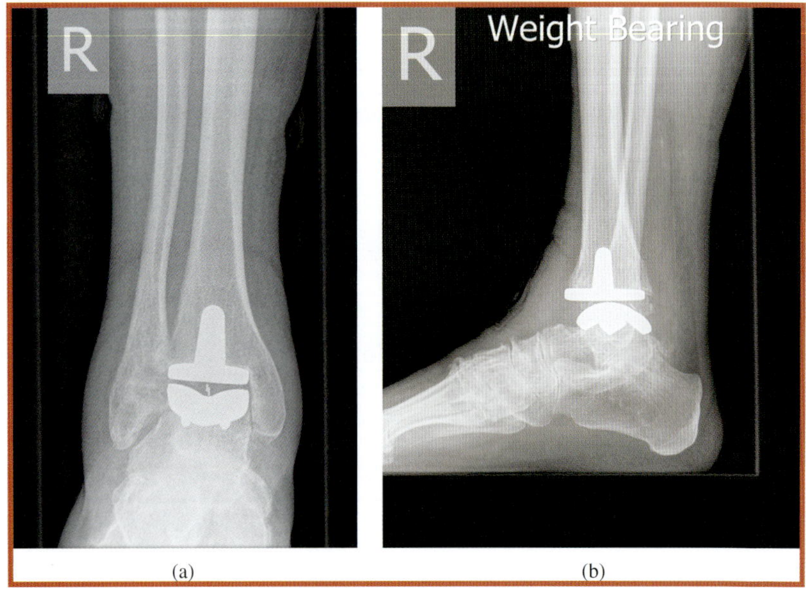

Figure 6. *(a) and (b) Mobility TAR in site. Radiologically no detectable abnormality but clinically ongoing pain.*

REVISION STRATEGIES

Aseptic Loosening

In cases of aseptic loosening where there is insufficient bone stock to allow a revisional ankle replacement then conversion to fusion is usually the only available option. In some instances, this can be achieved as an ankle fusion using screws with possible augmentation with a plate (Culpan *et al.*, 2007; Rippstein *et al.*, 2012; Gross *et al.*, 2015). If ankle fusion is possible, it has the advantage of preserving the subtalar joint, and when combined with structural tricortical iliac crest allograft, can help minimise leg shortening. High rates of union (94%) can be achieved (Culpan *et al.*, 2007). While tibiotalar fusion is therefore preferable as a fusion salvage option, in the authors experience, it is more common that after removal of the failed ankle replacement, there is often insufficient bone left on the talar side to achieve a solid ankle purchase with metalwork and therefore fusion, and a tibiotalar-calcaneal fusion is then required. This can be achieved with an intramedullary nail device (Hopgood *et al.*, 2006; Kotnis *et al.*, 2006) or with the use of fine wire external fixation (Carlsson *et al.*, 1998). Caution should be used when considering using external fixation in patients with rheumatoid arthritis, because of the high risk of pin site infections, and the longer rehabilitation time when compared to intramedullary nail fixation (Carlsson *et al.*, 1998). Intramedullary nails are the authors favoured option.

Bone graft is required to fill the large cavity left by the failed prosthesis to preserve limb length. Simple iliac crest harvesting usually will yield insufficient bone for this purpose, and options include void filling with fresh frozen femoral head allograft (authors favoured option), other bulk allograft, a Blair type sliding fusion, or demineralised bone matrix. Metallic spacer implants, either off the shelf or custom 3D printed, are also now available to fill spaces and offer structural support. Acute shortening can be performed, with consideration then for subsequent limb lengthening with a fine wire frame fixator.

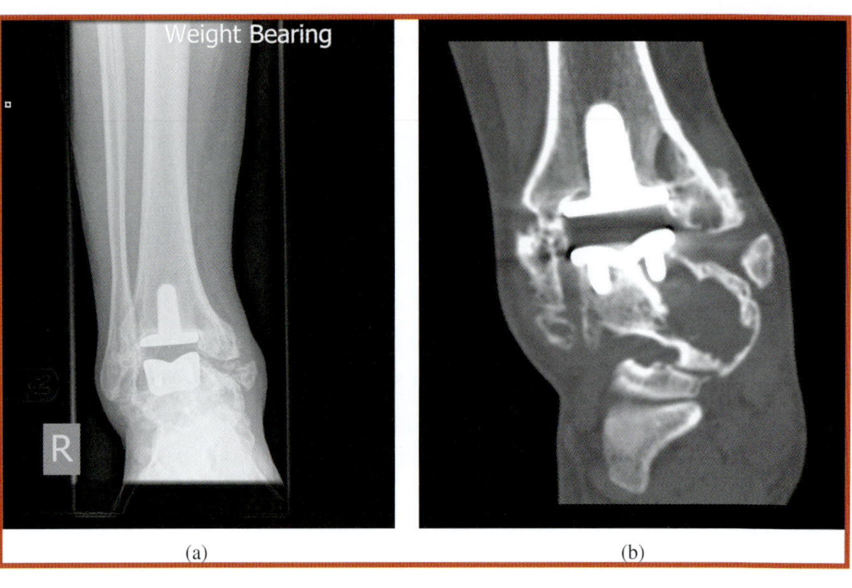

Figure 7. *(a) X-rays of a Mobility TAR with cyst in talus though it is difficult to define its full extent. (b) CT scans confirm full extent of huge cystic involvement of the medial side talus and medial malleolus. Extensive bone graft is required to fill this void.*

Often plain radiographs underestimate the size of the cyst involved in aseptic loosening and if suspicion exists, then preoperative CT scan should be performed to prevent any intraoperative surprises.

In cases therefore of aseptic loosening, the authors would try to decide preoperatively whether there is merely isolated cavitation, whether there is extensive loosening associated with sinkage/malposition of the components, or whether there is merely component demarcation (Figure 7).

If the components are aligned and not loose but there is isolated cavitation, the author's treatment would be to bone graft the cavity, replace any loose components, and change the polyethylene bearing.

If the components are loose and the cavity is extensive, there will often be associated component sinkage or malposition (Figure 9).

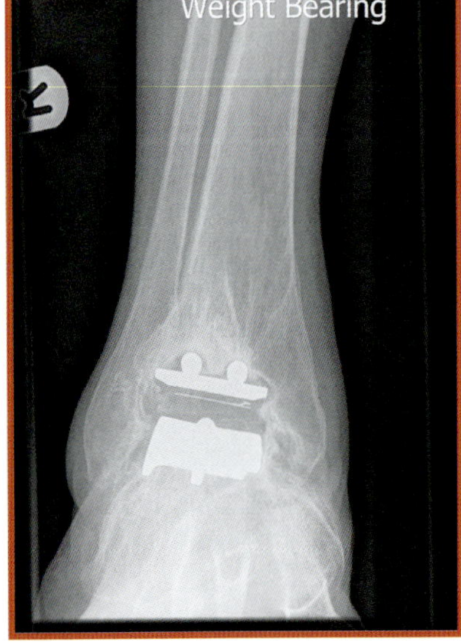

Figure 8. *A STAR prosthesis showing non-progressive demarcation to the tibial component. Treated with close clinical and radiological observation.*

For this, the authors favoured treatment would be as follows:

- Bone graft the defect.
- Conversion to fusion (tibiotalar joint only, if possible, but more commonly tibiotalarcalcaneal (Figure 10)).

If there is merely component demarcation, the authors favoured treatment would be:

- Close clinical and radiological review.
- Surgery only on clinical symptoms or progressive and worrying radiological features. It is the author's experience that in the absence of infection, simple demarcation of the components is non-progressive, is often minimally symptomatic, and can be treated conservatively and expectantly (see Figure 8).

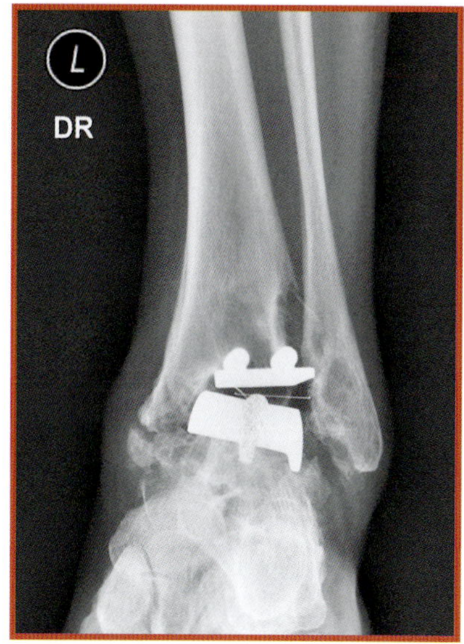

Figure 9. *Cavitation between the tibial pegs of STAR implant.*

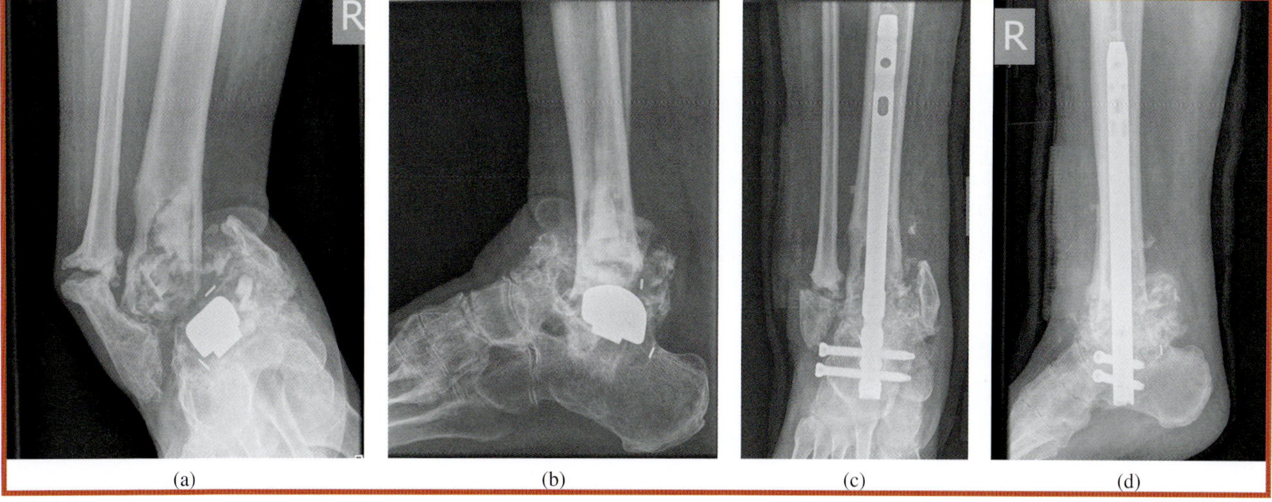

Figure 10. *(a)–(d) Extensive osteolysis with sinkage ((a) and (b), as seen in Figure 1). Conversion to hindfoot intramedullary nail fusion ((c) and (d)) with femoral head allograft was required.*

Component Malposition

If appears early, this is usually due to technical error at the time of component implantation, and can often be corrected with revisional ankle replacement. However, if revisional replacement is undertaken, one should not have a patient in a position whereby amputation would then be the only further option should the revisional replacement fail, in either the early or longer term.

If the components were initially well-aligned, but then over the years, subsequent X-rays confirm progressive component malposition, this is due to component subsidence. This often happens in association with one of the other failure mechanisms described above (usually aseptic loosening and/or recurrent edge loading), and revision strategies are described in these subsections (Figure 11).

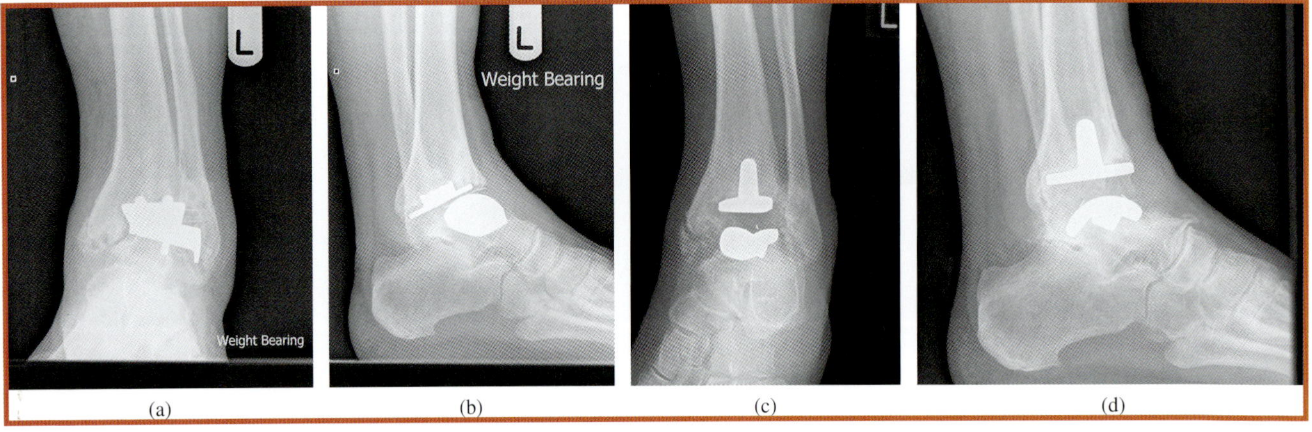

Figure 11. *(a)–(d) Component malposition either from intraoperative technical error with implantation ((a) and (b)) or from subsidence ((c) and (d)).*

Recurrent Edge Loading

Together with aseptic loosening, this is probably the most common cause of TAR failure. Preoperative varus or valgus deformity can be difficult to release and fully correct, and seems to recur over time, which if not addressed can lead to early failure of the implant (Wood *et al.*, 2010; McInnes *et al.*, 2014). The author's management strategy would be defined as follows:

- If the recurrent drift is not severe (that is caught early), but is progressing:
  — Correct malalignment — os calcis osteotomy, lateral ligament reconstruction, fibular shortening osteotomy, deltoid ligament release, tibialis posterior tendon release.
  — This should all be combined with polyethylene exchange if possible (Figure 12).

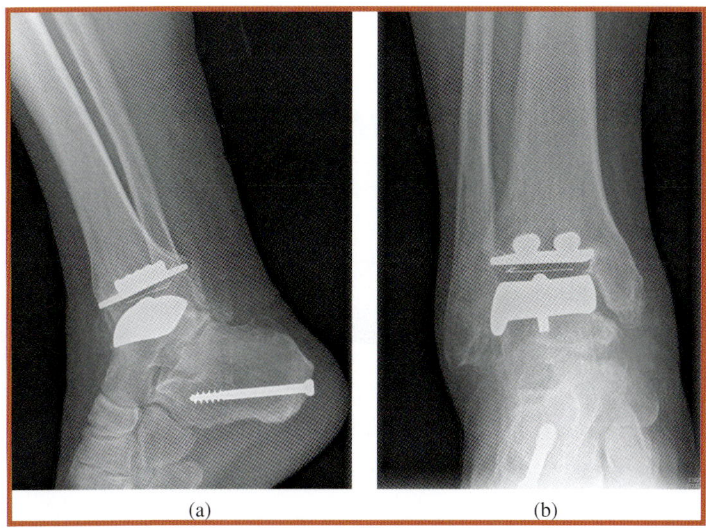

Figure 12. *(a) and (b) Malalignment correction with os calcis osteotomy and change of polyethylene bearing.*

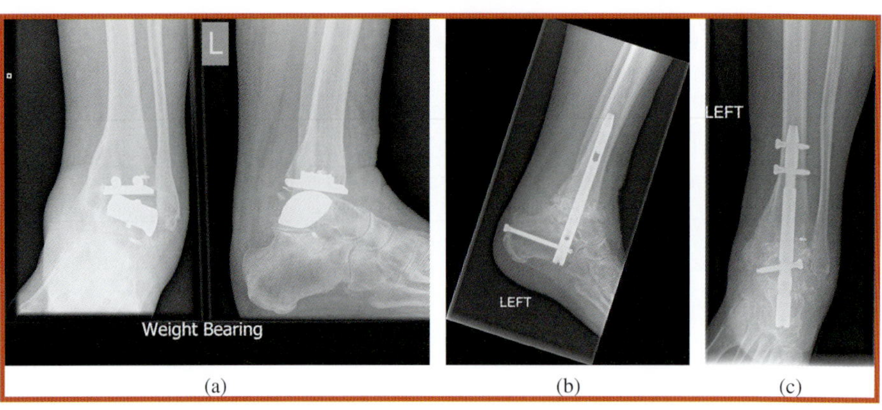

Figure 13. *(a)-(c) Severe recurrent edge loading with unstable lateral ligament complex. Elected for conversion to intramedullary nail fusion.*

- If the drift is severe — then this is often associated with some component loosening (Figure 13):
  - Hindfoot nail.
  - Bone graft (femoral head allograft).

Malleolar Fracture

The overall incidence of malleolar fracture varies according to surgeon experience, rheumatoid status, concomitant osteoporosis, and presence of hindfoot malalignment. Malleolar fractures need to be treated with great caution, as the loss of peripheral constraint to the ankle with a malleolar fracture can lead to drift of the heel, malalignment and maltracking of the component, and early failure. The authors have noted these fractures to occur either early (intraoperative or perioperative) or late.

Early fractures — can be subgrouped into intraoperative and perioperative (within the first 3 months).

Intraoperative — if recognised, it is the authors favoured option to surgically stabilise the fracture. The fracture heals rapidly and does not significantly alter the postoperative rehabilitation.

Medial malleolus fractures can either be caused with the saw blade, or as a blow-off fracture with the use of a laminar spreader distractor intraoperatively. They should be stabilised with screw fixation. A transverse fracture of the lateral malleolus can be caused by the saw blade when cutting the distal tibia. If this occurs, it requires fixation with a plate and screws using a separate lateral incision over the fibula.

Perioperative — within the first 3 months. The management of this complication is controversial. Most favour a conservative approach with a boot or plaster immobilisation. However, extreme caution and close monitoring need to be performed and any sign of progressive drift should then be treated aggressively with surgical fixation, as it is the authors experience that once drift starts, with continued conservative management it often progresses, causing subsequent component malalignment, maltracking, and early failure. Fixation for the medial and lateral malleolus, can be easily treated with screw fixation and neutralisation plate (providing the drift is minimal and acceptable) (Figure 14).

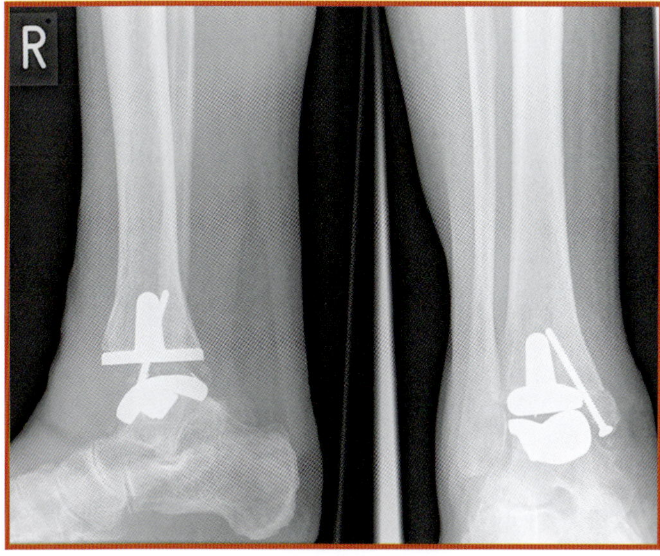

Figure 14. *ORIF medial malleolus.*

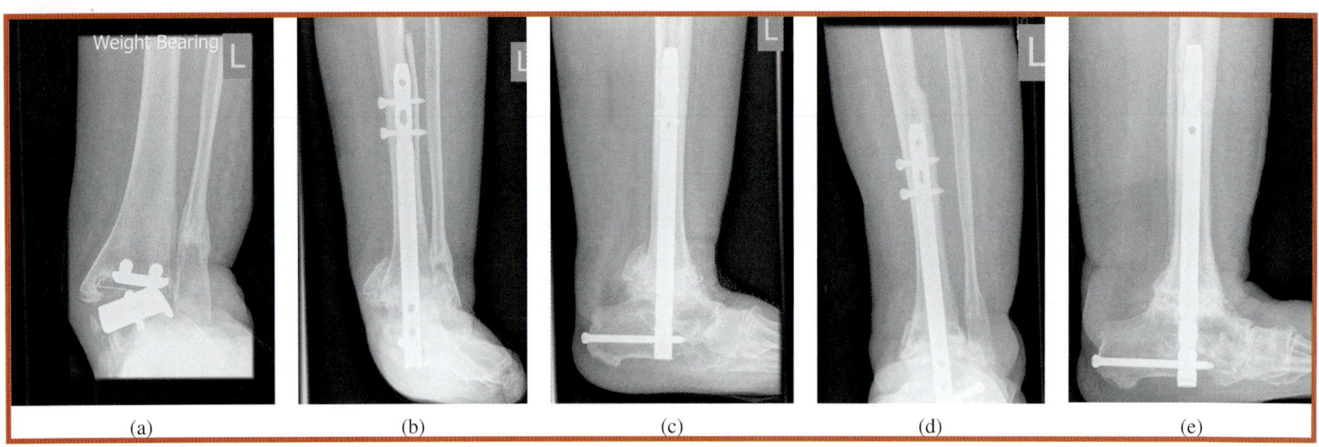

Figure 15. *(a)–(e) Late malleolar fracture in a STAR implant (a) should be considered sinister. Associated with recurrent edge loading. Required conversion to IM nail ((b) and (c)). Intraoperative split of the tibia with nail insertion noted (b) and treated conservatively. Full union in maintained position obtained ((d) and (e)).*

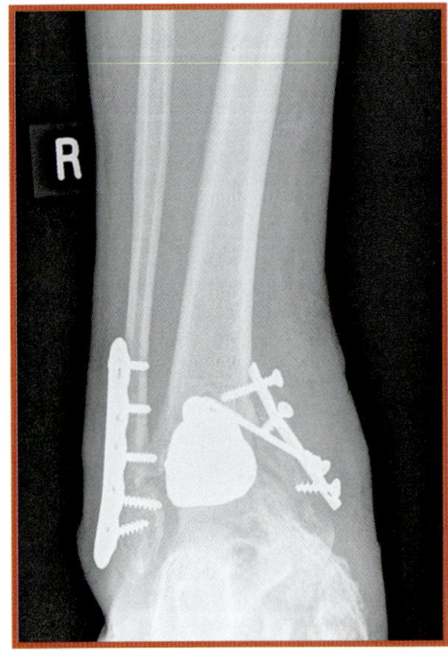

Figure 16. *Failure of initial malleolar fracture fixation leads to loss of construct stability and progressive drift. Required conversion to IM nail.*

Late — These are sinister complications, usually stress fractures from recurrent heel drift, and can be the first sign of eventual failure from varus/valgus recurrence. Conservative treatment will heal the stress fracture (Figure 15) , but consideration should then be made as to whether the alignment can be salvaged back to neutral, often by corrective osteotomy (see Recurrent edge loading above) or whether the components are already loose or the drift is severe, in which case the TAR may be doomed (Figure 15). If an aggressive approach is not adopted, then unfortunately catastrophic failure may well ensue (Figures 16 & 19).

If an aggressive approach is not adopted, then unfortunately catastrophic failure may well ensue.

Infection

Deep TAR infection, like that of hip or knee arthroplasty, can have depressing and catastrophic results for all parties (Patton *et al.*, 2015) (Figure 17). The authors advocate the Oxford treatment algorithm

for the management of this complication (Kotnis *et al.*, 2006; Patton *et al.*, 2015), which is as follows:

- Aspirate the joint for culture and sensitivities. Some argue this has little place in the management of ankle infections and hence if negative, consider open biopsy for confirmation.
- Two-stage revision.
- Multiple deep biopsies sent for microbiology and histology.
- Antibiotic impregnated fashioned cement spacer.
- Minimum 8 weeks antibiotic phase.
- Monitor inflammatory blood markers (ESR, CRP, WCC, antiStaph titres).
- Attempt second-stage revision, but in the authors experience more often than not, there is insufficient bone usually on the talus, and conversion to a fusion with bone grafting would then be recommended (Figure 17).

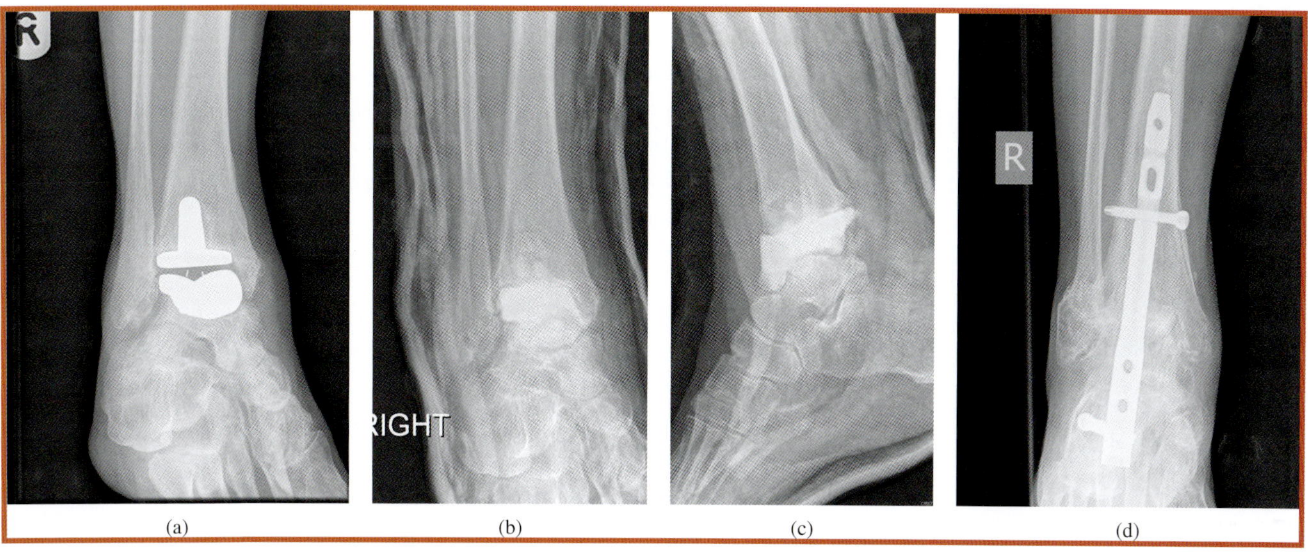

Figure 17. *(a)–(d) Infected TAR with two-stage revision, using femoral head allograft to provide bone graft and maintain limb length.*

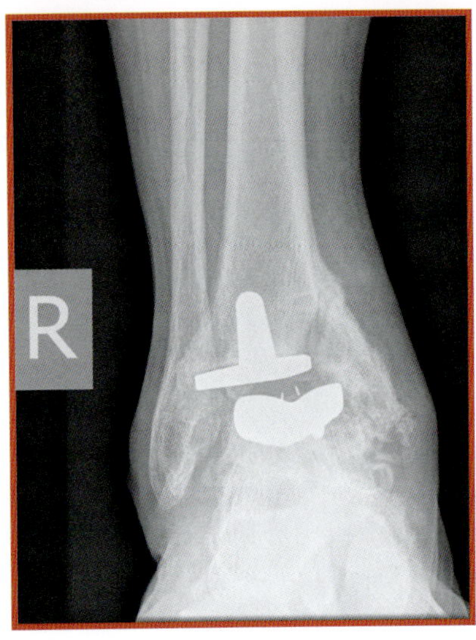

Figure 18. *Patient with combined failure of medial malleolar fracture and component malalignment. A cautious conservative approach was initially adopted to obtain fracture union (Figure 19).*

Combined Modes of Failure

In those patients with combined modes of failure, these need to be carefully identified and individually assessed. For example in Figure 18, a patient with component malalignment has developed a fracture of the medial malleolus. Although healed with conservative treatment, the underlying cause was not addressed leading to failure and the necessity to convert this patient to a TTC nail (Figure 19).

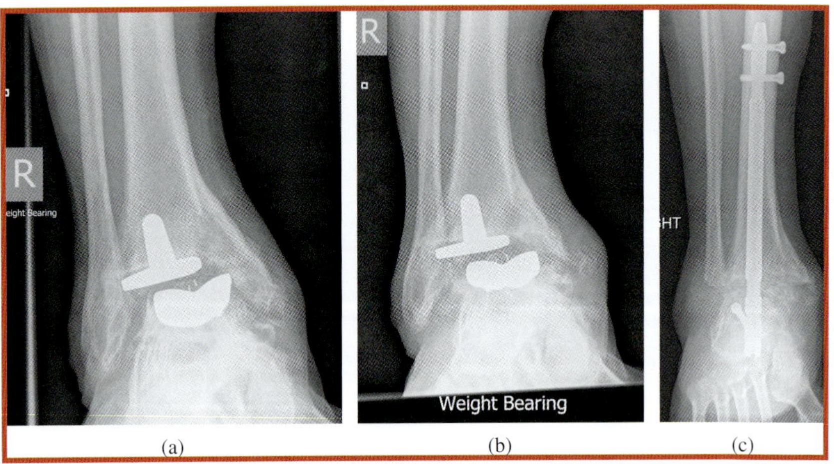

Figure 19. *(a)–(c) Following medial malleolar fracture union, the ankle however continued to drift and had to be revised by conversion to hindfoot intramedullary nail fusion.*

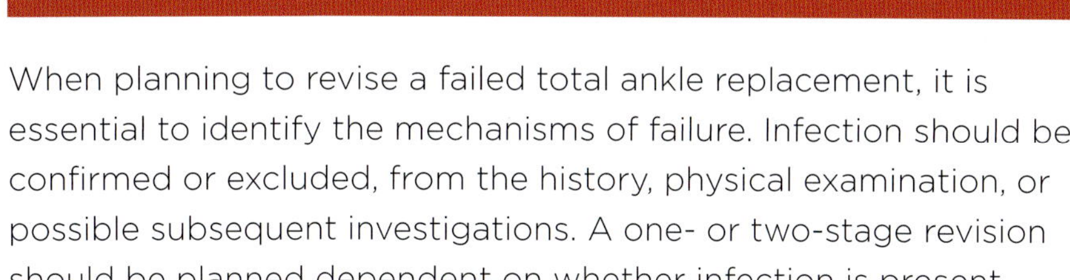

CONCLUSIONS

When planning to revise a failed total ankle replacement, it is essential to identify the mechanisms of failure. Infection should be confirmed or excluded, from the history, physical examination, or possible subsequent investigations. A one- or two-stage revision should be planned dependent on whether infection is present.

The authors recommend assessing for bone defects and the size of osteolytic cavities preoperatively with a CT scan. In the majority of cases, the authors have found it is not possible to convert a failed ankle replacement into a revision replacement, and a fusion is required. An ankle fusion and bone graft (preserving the subtalar joint) should preferentially be performed if there is enough talar bone stock to achieve a rigid fixation. However in the authors experience, in most cases there is insufficient bone stock on the talus to allow this and a tibiotalarcalcaneal fusion using an intramedullary nail with bone graft is required in the majority of cases. External fixation with a fine wire frame can be used as an alternative to intramedullary nail fixation for tibiotalocalcaneal fusion, but is not recommended for patients with rheumatoid arthritis.

REFERENCES

Besse, J. L., Colombier, J. A., Asencio, J., Bonnin, M., Gaudot, F., Jarde, O., Judet, T., Maestro, M., Lemrijse, T., Leonardi, C., Toullec, E. & L'afcp 2010. Total ankle arthroplasty in France. *Orthop Traumatol Surg Res*, 96, 291–303.

Borenstein, T., Thordarson, D. B., Charlton, T. P., & Chen, S. 2017. Perioperative complications of outpatient total ankle arthroplasty. *Foot & Ankle Orthopaedics*. https://doi.org/10.1177/2473011417S000122.

Buechel Sr, F. F., Buechel, F. F., Jr. & Pappas, M. J. 2004. Twenty-year evaluation of cementless mobile-bearing total ankle replacements. *Clinical Orthop Relat Res*, 424, 19–26.

Carlsson, A. S., Montgomery, F. & Besjakov, J. 1998. Arthrodesis of the ankle secondary to replacement. *Foot Ankle Int*, 19, 240–245.

Clough T. M., Alvi, F. & Majeed, H. 2018. Total ankle arthroplasty: What are the risks? *Bone Joint Journal*, 100-B, 1352–1358.

Clough, T. M., Bodo K., Majeed H., Davenport J. & Karski, M. 2019. Survivorship and long-term outcome of a consecutive series of 200 Scandinavian Total Ankle Replacement (STAR) implants. *Bone Joint Journal*, 101-B(1), 47–54.

Cooke, P. H. 2007. *Re: Personal Communication.*

Culpan, P., Le Strat, V., Piriou, P. & Judet, T. 2007. Arthrodesis after failed total ankle replacement. *J Bone Joint Surg Br*, 89, 1178–1183.

Di Iorio, A., Viste, A., Fessy, M. H. & Besse, J. L. 2017. The AES total ankle arthroplasty analysis of failures and survivorship at ten years. *Int Orthop*, 41, 2525–2533.

Fevang, B. T., Lie, S. A., Havelin, L. I., Brun, J. G., Skredderstuen, A. & Furnes, O. 2007. 257 Ankle arthroplasties performed in Norway between 1994 and 2005. *Acta Orthop*, 78, 575–583.

Frigg, A., Germann, U., Huber, M. & Horisberger, M. 2017. Survival of the Scandinavian total ankle replacement (STAR): Results of ten to nineteen years follow-up. *Int Orthop*, 41, 2075–2082.

Gauvain, T. T., Hames, M. A. & Mcgarvey, W. C. 2017. Malalignment correction of the lower limb before, during, and after total ankle arthroplasty. *Foot Ankle Clin*, 22, 311–339.

Gross, C., Erickson, B. J., Adams, S. B. & Parekh, S. G. 2015. Ankle arthrodesis after failed total ankle replacement: A systematic review of the literature. *Foot Ankle Spec*, 8, 143–151.

Haddad, S. L., Coetzee, J. C., Estok, R., Fahrbach, K., Banel, D. & Nalysnyk, L. 2007. Intermediate and long-term outcomes of total ankle arthroplasty and ankle arthrodesis: A systematic review of the literature. *J Bone Joint Surg Am*, 89, 1899–1905.

Hamblen, D. L. 1985. Can the ankle joint be replaced? *J Bone Joint Surg Br*, 67, 689–690.

Haskell, A. & Mann, R. A. 2004. Ankle arthroplasty with preoperative coronal plane deformity: Short-term results. *Clin Orthop Relat Res*, 424, 98–103.

Henricson, A., Skoog, A. & Carlsson, A. 2007. The Swedish ankle arthroplasty register: An analysis of 531 arthroplasties between 1993 and 2005. *Acta Orthop*, 78, 569–574.

Hobson, S. A., Karantana, A. & Dhar, S. 2009. Total ankle replacement in patients with significant pre-operative deformity of the hindfoot. *J Bone Joint Surg Br*, 91, 481–486.

Hopgood, P., Kumar, R. & Wood, P. L. 2006. Ankle arthrodesis for failed total ankle replacement. *J Bone Joint Surg Br*, 88, 1032–1038.

Hosman, A. H., Mason, R. B., Hobbs, T. & Rothwell, A. G. 2007. A New Zealand National Joint Registry review of 202 total ankle replacements followed for up to 6 years. *Acta Orthop*, 78, 584–591.

Knecht, S. I., Estin, M., Callaghan, J. J., Zimmerman, M. B., Alliman, K. J., Alvine, F. G. & Saltzman, C. L. 2004. The agility total ankle arthroplasty. seven to sixteen-year follow-up. *J Bone Joint Surg Am*, 86-A, 1161–1171.

Koivu, H., Kohonen, I., Sipola, E., Alanen, K., Vahlberg, T. & Tiusanen, H. 2009. Severe periprosthetic osteolytic lesions after the ankle evolutive system total ankle replacement. *J Bone Joint Surg Br*, 91, 907–914.

Koivu, H., Kohonen, I., Mattila, K., Loyttyniemi, E. & Tiusanen, H. 2017. Medium to long-term results of 130 ankle evolutive system total ankle replacements-inferior survival due to peri-implant osteolysis. *Foot Ankle Surg*, 23, 108–115.

Kotnis, R., Pasapula, C., Anwar, F., Cooke, P. H. & Sharp, R. J. 2006. The management of failed ankle replacement. *J Bone Joint Surg Br*, 88, 1039–1047.

Mcgarvey, W. C., Clanton, T. O. & Lunz, D. 2004. Malleolar fracture after total ankle arthroplasty: A comparison of two designs. *Clin Orthop Relat Res*, 104–110.

Mcinnes, K. A., Younger, A. S. & Oxland, T. R. 2014. Initial instability in total ankle replacement: A cadaveric biomechanical investigation of the star and agility prostheses. *J Bone Joint Surg Am*, 96, E147.

Palanca, A., Mann, R. A., Mann, J. A. & Haskell, A. 2018. Scandinavian total ankle replacement: 15-year follow-up. *Foot Ankle Int*, 39, 135–142.

Patton, D., Kiewiet, N. & Brage, M. 2015. Infected total ankle arthroplasty: Risk factors and treatment options. *Foot Ankle Int*, 36, 626–634.

Rippstein, P. F., Huber, M., Coetzee, J. C. & Naal, F. D. 2011. Total ankle replacement with use of a new three-component implant. *J Bone Joint Surg Am*, 93, 1426–1435.

Rippstein, P. F., Huber, M. & Naal, F. D. 2012. Management of specific complications related to total ankle arthroplasty. *Foot Ankle Clin*, 17, 707–717.

Skytta, E. T., Koivu, H., Eskelinen, A., Ikavalko, M., Paavolainen, P. & Remes, V. 2010. Total ankle replacement: A population-based study of 515 cases from the Finnish arthroplasty register. *Acta Orthop*, 81, 114–118.

Tomlinson, M. & Harrison, M. 2012. The New Zealand Joint Registry: Report of 11-year data for ankle arthroplasty. *Foot Ankle Clin*, 17, 719–723.

Wood, P. L. & Deakin, S. 2003. Total ankle replacement. The results in 200 ankles. *J Bone Joint Surg Br*, 85, 334–341.

Wood, P. L., Clough, T. M. & Smith, R. 2008a. The present state of ankle arthroplasty. *Foot Ankle Surg*, 14, 115–119.

Wood, P. L., Prem, H. & Sutton, C. 2008b. Total ankle replacement: Medium-term results in 200 scandinavian total ankle replacements. *J Bone Joint Surg Br*, 90, 605–609.

Wood, P. L., Karski, M. T. & Watmough, P. 2010. Total ankle replacement: The results of 100 mobility total ankle replacements. *J Bone Joint Surg Br*, 92, 958–962.

Zaidi, R., Cro, S., Gurusamy, K., Siva, N., Macgregor, A., Henricson, A. & Goldberg, A. 2013. The outcome of total ankle replacement: A systematic review and meta-analysis. *Bone Joint J*, 95-B, 1500–1507.

Zeng, Y., Shen, B., Yang, J., Zhou, Z. K., Kang, P. D. & Pei, F. X. 2013. Is there reduced polyethylene wear and longer survival when using a mobile-bearing design in total knee replacement? A meta-analysis of randomised and non-randomised controlled trials. *Bone Joint J*, 95-B, 1057–1063.

CHAPTER
15

REVISION TOTAL ANKLE REPLACEMENT

S. Dhar, D. Sunderamoorthy and H. Majeed

Summary

As outcomes of the latest generation of mobile-bearing total ankle replacements (TARs) have improved and become increasingly predictable, indications have been extended and TARs are now being done in patients younger than 50 years of age, in ankles that are considerably deformed, in neuromuscular conditions and in ankles with patchy AVN (Hobson *et al.*, 2009; Kofoed and Lundberg-Jensen, 1999). With increasing numbers of operations being performed, there are going to be an increasing number of inevitable failures. Failure of ankle replacements results in significant discomfort and disability, and affects the functional outcome of the patients.

Unlike the knee and hip replacement literature, much less is published regarding failure of TARs. Nevertheless, the cumulative overall survival rate of TAR from published data seems to be approximately 89% at 10 years, with a cumulative annual failure rate of up to 1.9% (Zaidi *et al.*, 2013). There is variation between different centres (Wood, 2002, Henricson, 2007, Hosman, 2007, Fevang, 2007, Gougoulias, 2009). As with other joint replacements, failure of TARs usually appears to be due to numerous factors that may be patient, surgeon or implant related or indeed a combination of these. Patient-related factors include manual work, obesity, significant ankle deformity, poor compliance, and co-morbidities. Surgeon factors include improper patient selection, learning curve, poor implant positioning or technique; and implant factors include implant design (some implants such as the AES and Mobility have been withdrawn), along with poor instrumentation and surgical guidance.

Associated contributory problems may include wound dehiscence, deep infection, instability, fractures, tendon disorders, aseptic loosening, subsidence, malleolar impingement, and pain (Kofoed and Lundberg-Jensen, 1999; Helm and Stevens, 1986; Buechel and Pappas, 1992; Pyevich *et al.*, 1998; Anderson *et al.*, 2003; Wood and Deakin, 2003; Wood *et al.*, 2008; Buechel Sr *et al.*, 2003; Morgan *et al.*, 2010; Wood, 2002; Haddad *et al.*, 2007; Kotnis *et al.*, 2006; Barg *et al.*, 2013; Borenstein *et al.*, 2018; Gross *et al.*, 2017; Overley and Beideman, 2015).

One of the commonest modes of failure of TARs is aseptic loosening. Aseptic loosening may be associated with extensive bone loss, especially in cases of osteoporotic bone. Barg *et al.* (2013) have defined loosening of the tibial component as a change in the position of the flat base by more than 2° relative to the long axis of the tibia and/or a progressive radiolucency of more than 2 mm on the AP and/or lateral radiograph. Loosening of the talar component, as seen on the lateral radiograph, was defined as subsidence into the talus by more than 5 mm or a change in position of more than 5° relative to a line drawn from the top of the talonavicular joint to the tuberosity of the calcaneus.

SURGICAL STRATEGIES

Surgical intervention for failed ankle replacement is aimed towards restoring alignment, stability, and function of the joint. Factors such as infection, loss of bone stock, soft tissue instability, distorted soft tissue envelope, fracture of malleoli, subtalar stiffness, and the poor availability of revision implants make revision TAR challenging (Barg *et al.*, 2013; Haddad *et al.*, 2007; Hopgood *et al.*, 2006; Wapner, 2002).

Kotnis *et al.* (2006) have published their protocol for the management of failed TAR. The deciding factor is whether the failure is due to infection or not. For a failed TAR due to infection, they advise a two-stage salvage procedure. The first stage involves debridement and removal of the implants and insertion of a gentamicin-loaded cement spacer. Appropriate antibiotics are given for a minimum of 6 weeks after sampling. The second stage is usually an ankle fusion with a circular frame or, in extreme, resistant instances, a transtibial amputation. For non-infected TAR, a one-stage revision procedure is planned to either a revision TAR or arthrodesis.

Traditionally, revision of the failed TAR to arthrodesis is considered to be the main option, the "gold standard" treatment for the salvage of the failed prostheses. However, these are technically demanding procedures and functional limitations following arthrodesis may include walking with a limp, difficulty in walking on uneven surfaces, while climbing stairs, and when running. Revision joint replacement has the advantages of maintaining some range of movement and restoring the normal kinematics in order to achieve better functional outcome and prevent degeneration of the neighbouring joints (Haddad *et al.*, 2007). However, revision TAR is also technically demanding with higher risk of further failure (Bonnin *et al.*, 2011; Williams *et al.*, 2015). Revision to another TAR is contraindicated in the presence of active infection and poor vascular supply, and is less commonly undertaken in the presence of large bony defects, which increase the chances of malalignment and instability of the prosthesis with resultant early failure (Kotnis *et al.*, 2006).

The choice of salvage/revision procedure is complex and depends on the cause of failure, the individual patients' circumstances, and the experience of the treating surgeon. It requires thorough discussion between the surgeon and the patient, addressing their expectations, and the objectives of further surgery (Haddad *et al.*, 2007).

WHAT IS A REVISION TAR?

The definition of the term "revision" lacks consensus and creates confusion. Primary TAR is not infrequently part of a series of procedures to address foot and ankle pathology or itself results in a number of secondary procedures that have been interchangeably named "revisions", "reoperations", or "additional procedures" (Henricson *et al.*, 2011).

All revisions in the UK require the completion of a *pro forma* for a revision ankle replacement which is submitted to the National Joint Registry (NJR, 2010–2018). This also applies to cases in which the ankle replacement implant is removed and a fusion or amputation is performed.

Henricson *et al.* (2011) proposed a definition "— removal or exchange of one or more of the prosthetic components with the exception of incidental exchange of the polyethylene insert." Definition of Revision TAR (Henricson *et al.*, 2011). This definition is used by the Swedish National Ankle Register. The UK NJR for ankle replacements has since updated its guidance and now considers any procedure where an implant is removed or exchanged as a revision procedure (NJR 15th Annual Report 2018).

Procedures where any of the components of the implant are not removed or exchanged are described as "reoperations other than revisions". Examples being gutter debridement or midfoot arthrodesis, assuming no TAR components are removed or exchanged.

The most controversial definition pertains to a procedure for an infected TAR in which the components are left *in situ*. Therefore, for early deep infection where debridement, antibiotics, and implant retention (also known as a DAIR procedure) takes place, the UK NJR recommends that this be recorded as a revision even if the meniscus is retained, as this is in line with how hip and knee prosthetic infections are reported.

One of the commonest "revision" procedures is an exchange of the UHMWPE insert in mobile-bearing implants. The polyethylene insert may require an exchange for many reasons, the most common being fracture or wear (Figure 1). Exchange of the polyethylene insert due to fracture or wear is considered a revision (Figure 2) (Carlsson *et al.*, 1998; Wood *et al.*, 2009; Henricson *et al.*, 2011; Anderson *et al.*, 2003) and is defined as a revision by the UK NJR.

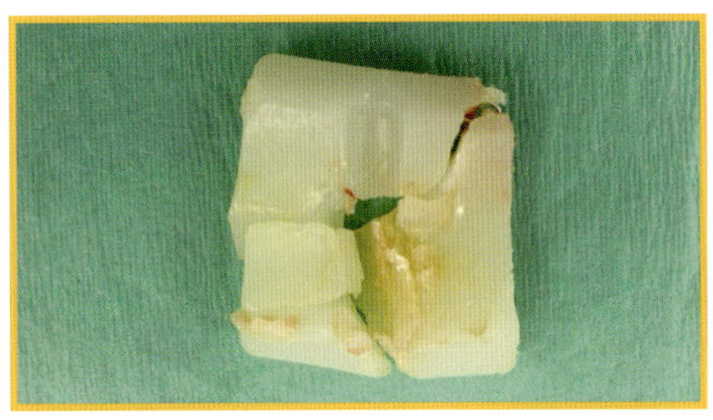

Figure 1. *Photograph of a fractured polyethylene insert of an STAR prosthesis.*

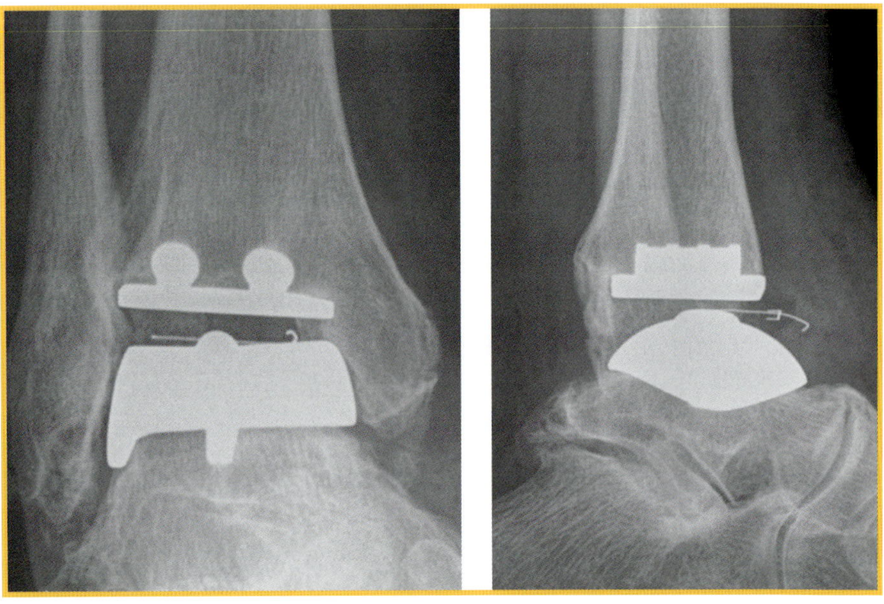

Figure 2. *A 65 Radiograph of an STAR implant in a patient with varus edge loading and a fractured meniscal insert, 82 months from primary TAR.*

THE NOTTINGHAM EXPERIENCE

In one of our series from Nottingham University Hospitals, UK, between 1999 and 2006, the senior author (Sunil Dhar) had performed 213 primary Scandinavian TARs (STARs). Out of the STARs performed, 27 (12%) had been revised at an average duration of 6.6 years (1–13 years) from the primary surgery. The average age was 68 years (44–86) with 22 male and 5 female patients. The mean follow up after revision surgery was 33 months (range: 6–57 months).

Fourteen patients had revision surgery for fractured polyethylene inserts, six patients had aseptic loosening and seven patients had failed implants due to instability or deformity of the ankle. None of the patients had infected loosening. We divided the patients into two groups — Group A with fractured insert (14 patients) and Group B with the insert intact (aseptic loosening, instability, deformity) (13 patients). The average time from primary surgery to revision surgery was 66 months (range: 12–154) in Group A and 80 months (range: 12–156) in Group B. All patients in Group A underwent exchange of the polyethylene insert. Revision procedures performed in Group B included revision of the tibial component ($n = 3$), revision of the talar component ($n = 2$), revision of all components ($n = 2$), revision to fusion using hind-foot nail ($n = 4$), and fusion using Ilizarov frame ($n = 2$). Some additional procedures were performed in order to achieve ankle stability or correct the deformity either at the time of revision surgery or at a later stage. These included lateral ligament reconstruction, Achilles tendon lengthening, tibialis posterior lengthening in combination with complete deltoid ligament release, and calcaneal osteotomy.

Pain was the main symptom in our patients. Prior to revision surgery, the majority of our patients had moderate pain but after undergoing revision surgery four patients in each group had mild pain and the rest were found to be pain-free at latest review.

Four patients developed superficial wound infection after revision surgery, which were treated successfully with antibiotics.

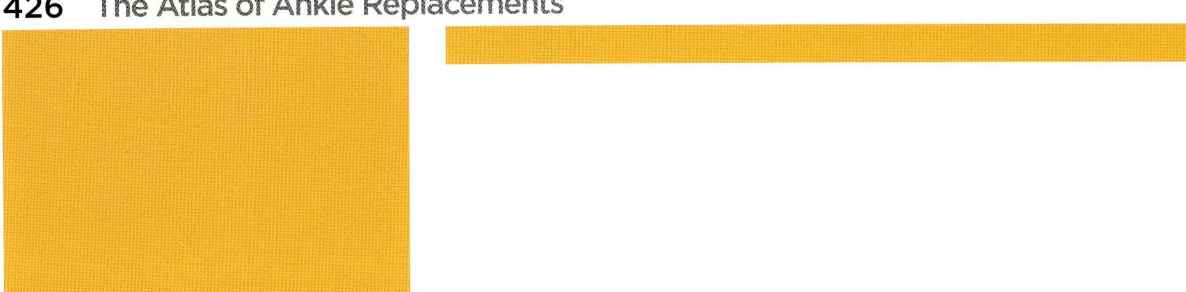

Seven patients underwent second revision surgery with an average duration of 42 months from their first revision (25–65 months) and included exchange of inserts ($n = 4$) and tibiotalocalcaneal (TTC) fusion ($n = 2$). One patient developed deep infection and the ankle was revised to fusion with Ilizarov frame in a two-stage procedure.

CHOICE OF THE REVISION IMPLANT

Standard Components

Up until recently the options were standard components or ordering custom implants due to a paucity of revision systems on the market. Hintermann *et al.* (2013) suggested the use of a standard talar component for bone defects less than 18 mm with the talar body preserved. For bone defects between 19 and 24 mm with partially destroyed talar body, a revision component was advised, and for bone defects over 25 mm with destroyed talar body, a custom-made component was recommended. Most primary TAR prostheses do not have a revision counterpart and custom implants can be very expensive and difficult to obtain. Therefore, till recently, standard implants were used for revision purposes, often with the additional use of bone cement, as shown in the following example.

The example is of a 72-year-old lady in good health who had a TAR 4 years earlier but a poor outcome because of poor surgical technique and incorrect placement of implants (Figure 3). She went onto have a successful revision (Figures 4 and 5).

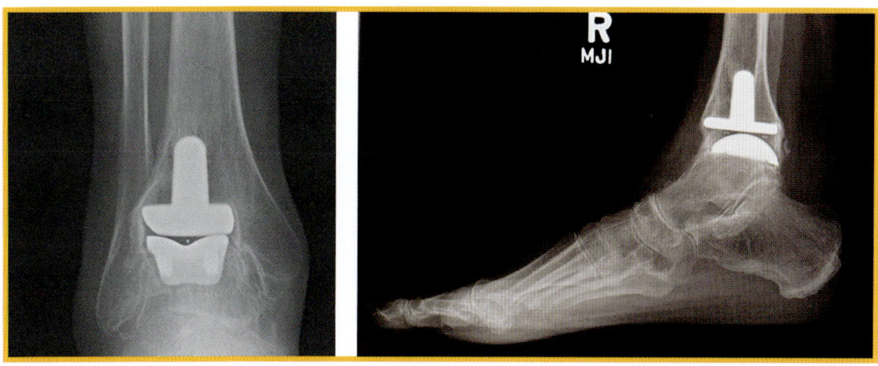

Figure 3. *AP and Lateral radiographs of a 72-year-old lady with a TAR in situ done 4 years earlier. The ankle was rigid, in considerable equinus and painful.*

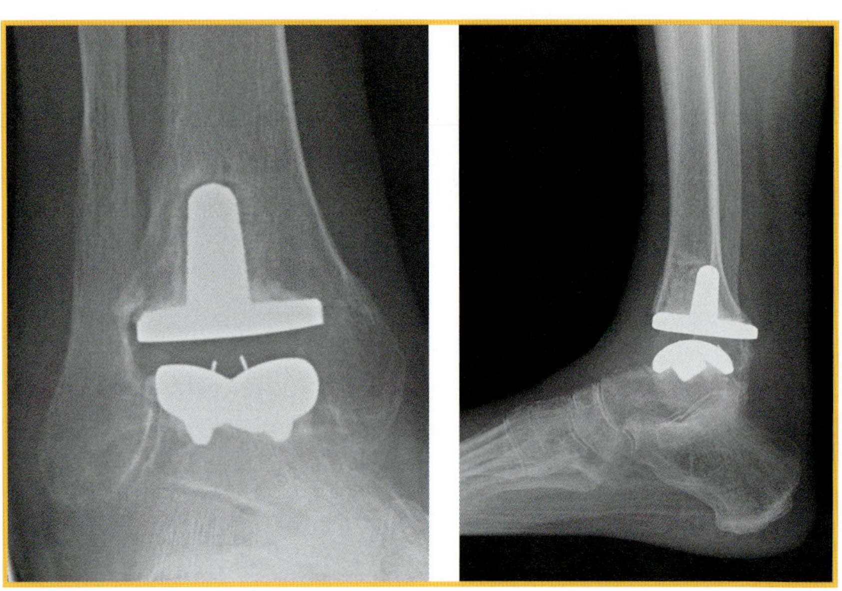

Figure 4. *Revision TAR of ankle given in Figure 3. Note the correction of deformity. There is a 20° arc of motion and no pain. The implant was cemented in.*

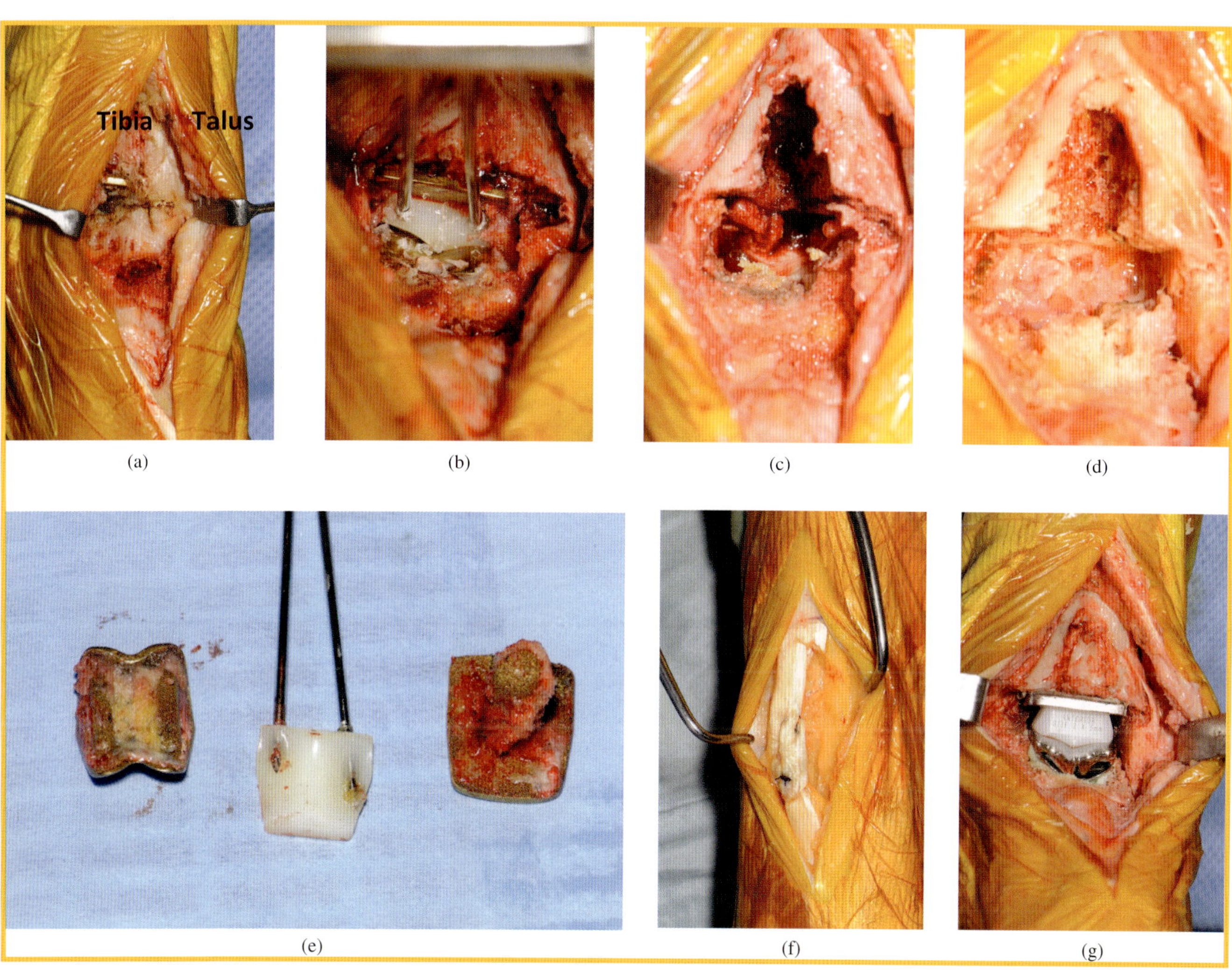

Figure 5. *(a–g) Photographs of the 72-year-old patient's revision mentioned in Figure 4. (a) Showing complete ectopic bony coverage of prosthesis anteriorly; (b) the components come into view after removal of bone — threaded inserts are used to remove the meniscus; (c) prosthesis removed to show posterior ectopic bone and overgrowth of the gutters medially and laterally; (d) thoroughly debrided joint; (e) removed prosthesis; (f) Achilles tendon Z lengthening via separate posterior incision; and (g) the new mobility prosthesis cemented in.*

INBONE II

More recently the INBONE II™ TAR (Wright Medical) has been utilised increasingly as a revision implant. It uses intramedullary instrumentation and is perceived to provide improved stability and the ability to deal with considerable bone loss on both the tibial and talar sides. There is little data regarding the use of INBONE II as a revision prosthesis but initial impressions are favourable. Figures 6 and 7 demonstrate radiographs of a patient with aseptic loosening in a mobile-bearing implant 3 years post surgery that was revised to an INBONE II in a single procedure with a good outcome, eliminating pain and enabling full function.

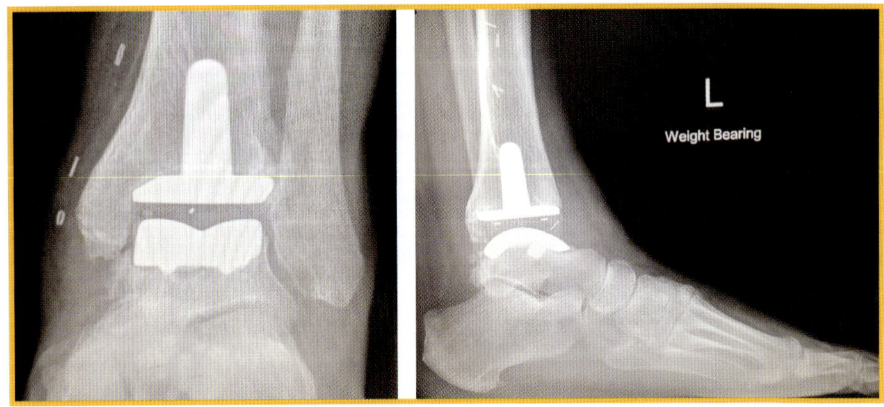

Figure 6. *Radiographs of a 3-year-old Zenith TAR, which is painful on weight bearing. SPECT CT suggested aseptic loosening.*

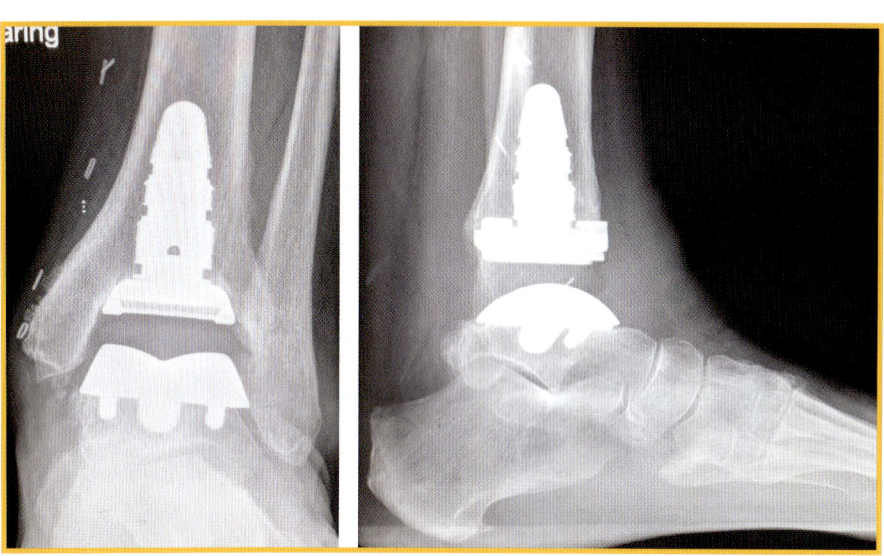

Figure 7. *Radiographs of the patient mentioned in Figure 6, 2 years following revision to an INBONE II prosthesis.*

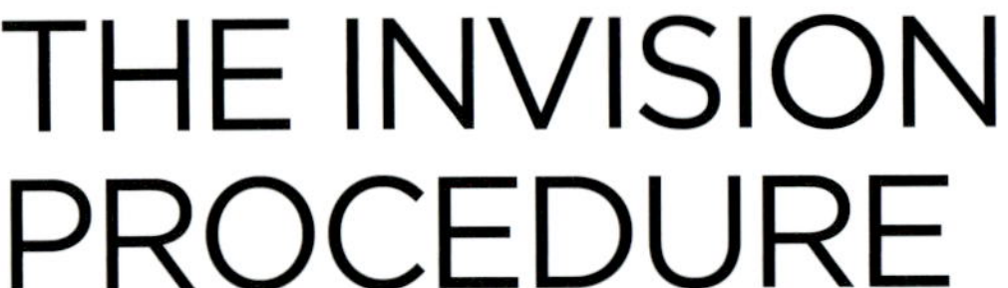

THE INVISION PROCEDURE

The INVISION (TM) Total Ankle Revision System developed by the Wright Medical Group (Memphis, Tennessee, USA) was designed in the main by the same design surgeons responsible for the Infinity & INBONE II prostheses. It utilises an INBONE tibial stem for proximal fixation of differing base tray heights and lengths to control bone loss in an attempt to avoid raising the joint line. The INVISION has a talar base plate to maximise cortical coverage after bone loss of the talus.

In the USA, the fixation of the talar base plate is with three pegs on the distal surface but in the rest of the world screw fixation is also possible. The base plate is manufactured from titanium alloy, and the inferior surface of the talar plate is coated to encourage bone on-growth. The talar dome implants are the INBONE II type manufactured from cobalt chrome (CoCr), and the implant fixes onto the base plate using a morse taper coupling.

The INVISION (TM) Total Ankle Revision System can be supplemented with Patient-Specific Instrumentation (known as PROPHECY (TM) system), which allows computer-generated images from preoperative CT scans of the patient. The first INVISION (TM) implant was performed in 2016 and hence no long-term data are available to assess the performance of this technology but short-term results have been encouraging (personal communication).

The following example is of a 59-year-old male who began to become symptomatic 8 years after a Mobility TAR for end-stage ankle arthritis, but developed pain and suspected aseptic loosening. X-rays showed rapid subsidence of the talar component (Figure 8) and CT confirmed this. There was little by way of clinical deformity and the mechanical axis of the limb was preserved. The patient was presented with various salvage options including conversion to hind-foot fusion or consideration of a revision ankle replacement. The patient being keen on movement preservation, he opted for the latter.

Given the amount of talar bone loss, the patient underwent an INVISION™ revision 10 years following the primary TAR (Figure 9).

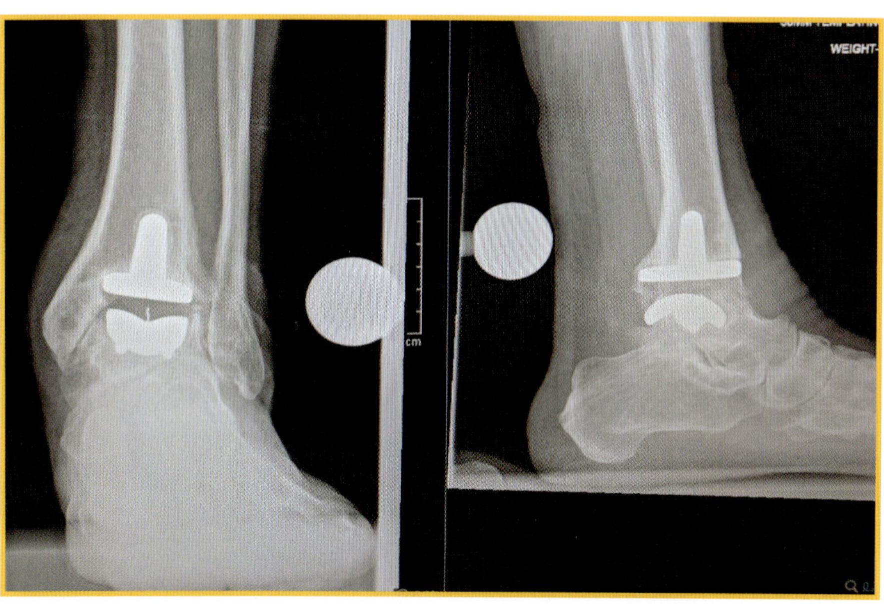

Figure 8. *AP and Lateral X-rays of a 59-year-old male with a TAR in situ done 10 years prior with subsidence of the talar component.*

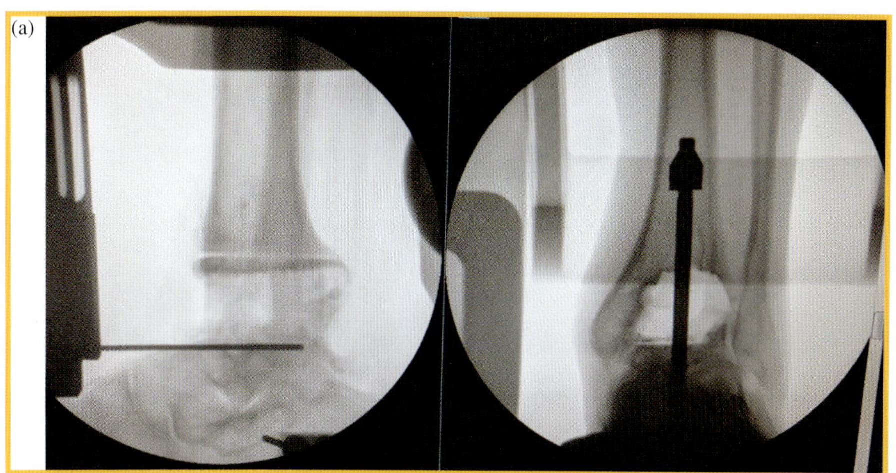

Figure 9. *INVISION Revision TAR of ankle in Figure 8. Note that the reaming was centrally located in the tibia. (a) Bone loss was on the lateral side of the tibia and hence when the base plate was impacted, the entire tibial stem drifted into valgus.*

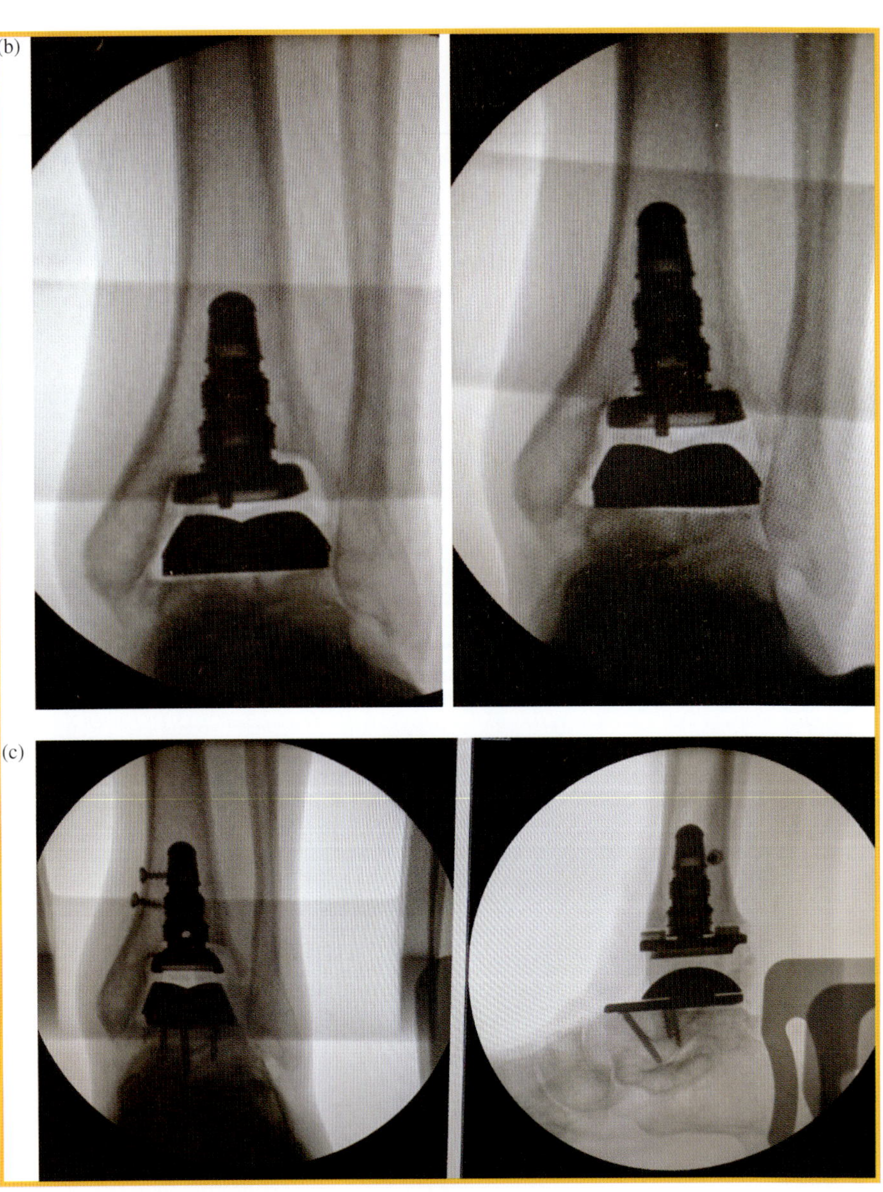

Figure 9 (Continued). *(b) Two screws were used to correct the alignment and as positioning screws, which have been maintained at the 12-month follow-up. (c) The talar base plate has room for two posterior screws which were not used due to lack of room without breaching the subtalar joint.*

During the procedure, the INBONE tibial stem drifted into valgus largely due to bone loss laterally and hence we used transtibial screws to straighten the stem and maintain its position, a technique we have found useful. At the 12-month follow–up, the patient was doing well and was pain-free but has not yet returned to any impact or sporting activity. Clearly long-term follow-up is necessary.

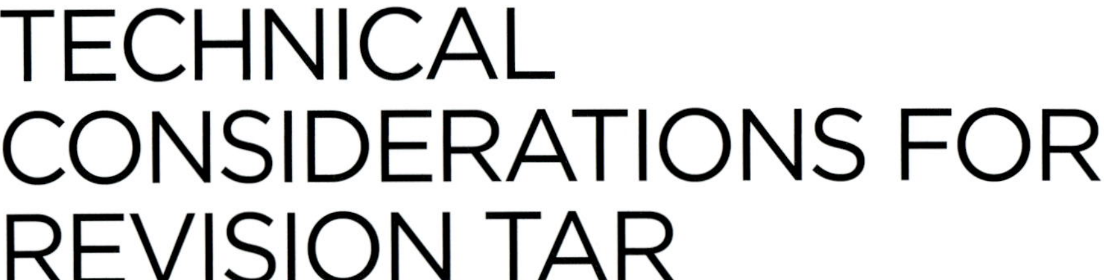

TECHNICAL CONSIDERATIONS FOR REVISION TAR

The principle technical considerations for a revision TAR include the following:

(1) The choice of surgical approach is usually anterior but may depend on pre-existing scarring and previous incisions.

(2) Implant removal should always be aimed at conserving the bone as far as possible for stable component implantation. It has been our impression that many current TARs have poor osseous integration of their bonding surfaces and technically therefore it is usually relatively straightforward to remove the non-cemented TAR.

(3) The joint should be thoroughly debrided by way of complete excision of biofilms, thickened capsule, thorough synovectomy and removal of any metallosis, and periarticular ossification in the gutters and posteriorly.

(4) Resection for the new components. Implants must be performed into healthy bones.

(5) Assessment of residual bone available for implantation and choice of revision implant.

(6) If reconstruction is considered impossible, an arthrodesis, with or without bone graft, should be planned (Besse *et al.*, 2010).

RESULTS OF REVISION ANKLE REPLACEMENT

There are very few studies that have reported the outcomes after revision of a failed TAR to another TAR (Kotnis *et al.*, 2006; Spirt *et al.*, 2004; Johl *et al.*, 2006; Williams *et al.*, 2015; Kamrad *et al.*, 2015; Lai *et al.*, 2018; Hordyk *et al.*, 2018; Lachman *et al.*, 2019).

Williams *et al.* (2015) described the revision of 35 Agility TAR to INBONE II. Revision TAR was indicated due to mechanical loosening, osteolysis, periprosthetic fracture, and a dislocated prosthesis. Adjunctive procedures were performed in 31 of 35 cases. There were six intraoperative and five acute postoperative complications, leading to an overall complication rate of 31.4%. There was one patient with continued pain postoperatively who underwent a second revision of the INBONE II, 20 months postoperatively.

Devries *et al.* (2011) reported retrospectively on five patients who underwent revision of a failed Agility total ankle arthroplasty to an INBONE total ankle arthroplasty. At 17 months, three patients required additional surgery, including one transtibial amputation and one TTC arthrodesis. Their early results demonstrated a high risk of early failure and complications.

Kharwadkar *et al.* (2009) have reported on the early results of two cases in which STARs were revised to hybrid Ankle Evolution System-STAR (AES-STAR) replacements for aseptic loosening of the tibial components. Ironically, the AES system has since been withdrawn from the market following unacceptably high reported failure rates.

Barg *et al.* (2013) reported the outcomes of their primary HINTEGRA three-component prosthesis over a period of 10 years. Sixty one ankles had a revision arthroplasty with 27 having both components revised, 13 had only the tibial component revised, 14 had only the talar component revised, and 7 were revised to arthrodesis. There were no polyethylene failures. The generation category of the prosthesis, the cause of ankle osteoarthritis, and the age of the patient were identified as independent risk factors for prosthesis failure.

In a study by Hintermann *et al.* (2013), the outcomes of revision TAR using HINTEGRA prosthesis as the revision implant were reported. Different types of primary TAR implants were revised to HINTEGRA implants. The authors reported on 117 cases of revision TAR. The reason for revision included failure of metallic components in 60 ankles (51%), the bone in 28 (24%), soft tissues in 20 (17%), and infection in 9 (8%) ankles. The talar component was revised in 104 ankles (89%) and the tibial component in 106 (91%). The mean follow-up was 6.3 years. The revision arthroplasty was considered successful in 109 (93%) of the 117 ankles. Standard components were used in 50% of the revised talar components and in 86% of the revised tibial components. Additional procedures to achieve a stable and balanced ankle were required in 57% patients. Components with a single HA coating performed worse than double-coated components with a loosening rate of 26% (compared to 5%). The medium-term results of revision arthroplasty after a failed total ankle arthroplasty were found to be similar to those after primary arthroplasty and the authors reported the key to success being firm anchorage of the components to the primary bone stock.

Many authors have reported variable revision rates of primary TAR to another TAR. For Agility prostheses, three different studies have described the outcomes of a total cohort of 234 ankle replacements with 16% failed prostheses, and 10% revisions to another TAR with average duration of 6.6 years after primary TAR (Hurowitz *et al.*, 2007; Knecht *et al.*, 2004; Kopp *et al.*, 2006). Four different studies have reported the results of a total cohort of 344 patients who underwent ankle replacements using STAR prostheses, with 13% failure rate, and 6% revisions to another TAR with an average duration of 6.3 years of follow-up (Kofoed, 2004; Valderrabano *et al.*, 2004; Wood *et al.*, 2009; Anderson *et al.*, 2003).

Three different studies have reviewed the results of patients with TAR using Buechel–Pappas prostheses and reported 7.5% failure rate on a total cohort of 105 ankles, of which 4% underwent revision of TAR prostheses, with an average duration of 5.5 years after primary surgery (Buechel *et al.*, 2004; Naal *et al.*, 2009; San Giovanni *et al.*, 2006).

Bonnin *et al.* (2011) reviewed the outcome of Salto Total Ankle Arthroplasty in 96 patients (98 ankles). There were a total of 18 revisions without arthrodesis. The polyethylene was exchanged secondary to fracture in five patients, between 72 and 122 months after the initial surgery (mean, 103 ± 19 months). This occurred only in patients in whom 3-mm polyethylene components were used. In one patient, concomitant revision of the tibial component was necessary owing to the development of osteolysis. Eight patients required reoperations for the development of symptomatic osteolytic cysts. The cysts were curetted and filled with cancellous autograft harvested from the ipsilateral iliac crest and the polyethylene was routinely exchanged.

Rippstein *et al.* (2011) have reported on 240 consecutive primary total ankle arthroplasties performed in 233 patients (115 women and 118 men; mean age: 61.6 years) between November 2003 and October 2007 with the Mobility prosthesis of which 233 were available for follow-up at a mean of 32.8 ± 15.3 months. A reoperation was necessary in 18 ankles (7.7%). Five arthroplasties (2.1%) failed at a mean of 27 months after surgery and revision TAR was performed in four patients.

A systematic review and meta-analysis of the outcome of TARs by Zaidi *et al.* (2013) has looked at the survivorship, outcome, complications, radiological findings, and range of movement in patients with end-stage osteoarthritis (OA) who underwent TAR. Despite an overall survivorship of 89% at 10 years, the quality of evidence was weak and fraught with biases. Long-term outcome data and high-quality randomised controlled trials were recommended.

CONCLUSION

Revision TAR surgery is going to be a major challenge for foot and ankle surgeons. With increasing numbers of primary TARs being carried out, failures are inevitable and therefore there is an urgent need for developing strategies based on sound science to deal with these complex cases. New revision implant systems will mean a shift from revision to fusion towards revision TAR and close follow-up is essential to demonstrate their utility and survivorship.

REFERENCES

Anderson, T., Montgomery, F. & Carlsson, A. 2003. Uncemented STAR total ankle prostheses: Three to eight-year follow-up of fifty-one consecutive ankles. *J Bone Joint Surg Am*, 85-A, 1321–1329.

Barg, A., Zwicky, L., Knupp, M., Henninger, H. B. & Hintermann, B. 2013. HINTEGRA total ankle replacement: Survivorship analysis in 684 patients. *J Bone Joint Surg Am*, 95, 1175–1183.

Besse, J. L., Colombier, J. A., Asencio, J., Bonnin, M., Gaudot, F., Jarde, O., Judet, T., Maestro, M., Lemrijse, T., Leonardi, C., Toullec, E. & L'AFCP. 2010. Total ankle arthroplasty in France. *Orthop Traumatol Surg Res*, 96, 291–303.

Bonnin, M., Gaudot, F., Laurent, J. R., Ellis, S., Colombier, J. A. & Judet, T. 2011. The Salto total ankle arthroplasty: Survivorship and analysis of failures at 7 to 11 years. *Clin Orthop Relat Res*, 469, 225–236.

Borenstein, T. R., Anand, K., Li, Q., Charlton, T. P. & Thordarson, D. B. 2018. A review of perioperative complications of outpatient total ankle arthroplasty. *Foot Ankle Int*, 39, 143–148.

Buechel, F. F. & Pappas, M. J. 1992. Survivorship and clinical evaluation of cementless, meniscal-bearing total ankle replacements. *Semin Arthroplasty*, 3, 43–50.

Buechel, F. F., SR., Buechel, F. F., JR. & Pappas, M. J. 2004. Twenty-year evaluation of cementless mobile-bearing total ankle replacements. *Clin Orthop Relat Res*, 19–26.

Buechel SR, F. F., Buechel JR, F. F. & Pappas, M. J. 2003. Ten-year evaluation of cementless Buechel-Pappas meniscal bearing total ankle replacement. *Foot Ankle Int*, 24, 462–472.

Carlsson, A. S., Montgomery, F. & Besjakov, J. 1998. Arthrodesis of the ankle secondary to replacement. *Foot Ankle Int*, 19, 240–245.

Devries, J. G., Berlet, G. C., Lee, T. H., Hyer, C. F. & Deorio, J. K. 2011. Revision total ankle replacement: An early look at agility to INBONE. *Foot Ankle Spec*, 4, 235–244.

Fevang, B. T., Lie, S. A., Havelin, L. I., Brun, J. G., Skredderstuen, A. & Furnes, O. 2007. 257 ankle arthroplasties performed in Norway between 1994 and 2005. *Acta Orthop*, 78, 575–583.

Gougoulias, N. E., Khanna, A. & Maffulli, N. 2009. How successful are current ankle replacements? A systematic review of the literature. *Clin Orthop Relat Res*, 468, 199–208.

Gross, C. E., Hamid, K. S., Green, C., Easley, M. E., Deorio, J. K. & Nunley, J. A. 2017. Operative wound complications following total ankle arthroplasty. *Foot Ankle Int*, 38, 360–366.

Haddad, S. L., Coetzee, J. C., Estok, R., Fahrbach, K., Banel, D. & Nalysnyk, L. 2007. Intermediate and long-term outcomes of total ankle arthroplasty and ankle arthrodesis: A systematic review of the literature. *J Bone Joint Surg Am*, 89, 1899–1905.

Helm, R. & Stevens, J. 1986. Long-term results of total ankle replacement. *J Arthroplasty*, 1, 271–277.

Henricson, A., Carlsson, A. & Rydholm, U. 2011. What is a revision of total ankle replacement? *Foot Ankle Surg*, 17, 99–102.

Henricson, A., Skoog, A. & Carlsson, A. 2007. The Swedish ankle arthroplasty register: An analysis of 531 arthroplasties between 1993 and 2005. *Acta Orthop*, 78, 569–574.

Hintermann, B., Zwicky, L., Knupp, M., Henninger, H. B. & Barg, A. 2013. HINTEGRA revision arthroplasty for failed total ankle prostheses. *J Bone Joint Surg Am*, 95, 1166–1174.

Hobson, S. A., Karantana, A. & Dhar, S. 2009. Total ankle replacement in patients with significant pre-operative deformity of the hindfoot. *J Bone Joint Surg Br*, 91, 481–486.

Hopgood, P., Kumar, R. & Wood, P. L. 2006. Ankle arthrodesis for failed total ankle replacement. *J Bone Joint Surg Br*, 88, 1032–1038.

Hordyk, P. J., Fuerbringer, B. A. & Roukis, T. S. 2018. Sagittal ankle and midfoot range of motion before and after revision total ankle replacement: A retrospective comparative analysis. *J Foot Ankle Surg*, 57(3), 521–526.

Hosman, A. H., Mason, R. B., Hobbs, T. & Rothwell, A. G. 2007. A New Zealand national joint registry review of 202 total ankle replacements followed for up to 6 years. *Acta Orthop*, 78, 584–591.

Hurowitz, E. J., Gould, J. S., Fleisig, G. S. & Fowler, R. 2007. Outcome analysis of agility total ankle replacement with prior adjunctive procedures: Two to six year followup. *Foot Ankle Int*, 28, 308–312.

Johl, C., Kircher, J., Pohlmannn, K. & Jansson, V. 2006. Management of failed total ankle replacement with a retrograde short femoral nail: A case report. *J Orthop Trauma*, 20, 60–65.

Kamrad, I., Henricsson, A., Karlsson, M. K., Magnusson, H., Nilsson, J. A., Carlsson, A. & Rosengren, B. E. 2015. Poor prosthesis survival and function after component exchange of total ankle prostheses. *Acta Orthop*, 86, 407–411.

Kharwadkar, N. & Harris, N. J. 2009. Revision of STAR total ankle replacement to hybrid AES-STAR total ankle replacement — A report of two cases. *Foot Ankle Surg*, 15, 101–105.

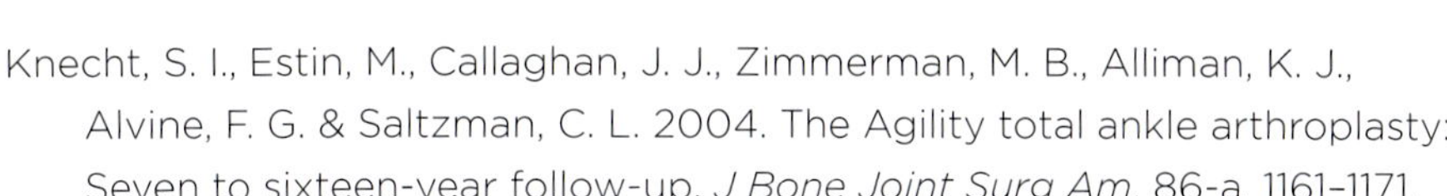

Knecht, S. I., Estin, M., Callaghan, J. J., Zimmerman, M. B., Alliman, K. J., Alvine, F. G. & Saltzman, C. L. 2004. The Agility total ankle arthroplasty: Seven to sixteen-year follow-up. *J Bone Joint Surg Am*, 86-a, 1161–1171.

Kofoed, H. 2004. Scandinavian total ankle replacement (STAR). *Clin Orthop Relat Res*, 73–79.

Kofoed, H. & Lundberg-Jensen, A. 1999. Ankle arthroplasty in patients younger and older than 50 years: A prospective series with long-term follow-up. *Foot Ankle Int*, 20, 501–506.

Kopp, F. J., Patel, M. M., Deland, J. T. & O'Malley, M. J. 2006. Total ankle arthroplasty with the Agility prosthesis: Clinical and radiographic evaluation. *Foot Ankle Int*, 27, 97–103.

Kotnis, R., Pasapula, C., Anwar, F., Cooke, P. H. & Sharp, R. J. 2006. The management of failed ankle replacement. *J Bone Joint Surg Br*, 88, 1039–1047.

Lachman, J. R., Ramos, J. A., Adams, S. B., Nunley, J. A., II, Easley, M. E. & DeOrio, J. K. 2019. Patient-reported outcomes before and after primary and revision total ankle arthroplasty. *Foot Ankle Int*, 40(1), 34–41. doi: 10.1177/1071100718794956. Epub Aug 30, 2018.

Lai, W. C., Arshi, A., Ghorbanifarajzadeh, A., Williams, J. R. & Soohoo, N. F. 2018. Incidence and predictors of early complications following primary and revision total ankle arthroplasty. *Foot Ankle Surg*, pii, S1268–S7731(18)30325–30334. doi: 10.1016/j.fas.2018.10.009.

Morgan, S. S., Brooke, B. & Harris, N. J. 2010. Total ankle replacement by the Ankle Evolution System: Medium-term outcome. *J Bone Joint Surg Br*, 92, 61–65.

2012–2018. National Joint Registry for England and Wales, 9–15th Annual Report.

Naal, F. D., Impellizzeri, F. M., Loibl, M., Huber, M. & Rippstein, P. F. 2009. Habitual physical activity and sports participation after total ankle arthroplasty. *Am J Sports Med*, 37, 95–102.

Overley, B. D., Jr. & Beideman, T. C. 2015. Painful osteophytes, ectopic bone, and pain in the malleolar gutters following total ankle replacement: Management and strategies. *Clin Podiatr Med Surg*, 32, 509–516.

Pyevich, M. T., Saltzman, C. L., Callaghan, J. J. & Alvine, F. G. 1998. Total ankle arthroplasty: A unique design — Two to twelve-year follow-up. *J Bone Joint Surg Am*, 80, 1410–1420.

Rippstein, P. F., Huber, M., Coetzee, J. C. & Naal, F. D. 2011. Total ankle replacement with use of a new three-component implant. *J Bone Joint Surg Am*, 93, 1426–1435.

Roukis, T. S. 2012. Incidence of revision after primary implantation of the Agility total ankle replacement system: A systematic review. *J Foot Ankle Surg*, 51, 198–204.

San Giovanni, T. P., Keblish, D. J., Thomas, W. H. & Wilson, M. G. 2006. Eight-year results of a minimally constrained total ankle arthroplasty. *Foot Ankle Int*, 27, 418–426.

Schuberth, J. M., Patel, S. & Zarutsky, E. 2006. Perioperative complications of the Agility total ankle replacement in 50 initial, consecutive cases. *J Foot Ankle Surg*, 45, 139–146.

Skytta, E. T., Koivu, H., Eskelinen, A., Ikavalko, M., Paavolainen, P. & Remes, V. 2010. Total ankle replacement: A population-based study of 515 cases from the Finnish Arthroplasty Register. *Acta Orthop*, 81, 114–118.

Spirt, A. A., Assal, M. & Hansen, S. T., JR. 2004. Complications and failure after total ankle arthroplasty. *J Bone Joint Surg Am*, 86-a, 1172–1178.

Valderrabano, V., Hintermann, B. & Dick, W. 2004. Scandinavian total ankle replacement: A 3.7-year average followup of 65 patients. *Clin Orthop Relat Res*, 47–56.

Wapner, K. L. 2002. Salvage of failed and infected total ankle replacements with fusion. *Instr Course Lect*, 51, 153–157.

Williams, J. R., Wegner, N. J., Sangeorzan, B. J. & Brage, M. E. 2015. Intraoperative and perioperative complications during revision arthroplasty for salvage of a failed total ankle arthroplasty. *Foot Ankle Int*, 36, 135–142.

Wood, P. L. 2002. Experience with the STAR ankle arthroplasty at Wrightington Hospital, UK. *Foot Ankle Clin*, 7, 755–764, vii.

Wood, P. L. & Deakin, S. 2003. Total ankle replacement: The results in 200 ankles. *J Bone Joint Surg Br*, 85, 334–341.

Wood, P. L., Prem, H. & Sutton, C. 2008. Total ankle replacement: Medium-term results in 200 Scandinavian total ankle replacements. *J Bone Joint Surg Br*, 90, 605–609.

Wood, P. L., Sutton, C., Mishra, V. & Suneja, R. 2009. A randomised, controlled trial of two mobile-bearing total ankle replacements. *J Bone Joint Surg Br*, 91, 69–74.

Zaidi, R., Cro, S., Gurusamy, K., Siva, N., Macgregor, A., Henricson, A. & Goldberg, A. 2013. The outcome of total ankle replacement: A systematic review and meta-analysis. *Bone Joint J*, 95-b, 1500–1507.

INDEX